Pathways to Quality Health Care

PERFORMANCE MEASUREMENT

Accelerating Improvement

Committee on Redesigning Health Insurance Performance Measures,
Payment, and Performance Improvement Programs

Board on Health Care Services

INSTITUTE OF MEDICINE
OF THE NATIONAL ACADEMIES

THE NATIONAL ACADEMIES PRESS
Washington, D.C.
www.nap.edu

THE NATIONAL ACADEMIES PRESS   500 Fifth Street, N.W.   Washington, DC 20001

NOTICE: The project that is the subject of this report was approved by the Governing Board of the National Research Council, whose members are drawn from the councils of the National Academy of Sciences, the National Academy of Engineering, and the Institute of Medicine. The members of the committee responsible for the report were chosen for their special competences and with regard for appropriate balance.

This study was supported by Contract No. HHSM-500-2004-00005C between the National Academy of Sciences and the U.S. Department of Health and Human Services through the Centers for Medicare and Medicaid Services. Any opinions, findings, conclusions, or recommendations expressed in this publication are those of the author(s) and do not necessarily reflect the view of the organizations or agencies that provided support for this project.

Library of Congress Cataloging-in-Publication Data

Performance measurement : accelerating improvement / Committee on
    Redesigning Health Insurance Performance Measures, Payment,
    and Performance Improvement Programs, Board on Health Care
    Services.
        p. ; cm. — (Pathways to quality health care)
    Includes bibiographical references.
    ISBN 0-309-10007-0 (hardback)
    1. Medical care—United States—Quality control. 2. Medical care
    —Standards—United States. 3. Performance—Measurement.
    I. Institute of Medicine (U.S.). Committee on Redesigning Health
    Insurance Performance Measures, Payment, and Performance
    Improvement Programs. II. Series.
    [DNLM: 1. Quality Assurance, Health Care—methods—United
    States. 2. Quality of Health Care—standards—United States.
    W 84 AA1 P32 2006]
    RA399.A3P44 2006
    362.1068—dc22
                                2005037405

Additional copies of this report are available from the National Academies Press, 500 Fifth Street, N.W., Lockbox 285, Washington, DC 20055; (800) 624-6242 or (202) 334-3313 (in the Washington metropolitan area); Internet, http://www.nap.edu.

For more information about the Institute of Medicine, visit the IOM home page at: **www.iom.edu.**

The serpent has been a symbol of long life, healing, and knowledge among almost all cultures and religions since the beginning of recorded history. The serpent adopted as a logotype by the Institute of Medicine is a relief carving from ancient Greece, now held by the Staatliche Museum in Berlin.

"Knowing is not enough; we must apply.
Willing is not enough; we must do."
—Goethe

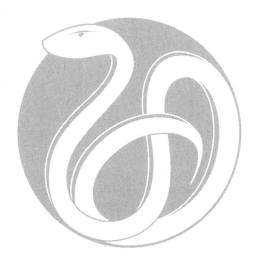

INSTITUTE OF MEDICINE
OF THE NATIONAL ACADEMIES

Advising the Nation. Improving Health.

THE NATIONAL ACADEMIES
Advisers to the Nation on Science, Engineering, and Medicine

The **National Academy of Sciences** is a private, nonprofit, self-perpetuating society of distinguished scholars engaged in scientific and engineering research, dedicated to the furtherance of science and technology and to their use for the general welfare. Upon the authority of the charter granted to it by the Congress in 1863, the Academy has a mandate that requires it to advise the federal government on scientific and technical matters. Dr. Ralph J. Cicerone is president of the National Academy of Sciences.

The **National Academy of Engineering** was established in 1964, under the charter of the National Academy of Sciences, as a parallel organization of outstanding engineers. It is autonomous in its administration and in the selection of its members, sharing with the National Academy of Sciences the responsibility for advising the federal government. The National Academy of Engineering also sponsors engineering programs aimed at meeting national needs, encourages education and research, and recognizes the superior achievements of engineers. Dr. Wm. A. Wulf is president of the National Academy of Engineering.

The **Institute of Medicine** was established in 1970 by the National Academy of Sciences to secure the services of eminent members of appropriate professions in the examination of policy matters pertaining to the health of the public. The Institute acts under the responsibility given to the National Academy of Sciences by its congressional charter to be an adviser to the federal government and, upon its own initiative, to identify issues of medical care, research, and education. Dr. Harvey V. Fineberg is president of the Institute of Medicine.

The **National Research Council** was organized by the National Academy of Sciences in 1916 to associate the broad community of science and technology with the Academy's purposes of furthering knowledge and advising the federal government. Functioning in accordance with general policies determined by the Academy, the Council has become the principal operating agency of both the National Academy of Sciences and the National Academy of Engineering in providing services to the government, the public, and the scientific and engineering communities. The Council is administered jointly by both Academies and the Institute of Medicine. Dr. Ralph J. Cicerone and Dr. Wm. A. Wulf are chair and vice chair, respectively, of the National Research Council.

www.national-academies.org

CHERYL M. SCOTT, President Emerita, Group Health Cooperative, Seattle, WA

STEPHEN M. SHORTELL, Blue Cross of California Distinguished Professor of Health Policy and Management and Dean, School of Public Health, University of California, Berkeley, CA

SAMUEL O. THIER, Professor of Medicine and Professor of Health Care Policy, Harvard Medical School and Massachusetts General Hospital, Boston, MA

GAIL R. WILENSKY, Senior Fellow, Project HOPE, Bethesda, MD

Study Staff

JANET CORRIGAN, Project Director[1]

ROSEMARY A. CHALK, Project Director[2]

KAREN ADAMS, Senior Program Officer, Lead Staff for the Subcommittee on Performance Measurement Evaluation

DIANNE MILLER WOLMAN, Senior Program Officer, Lead Staff for the Subcommittee on Quality Improvement Organizations Evaluation

CONTESSA FINCHER, Program Officer[3]

TRACY HARRIS, Program Officer

SAMANTHA CHAO, Senior Health Policy Associate

DANITZA VALDIVIA, Program Associate

MICHELLE BAZEMORE, Senior Program Assistant

Editorial Consultants

RONA BRIERE, Briere Associates, Inc.

ALISA DECATUR, Briere Associates, Inc.

---

[1]Served through May 2005.
[2]Beginning May 2005.
[3]Served through July 2005.

Reviewers

This report has been reviewed in draft form by individuals chosen for their diverse perspectives and technical expertise, in accordance with procedures approved by the National Research Council's (NRC's) Report Review Committee. The purpose of this independent review is to provide candid and critical comments that will assist the institution in making its published report as sound as possible and to ensure that the report meets institutional standards for objectivity, evidence, and responsiveness to the study charge. The review comments and draft manuscript remain confidential to protect the integrity of the deliberative process. We wish to thank the following individuals for their review of this report:

KATHLEEN O. ANGEL, Director of Global Benefits and International Compensation, Dell Computer Corporation, Round Rock, TX

ELIZABETH H. BRADLEY, Associate Professor of Public Health and Director of the Health Management Program in the Division of Health Policy and Administration, Yale School of Medicine, New Haven, CT

LINDA BURNES-BOLTON, Vice President and Chief Nursing Officer, Cedars-Sinai Medical Center, Los Angeles, CA

ROBERT GRAHAM, Professor of Family Medicine and a Robert and Myfanwy Smith Chair, University of Cincinnati College of Medicine, OH

STUART GUTERMAN, Senior Program Director of Medicare Future, Commonwealth Fund, New York, NY

DAVID A. KNAPP, Dean of the School of Pharmacy, University of Maryland, Baltimore, MD

STEVE LIPSTEIN, Chief Executive Officer, Barnes Jewish HealthCare, St. Louis, MO

HAROLD S. LUFT, Director and Caldwell B. Esselstyn Professor of Health Policy and Health Economics, The Institute of Health Policy Studies, University of California at San Francisco, San Francisco, CA

RICARDO MARTINEZ, Executive Vice President of Medical Affairs, The Schumacher Group, Kennesaw, GA

WALTER ORENSTEIN, Director of Vaccine Policy and Development and Associate Professor, Emory University School of Medicine, Atlanta, GA

L. GREGORY PAWLSON, Executive Vice President, National Committee on Quality Assurance, Washington, DC

PAMELA B. PEELE, Associate Professor and Vice Chair of Health Policy and Management, Graduate School of Public Health, University of Pittsburgh, PA

SARA ROSENBAUM, Chair of the Department of Health Policy, George Washington University, Washington, DC

TIM SIZE, Executive Director, Rural Wisconsin Health Cooperative, Sauk City, WI

SHOSHANNA SOFAER, Robert P. Luciano Professor of Health Care Policy, School of Public Affairs, Baruch College, New York, NY

ALAN M. ZASLAVSKY, Professor of Statistics, Department of Health Care Policy, Harvard Medical School, Boston, MA

Although the reviewers listed above have provided many constructive comments and suggestions, they were not asked to endorse the conclusions or recommendations nor did they see the final draft of the report before its release. The review of this report was overseen by coordinator **DONALD M. STEINWACHS, Ph.D.,** Professor and Chair, Johns Hopkins Bloomberg School of Public Health, Baltimore, MD, and monitor **HAROLD C. SOX, M.D., M.A.C.P.,** Editor, Annals of Internal Medicine, Philadelphia, PA. Appointed by the NRC, they were responsible for making certain that an independent examination of this report was carried out in accordance with institutional procedures and that all review comments were carefully considered. Responsibility for the final content of this report rests entirely with the authoring committee and the institution.

Preface

Performance Measurement: Accelerating Improvement is the first in a new series of reports by the Institute of Medicine (IOM), representing the latest phase of the ongoing IOM effort on health care quality. This report introduces a framework and implementation strategy for translating public and professional concerns about performance and accountability into measures of health care quality. In so doing, it builds upon central themes articulated in earlier IOM reports, including *To Err Is Human: Building a Safer Health System* and *Crossing the Quality Chasm: A New Health System for the 21st Century*. In particular, this report addresses one aspect of an overall strategy for implementing the six aims of the health care system articulated in the *Quality Chasm* report: health care should be safe, effective, patient-centered, timely, efficient, and equitable.

In its deliberations, the IOM Committee on Redesigning Health Insurance Performance Measures, Payment, and Performance Improvement Programs was struck by the energy and thoughtfulness displayed in multiple efforts to create health care quality improvement measures among public and private stakeholders and throughout the medical profession. These efforts represent important contributions to the development of new standards of accountability. However, the lack of connections and conceptual links among the performance measures put forth by different groups has created an administrative burden for providers, and is a significant barrier to moving the quality initiative forward to a new stage of development.

The time is ripe, therefore, for an informed national effort to standardize measures that can lay the foundation for a health care incentive system designed to reward the achievement of the six aims articulated in the *Qual-*

ity Chasm report. Such measures can be used for many purposes: data collection, public reports, provider awareness, quality improvement, purchaser benchmarks, and payment incentives. This report offers a set of measures to address these multiple goals. Some are ready to use now; others will require further research and dedicated effort in areas that are more difficult to address. Some measures will apply to multiple purposes and health care settings; others will require more selectivity and consideration. An oversight and coordinating system will be necessary to clarify the national goals for performance measurement, highlight ready-to-use measures, establish benchmarks, and allocate resources for the development of more robust measures that will be ready to use at a future time.

The IOM's health care quality reports have consistently sounded the call for evidence-based approaches and strategies formed by consensus that can change the health care environment and improve health outcomes for all. It is the committee's hope and expectation that this new series of reports will contribute to the development of consensus throughout the health care system regarding the basic performance measures, payment incentives, and quality improvement strategies that should be instituted now and in the future. The series builds on common ground but also offers a new vision in articulating where we must go and the pathways that offer the greatest promise in advancing the quality agenda.

This report is directed toward all concerned with improving the quality and performance of the nation's health care system in its multiple dimensions and in both the public and private sectors. The committee particularly encourages the U.S. Department of Health and Human Services to lay the groundwork for this effort within the Medicare system, setting an example through federal leadership that can strengthen the quality improvement process throughout the national health care environment. We recognize that such fundamental change in the health care system will not happen by itself. Therefore, we articulate the need for renewed effort, expanded resources, and an oversight and coordinating effort to guide the next stage of development. Creative partnerships will be necessary between the public and the private sectors, between Congress and health care leaders, between purchasers and providers, and between consumers and oversight groups. There will be a need for much good will to overcome personal interests in achieving shared goals that can serve the interests of multiple stakeholders and the common good.

As chairman of the committee, I thank the committee members and staff and the Subcommittee on Performance Measures for their generous contributions. They shared their time, their talent, and their expertise during many long sessions and deliberations. Our subcommittee cochairs, Don Berwick and Elliott Fisher, and IOM senior program officer Karen Adams, who directed this effort, deserve special recognition. It is my hope that this report reflects the integration of many voices that together can inform and advance the policy agenda to achieve the quality health care system envisioned in the *Quality Chasm* report.

Steven A. Schroeder, M.D.
Chairman
November 2005

Foreword

"We cannot wait any longer."

These were the closing words of the foreword to the report *To Err Is Human: Building a Safer Health System*, published almost 6 years ago by the Institute of Medicine (IOM). Indeed, a series of IOM reports over the past decade has consistently called for a comprehensive and strong response to improve the quality of health care in the United States.

The only way to know whether the quality of care is improving is to measure performance. Hundreds of proposed measures have emerged from many sources, including health professionals, care-giving institutions, employers, consumer groups, and insurers, among others. Progress in measurement has been uneven across different settings, populations, and health conditions. The task now is to develop a system of performance measurement that is more complete and reliable, that fills gaps in difficult-to-measure areas and for hard-to-reach populations.

Under the thoughtful direction of Chairman Steven A. Schroeder, the IOM Committee on Redesigning Health Insurance Performance Measures, Payment, and Performance Improvement Programs is developing a set of reports known as the *Pathways* series. The committee represents the collective wisdom of many leaders in the health care field and includes persons with experience and expertise in multiple health care settings. This first report highlights a set of foundational measures for quality improvement and calls attention to areas in which adequate measures do not yet exist. In addition, the report makes a compelling case for a more coherent system of measurement and reporting that can coordinate, guide, support, and enhance the multiple efforts now under way. Future reports will assess performance improvement initiatives in other arenas (with a special focus on Medicare's quality improvement organization programs) and formulate criteria that can guide payment strategies. We anticipate that the *Pathways* series will complement and extend the earlier *Quality Chasm* series of IOM reports. In short, we are moving from the "what" of quality improvement to the "how."

This series is part of a larger effort at the IOM to remedy flaws in our health care system, enhance the quality of services, reduce waste and inefficiency, promote patient safety and beneficiary protections, ensure that public and private purchasers obtain value for their dollars, and foster equity. These are the right goals to pursue, and we cannot wait any longer to undertake that crucial effort.

Harvey V. Fineberg, M.D., Ph.D.
President, Institute of Medicine
October 2005

Acknowledgments

Performance Measurement: Accelerating Improvement benefited from the contributions of many individuals. The committee takes this opportunity to recognize those who so generously gave their time and expertise to inform its deliberations.

The committee wishes to acknowledge the members of the Subcommittee on Performance Measurement and the outstanding leadership of co-chairs Don Berwick (Institute for Healthcare Improvement) and Elliott S. Fisher (Dartmouth Medical School). Subcommittee members included Patricia Gabow (Denver Health and Hospital Authority), Lillee Gelinas (VHA, Inc.), Margarita Hurtado (American Institutes for Research), George Isham (HealthPartners, Inc.), Brent James (Intermountain Health Care), Arthur Levin (Center for Medical Consumers), Glen Mays (University of Arkansas for Medical Sciences), Elizabeth McGlynn (RAND Corporation), Arnold Milstein (Pacific Business Group on Health), Sharon-Lise Normand (Harvard Medical School), Barbara Paul (Beverly Enterprises, Inc.), Samuel Thier (Harvard Medical School and Massachusetts General Hospital), and Paul Wallace (Kaiser Permanente Care Management Institute).

The committee commissioned several papers to provide background information for its deliberations and to synthesize the evidence on particular issues. These papers are included as appendixes to this report. We thank John D. Birkmeyer, Eve A. Kerr, and Justin B. Dimick of the University of Michigan for their paper on "Improving the Quality of Quality Improvement"; Eric M. Coleman of the University of Colorado Health Science Center for his paper on "Transitional Care Performance Measurement"; Kyle L. Grazier of the University of Michigan, School of Public Health, for her paper on "Efficiency/Value Based Measures for Services, Defined Populations, Acute Episodes and Chronic Conditions"; and Sydney Dy of the Johns Hopkins Bloomberg School of Public Health and Joanne Lynn of the Washington Home for Palliative Care Studies for their paper on "Palliative Care/End of Life Measures."

We also wish to acknowledge the input received from several experts who participated in the Performance Measurement Subcommittee Workshop held on December 1, 2004, in Washington, DC: R. Adams Dudley of the University of California, San Francisco; Robert Krughoff of the Center for the Study of Services; Tom Lee of Partners HealthCare System, Inc.; Mary Naylor of the University of Pennsylvania School of Nursing; Judy Hibbard of the University of Oregon; Al Mulley of the Massachusetts General Hospital; Dana Gelb Safran of the Health Institute at Tufts-New England Medical Center; Gail Amundson of HealthPartners, Inc.; Eugene C. Nelson of Dartmouth Medical Center; David Wennberg of the Health Dialog Data Service; and Mark E. Miller and Karen Milgate of MedPAC.

The committee appreciates the valuable feedback received from the case study participants: Community Medical Associates, San Antonio, Texas, GreenfieldHealth, Portland, Oregon; HealthPartners, Inc., Minneapolis, Minnesota; North Texas Medical Group, Plano, Texas; Primary Care Family Practice, Clinton, Oklahoma; Rochester Individual Practice Association, Rochester, New York; and Internal Medicine Solo Practice, Fort Walton Beach, Florida.

The committee would also like to acknowledge organizations that provided us feedback on various topics: Agency for Healthcare Research and Quality; Ambulatory care Quality Alliance; Centers for Medicare and Medicaid Services; Denver Health and Hospital Authority; Hospital Quality Alliance; Joint Commission on Accreditation of Healthcare Organizations; Kaiser Permanente Care Management Institute; Leapfrog Group; National Committee for Quality Assurance; National Quality Forum; Partners Health Care; Physician Consortium of the American Medical Association; and VHA, Inc.

The committee would also like to thank Tyjen Tsai and Shari Erickson of the Institute of Medicine staff for their additional support towards the completion of this report.

Finally, the committee gratefully acknowledges the U.S. Department of Health and Human Services through the Centers for Medicare and Medicaid Services, whose funding supported this congressionally mandated study.

Contents

APPENDIXES

Tables, Figures, and Boxes

TABLES

xx

Performance Measurement

Executive Summary

The past decade has seen an unprecedented level of concern and action focused on improving the quality of American health care. Catalyzed in part by two Institute of Medicine (IOM) reports—*To Err Is Human: Building a Safer Health System* (IOM, 2000) and *Crossing the Quality Chasm: A New Health System for the 21st Century* (IOM, 2001)—organizations, professional associations, payers, regulators, accrediting bodies, and consumer groups have begun to make significant changes in their respective agendas and investments, all designed to achieve better safety, effectiveness, patient-centeredness, timeliness, efficiency, and equity—the six aims for quality improvement specified in the *Quality Chasm* report. Initiatives undertaken include quality improvement collaboratives and other change programs; explorations of pay for performance; the development of early formats for public reporting on performance; and, most important, efforts to devise better ways to measure quality in nearly all of its dimensions.

Despite these investments, however, progress continues to be slow, lessons learned are fragmented, and little effort is being devoted to evaluating the impact of these improvement initiatives so future efforts can be guided more by evidence than by anecdote (Jencks et al., 2000; Leatherman and McCarthy, 2002, 2004, 2005). In short, the quality chasm in health care remains wide. On average, adults in the United States fail to receive almost half of the clinical services from which they would likely benefit (McGlynn et al., 2003). And while per capita health care spending in the United States greatly exceeds that in other industrialized countries, cross-national comparisons of health care quality reveal that other countries achieve better performance on many measures (Hussey et al., 2004; Reinhardt et al.,

2004). Similarly, spending levels vary widely among U.S. regions, yet there is no evidence that more expensive regions have either better quality or improved health outcomes (Baicker and Chandra, 2004; Fisher et al., 2003a,b). Racial, ethnic, and class disparities are pervasive; moreover, the numbers of uninsured are rising, currently making up more than 15 percent of the population (IOM, 2002, 2004). For the sizable investments being made in health care services, Americans should be getting much greater value from the care they receive.

There are many obstacles to rapid progress in improving the quality of health care, but none exceeds the fact that the nation still lacks a coherent, goal-oriented, consistent, and efficient system for assessing and reporting on the performance of the health care system. Thus if quality improvement initiatives are to achieve their full potential, a concerted national effort to consolidate health care performance measurement and reporting activities will be essential.

THE REDESIGNING HEALTH INSURANCE PROJECT

In September 2004, the IOM launched the Redesigning Health Insurance Performance Measures, Payment, and Performance Improvement Project in response to two congressional mandates in the Medicare Prescription Drug, Improvement, and Modernization Improvement Act of 2003 (Public Law 108-173, Section 109). The committee empaneled by the IOM to carry out this project is producing three reports for Congress, the Centers for Medicare and Medicaid Services (CMS), and other public and private purchasers on strategies for accelerating the diffusion and pace of quality improvement efforts in the United States (see Table ES-1).

Each of these reports, known collectively as the *Pathways to Quality Health Care* series, is focused on a specific policy approach to improving the quality of health care: (1) measurement and reporting of performance data, (2) payment incentives, and (3) quality improvement initiatives. All three approaches depend upon the availability of accurate, reliable, and valid performance measures. Performance measures can serve as the foundation for public reporting programs intended to promote accountability among providers and to aid consumers in making informed choices, serve as the basis for payment incentives that reward providers who deliver more effective and efficient care, and guide and inform clinicians and organizations in their quality improvement initiatives.

This first report in the *Pathways* series focuses on the selection of measures to support the quality improvement efforts of a diverse set of stakeholders, and on the creation of a common infrastructure for guiding and managing a consistent set of such measures nationally and regionally. Future reports, to be released in 2006, will address payment incentive strategies that incorporate these measures and offer an evaluation of the Quality Improvement Organizations that work under contracts with Medicare.

NEED FOR A NATIONAL SYSTEM FOR PERFORMANCE MEASUREMENT AND REPORTING

Congress, the public, and numerous other stakeholders concerned about the persistent quality gaps and rapidly rising costs of health care in the United States have high expectations that public reporting, pay for performance, and quality improvement initiatives can help realize the transformational change envisioned in the *Quality Chasm* report. As noted above, however, the full potential of these initiatives cannot be realized without a coherent, robust, integrated performance measurement system that is purposeful, comprehensive, efficient, and transparent. Such a system should link performance measures directly to explicit national goals for improvement. The performance measurement process should include audits to ensure the measures themselves are sufficiently accurate and reliable to yield credible data. The measurement process should also be streamlined to improve its value while reducing its costs. Its results should be open and available to all stakeholders.

The committee fully recognizes that many public- and private-sector initiatives have made substantial progress in developing, implementing, and reporting on measures of provider performance. These efforts have yielded a laudable array of assets for performance measurement. However, the committee believes a well-functioning national system that can meet the need for performance measurement and reporting is unlikely to emerge from current voluntary, consensus-based efforts, which are often fragmented and lack a consistent connection to explicit, overarching national goals for health care improvement. In short, while recent efforts offer some promise, the committee believes a bolder national initiative is required.

The current approach to quality measurement in the United States is unlikely to evolve on its own into an effective national system for performance measurement and reporting for the following reasons, among others:

- National goals are unlikely to be set and translated into measures, since existing entities have neither the authority nor the overarching leadership required to formulate such goals.
- Gaps in performance measurement, such as the capacity to measure equity and access, are unlikely to be filled because of the lack of clear ownership of these aspects of the nation's quality improvement agenda.
- Wasteful duplication and inconsistencies among measures will continue, since no single stakeholder group has the standing to require others to use specific, standardized definitions and measurements.

TABLE ES-1 Mapping of IOM Reports of the Committee on Redesigning Health Insurance to Congressional Mandates

P.L. 108-173 Section 238
EVALUATION-
  (1) IN GENERAL-Not later than the date that is 2 months after the date of the enactment of this Act, the Secretary shall enter into an arrangement under which the Institute of Medicine of the National Academy of Sciences (in this section referred to as the 'Institute') shall conduct an evaluation of leading health care performance measures in the public and private sectors and options to implement policies that align performance with payment under the Medicare program under title XVIII of the Social Security Act (42 U.S.C. 1395 et seq.).
  (2) SPECIFIC MATTERS EVALUATED-In conducting the evaluation under paragraph (1), the Institute shall—
    (A) catalogue, review, and evaluate the validity of leading health care performance measures;
    (B) catalogue and evaluate the success and utility of alternative performance incentive programs in public or private sector settings; and
    (C) identify and prioritize options to implement policies that align performance with payment under the medicare program that indicate—
      (i) the performance measurement set to be used and how that measurement set will be updated;
      (ii) the payment policy that will reward performance; and
      (iii) the key implementation issues (such as data and information technology requirements) that must be addressed.
  (3) SCOPE OF HEALTH CARE PERFORMANCE MEASURES-The health care performance measures described in paragraph (2)(A) shall encompass a variety of perspectives, including physicians, hospitals, other health care providers, health plans, purchasers, and patients.

P.L. 108-173 Section 109
IOM STUDY OF QIOs-
  (1) IN GENERAL-The Secretary shall request the Institute of Medicine of the National Academy of Sciences to conduct an evaluation of the program under part B of title XI of the Social Security Act. The study shall include a review of the following:
    (A) An overview of the program under such part.
    (B) The duties of organizations with contracts with the Secretary under such part.
    (C) The extent to which quality improvement organizations improve the quality of care for Medicare beneficiaries.
    (D) The extent to which other entities could perform such quality improvement functions as well as, or better than, quality improvement organizations.
    (E) The effectiveness of reviews and other actions conducted by such organizations in carrying out those duties.
    (F) The source and amount of funding for such organizations.
    (G) The conduct of oversight of such organizations.

Performance Measurement Report

This report will address issues related to the promulgation and use of standardized performance measures for payment, public reporting, and performance improvement. Specifically, it will do the following:

- Catalogue, review, and evaluate the validity of leading health care performance measures.
- Recommend a process for the ongoing promulgation and maintenance of performance measures, the submission of data by providers, and public reporting of performance information.

Payment Incentives Report

This report will identify and analyze options for aligning Medicare payment policies with provider performance in the original fee-for-service program (under parts A and B of Title XVIII of the Social Security Act), the new Medicare Advantage program (under Part C), and other programs (under Title XVIII). Specifically, it will do the following:

- Select and weight of health care performance measures for use in payment programs.
- Catalogue and evaluate the success and utility of alternative performance incentive programs in public- and private-sector settings.
- Identify and prioritize options for implementing policies that align performance with payment under the Medicare program, indicating:
  - The performance measurement set to be used and how that measurement set will be updated.
  - The payment policy that will reward performance.
  - The key implementation issues (such as data and information technology requirements) that must be addressed.

Performance Improvement Report

This report will provide an evaluation of Medicare's quality improvement program (under Part B of Title XI of the Social Security Act). Specifically, it will provide the following:

- An overview of the quality improvement program, including a description of the duties of private-sector organizations (known as quality improvement organizations, or QIOs) that have contracts with the Secretary under this program, and the source and amount of funding for QIOs.
- An assessment of the effectiveness of reviews and other actions conducted by QIOs, and the extent to which QIOs improve the quality of care for Medicare beneficiaries.
- An assessment of the extent to which other entities could perform such quality improvement functions as well as, or better than, QIOs.
- An assessment of the conduct of CMS oversight of QIOs.

• Measures may not be viewed as authoritative, credible, or objective since the measures developed by most stakeholders are more apt to reflect the interests of their constituencies than those of others.

• Public goods, such as investments in better risk adjustment methodologies and data aggregation methods, are unlikely to be addressed adequately in a competitive market among current developers of measures.

• Making all information fully transparent and available to the public is unlikely, since much of the technology and data on performance measurement is currently held as proprietary.

Creating a coherent national system that strengthens current performance measurement efforts by enabling those involved to work more effectively toward a common, clearly articulated set of goals is a major challenge. Strong, independent leadership is needed to coordinate and guide existing efforts and to broaden the scope of measurement to overcome existing gaps. Moreover, sustained, adequate funding is needed for a structure capable of encouraging multiple initiatives, withstanding pressures from narrow stakeholder interests, and sustaining patients' interests as the primary objective. And a social investment in learning is necessary to understand, as a matter of public good, how measurement can best accelerate improvement.

The factors cited above, along with the long history of multiple, sometimes competing efforts to promulgate and report on performance measures, convinced the committee that current initiatives are unlikely to evolve into the well-functioning national system required to achieve the six quality aims set forth in the *Quality Chasm* report. The committee believes federal leadership is necessary to overcome these limitations, to ensure that a viable national system does emerge, and to incorporate the public-good dimensions of performance measurement in the American health care enterprise. Such leadership should ensure the creation and maintenance of a robust system for performance measurement and reporting with at least the following functions: (1) establishing national health care improvement goals and priorities, (2) setting standards for measurement, and (3) ensuring a level playing field through oversight and public reporting.

RECOMMENDATIONS FOR ACHIEVING A NATIONAL PERFORMANCE MEASUREMENT AND REPORTING SYSTEM

Based on its careful analysis of alternatives for achieving a national performance measurement and reporting system, the committee recommends the establishment of a new independent board, the National Quality Coordination Board (NQCB), which would be recognized by all public and private stakeholders as the lead agency responsible for ensuring the creation of a national system for performance measurement and reporting. In addition to carrying out general management and coordinating functions, the board would provide leadership and policy guidance that would support existing efforts, and seek to align those efforts with national health goals through contractual agreements, educational programs, and consensus-building initiatives.

Recommendation 1: Congress should establish a National Quality Coordination Board (NQCB) with seven key functions:

- Specify the purpose and aims for American health care.
- Establish short- and long-term national goals for improving the health care system.
- Designate, or if necessary develop, standardized performance measures for evaluating the performance of current providers, and monitor the nation's progress toward these goals.
- Ensure the creation of data collection, validation, and aggregation processes.
- Establish public reporting methods responsive to the needs of all stakeholders.
- Identify and fund a research agenda for the development of new measures to address gaps in performance measurement.
- Evaluate the impact of performance measurement on pay for performance, quality improvement, public reporting, and other policy levers.

The NQCB should produce useful information for three purposes that address different audiences:

- *Accountability*—Information should be available to assist stakeholders in making choices about providers. These stakeholders include patients identifying a clinician, hospital, or other provider from which to seek services; purchasers and health plans selecting providers to include in their health insurance networks; and quality oversight organizations making accreditation and certification decisions.
- *Quality improvement*—The information provided should be of value to stakeholders responsible for improving the quality of care, including clinicians, and administrators and governing board members of health care organizations.
- *Population health*—The information should be useful for stakeholders making decisions about access to services (e.g., public insurance benefits and coverage); those involved in communitywide programs and efforts to address racial and ethnic disparities and promote healthy behav-

iors; and public officials responsible for disease surveillance and health protection.

> **Recommendation 2: The NQCB's membership and procedures should be designed to ensure that the board has structural independence, protection from undue special interests, substantive expertise drawn from the public and private sectors (including not-for-profit entities), contract authority, standards-setting authority, financial strength, and external accountability.**

The committee believes that an NQCB without adequate authority and protection cannot succeed in this endeavor. Therefore, the committee proposes that the NQCB be armed with at least the following attributes:

- *Structural independence.* The NQCB should have the capacity to move the health care system beyond the status quo. The committee recommends that the board be housed within the U.S. Department of Health and Human Services (DHHS) and report directly to the Secretary.
- *Protection from undue influence.* The membership of the NQCB should be appointed by the President, with terms that are staggered and long enough to protect the board against short-term political influence and major stakeholder interests.
- *Substantive expertise.* The committee's intention is not to supplant or duplicate the often outstanding work of the many organizations currently involved in developing, evaluating, vetting, and implementing performance measures in health care. Rather, the goal is to accelerate progress through coordination and direct financial support for these current activities. Thus the membership of the NQCB should encompass the technical competence needed to assess and guide that work.
- *Contract authority.* In the event that the major organizations currently engaged in measurement development, implementation, and reporting prove unwilling or unable to undertake the activities outlined by the NQCB or to deliver under contract the required levels of standardization, analysis, and reporting, the board should have the backup authority and sufficient funding to broaden the array of contractors through which it can execute its key functions.
- *Standards-setting authority.* The Secretary of DHHS should direct CMS (including Medicare, Medicaid, and the State Children's Health Insurance Program), the Health Resources and Services Administration, and the Agency for Healthcare Research and Quality (AHRQ) to focus on the achievement of all applicable national goals established by the NQCB through public reporting, payment reform, and other incentives such as health care improvement programs, benefit design, health professions edu-

cation, and organizational and systems capacity building. The Secretary should also direct CMS to require that providers submit to the NQCB (or its designee) performance data that can be used by Medicare for public reporting and quality improvement activities or as a basis for payment. In addition, Congress should activate an interagency task force to explore mechanisms for aligning other government health care programs with these efforts—including the Department of Defense (DoD) TRICARE program and DoD-operated clinical facilities, the Federal Employees Health Benefits Program, and the programs of the Veterans Health Administration and the Indian Health Service.

- *Financial strength.* The NQCB should have sufficient, stable funding to contract for services with outside groups and organizations so it can perform its designated functions effectively. The board should be funded directly from the Medicare Trust Fund and have bypass authority to request an appropriation directly from Congress. This bypass authority would free the NQCB from the unpredictable budgetary cycles commonly associated with preparing discretionary budgets that are subject to review and modification on the basis of other departmental, executive, and legislative priorities. Congress should authorize and appropriate funds to support the work of the NQCB and to implement its recommendations in Medicare and other government programs by the end of fiscal year 2007. More specifically, Congress should authorize an annual allocation from the Medicare Trust Fund, initially in the range of $100–200 million. This level of investment is based on an analysis of resources that currently support related but more limited activities within the National Quality Forum, the National Committee for Quality Assurance, and the Joint Commission on Accreditation of Healthcare Organizations. This figure constitutes approximately 0.1 percent of the Medicare annual budget,[1] a relatively small investment with great potential to enhance value and improve efficiency throughout the health care delivery system. The committee envisions substantial staff requirements to support the functions of the board delineated in Recommendation 1 and substantial costs related to contracts with existing entities to carry out tasks pursuant to the mission of the board. Although the federal government should provide up front the funding needed for the NQCB to become fully operational, particularly with regard to its public-good functions, public–private partnerships could be formed over time to support this ongoing work.

- *External accountability.* The NQCB should be required to provide an annual report to Congress on its progress toward implementing an effective quality measurement and reporting system. In addition, the board

---

[1] $278 billion in 2003 (CMS, 2004).

should undergo periodic independent assessments performed by an external organization such as the Medicare Payment Advisory Commission, the IOM, or the Government Accountability Office.

The health care system in the United States is fundamentally a local enterprise. The operations of the NQCB should therefore be sensitive and responsive to local goals and improvement priorities and create mechanisms for broad input from national and local stakeholders into the agenda-setting process. The national goals to be established by the NQCB should build upon earlier statements of purpose and aims of the health care system, as articulated by both the President's Advisory Commission on Consumer Protection and Quality in the Health Care Industry (1998) and the IOM (IOM, 1990, 2001). The national goals and performance measures articulated by the NQCB should provide a benchmark for an acceptable, minimum set of performance measures and an agenda for improvement on the part of each community, but these leadership activities should in no way preclude communities or states from establishing additional, locally relevant goals. Indeed, the NQCB should encourage widespread local innovation to improve health care, and standards setting by government should both build upon measures that are widely accepted in many sectors and promote local experimentation with innovative measures, from which all can learn.

> **Recommendation 3: Local innovation in pursuit of national goals for improving health care quality should be encouraged. Performance measurement, improvement, and reporting activities— including those of public and private purchasers; accreditation and certification entities; and federal, state, and local government programs—should be substantially aligned with the national goals and standardized measures established by the NQCB, but local communities should also be encouraged to identify and pursue local priorities, in addition to helping to achieve national goals.**

A RECOMMENDED STARTER SET OF PERFORMANCE MEASURES

The committee recommends that the NQCB build upon the substantial scientifically grounded gains that have already been made by various stakeholder groups committed to the development and promulgation of performance measures by immediately upon its inception endorsing the leading measure sets listed in Table ES-2 as national standards. The NQCB should ensure the reliable collection and national reporting of these measures through a data repository system that includes auditing functions and public reporting methods. During the first phase of implementation, providers

TABLE ES-2 Recommended Starter Set of Performance Measures

Ambulatory Care	**Ambulatory care Quality Alliance (26)** Prevention measures[a] (7), coronary artery disease[a] (3), heart failure[a] (2), diabetes[a] (6), asthma[a] (2), depression[a] (2), prenatal care[a] (2), quality measures addressing overuse or misuse (2) **Ambulatory Care Survey** CAHPS Clinician and Group Survey: getting care quickly, getting needed care, how well providers communicate, health promotion and education, shared decision making, knowledge of medical history, how well office staff communicate
Acute Care	**Hospital Quality Alliance (20)** Acute coronary syndrome[a] (7), heart failure[a] (3), pneumonia[a] (5), smoking cessation[a] (3), surgical infection prevention[a] (from the Surgical Care Improvement Project) (2) **Structural Measures** (computerized provider order entry, intensive care unit intensivists, evidence-based hospital referrals) **Hospital CAHPS** Patient communication with physicians, patient communication with nurses, responsiveness of hospital staff, cleanliness/noise level of physical environment, pain control, communications about medicines, discharge information
Health Plans and Accountable Health Organizations	**Health Plan Employer Data and Information Set (HEDIS) (61)** Integrated delivery systems (health maintenance organizations): effectiveness (26), access/availability of care (8), satisfaction with the experience of care (4), health plan stability (2), use of service (15), cost of care, informed health care choices, health plan descriptive information (6) Preferred provider organizations within Medicare Advantage: selected administrative data and hybrid measures **Ambulatory Care Survey** CAHPS Health Plan Survey: getting care quickly, getting needed care, how well providers communicate, health plan paperwork, health plan customer service
Long-Term Care	**Minimum Data Set (15)** Long-term care (12), short-stay care (3) **Outcome and Assessment Information Set (11)** Ambulation/locomotion (1), transferring (1), toileting (1), pain (1), bathing (2), management of oral medications (1), acute care hospitalization (1), emergent care (1), confusion (1)
End-Stage Renal Disease	**National Healthcare Quality Report (5)** Transplant registry and results (2), dialysis effectiveness (2), mortality (1)
Longitudinal Measures of Outcomes and Efficiency	1-year mortality, resource use, and functional status (SF-12) after acute myocardial infarction

[a]The committee recommends the aggregation of individual measures to patient-level composites for these areas.

should also be encouraged to invest in electronic health records if they have not already done so. Although most providers will be able to meet data reporting requirements during this first phase by abstracting samples of medical records and culling information from administrative files, this practice will be economically unsustainable as the NQCB moves toward more comprehensive measurement. Providers who have made concerted efforts to modernize information and communications technologies in their practice settings should be encouraged in these investments, and should be given additional latitude to customize their measurement systems in accordance with general guidelines from the NQCB.

> **Recommendation 4: The NQCB should promulgate measure sets that build on the work of key public- and private-sector organizations. Specifically, the NQCB should:**
>
> • As a starting point, endorse as national standards performance measures currently approved through ongoing consensus processes led by major stakeholder groups.
> • Ensure that a data repository system[2] and public reporting program capable of data collection at the individual patient level are established and open to participation by all payers and providers.
> • Ensure that technical and financial assistance is available to all providers who need help in establishing performance measurement and improvement capabilities.

The committee also believes that while the leading measure sets provide an excellent springboard, they are inadequate to drive the health sector toward the transformational changes envisioned in the *Quality Chasm*. The committee identified several serious limitations of currently available performance measures, and proposes complementary approaches to overcome these shortfalls:

> • *Lack of comprehensive measures.* The committee recommends broadening the limited scope of current measures to address important domains of quality, most notably the IOM aims of efficiency, equity, and patient-centeredness.

---

[2]The data repository system would collect, validate, and aggregate provider performance data (see Recommendation 1).

• *Narrow time window.* In general, most performance measures assess care at only one point in time. The committee recommends measuring the quality, costs, and outcomes of care over a longer time frame. Doing so will necessitate further development of longitudinal measures that can capture the performance of multiple providers caring for a patient; examine how well care is provided across transitions to different settings (e.g., hospital to nursing home); and, most important, evaluate patient outcomes over time. The committee believes that focusing on chronic illness, care across time and locations, and clinical and functional outcomes will move performance measurement much closer to a patient-centered perspective.

• *Provider-centric focus.* Current measures tend to focus on specific settings of care, so that measure specifications are applicable to only one setting, such as a physician office or hospital. The committee recommends moving toward individual patient-level measurement, even for the starter set of measures, because of the markedly increased value and flexibility offered by this approach. This approach to data collection would allow for aggregation along three important dimensions: (1) *composite measures* that can document whether a patient received all recommended services for a given condition within a specified time window; (2) *population-based measures*, whose aggregation for defined strata of the population on the basis of socioeconomic status, race, and ethnicity would allow for assessment of disparities in treatment at the provider, system, or community level; and (3) *systems-level measures* that can characterize the overall performance of an organization or entity across conditions and service lines, and can better identify gaps in performance and foster accountability at each level of care, from the individual clinician to the community. The committee strongly recommends that data collection protocols be planned and implemented to support such reporting.

• *Narrow focus of accountability.* The committee endorses the principle of shared accountability among all providers involved in a patient's care. This strategy represents perhaps the most significant explicit departure from a traditional guideline for selecting performance measures—that a responsible entity or person be known at the outset. The committee believes that shared accountability can be achieved both by reporting specific measures that are not uniquely the responsibility of a single provider (e.g., care transitions) and by aggregating patient-level measures. In short, the committee recommends that certain important aspects of care be measured even when no single entity can be held accountable for the results. Qualities such as population mortality rates, efficiency through time, chronic disease complication rates, and measures of oversupply of services may be among the most important of these aspects from the viewpoint of patients and society. Left unmeasured, they are certain to be left unaddressed.

A RECOMMENDED RESEARCH AGENDA

A key function of the NQCB would be to work collaboratively with stakeholder groups to develop, implement, and fund a research agenda that can support national goals and improve the measurement and reporting enterprise itself. The committee recommends four areas of focus for such a research agenda: (1) development, implementation, and evaluation of new measures to address current gaps; (2) applied research to address underlying methodological issues; (3) design and testing of reporting formats that will be helpful to different end-users; and (4) evaluation of the performance measurement and reporting system with regard to intended and unintended consequences for cost and care.

> Recommendation 5: The NQCB should formulate and promptly pursue a research agenda to support the development of a national system for performance measurement and reporting. The board should develop this agenda in collaboration with federal agencies and private-sector stakeholders. The agenda should address the following:
>
> - Development, implementation, and evaluation of new measures to address current gaps in performance measurement.
> - Applied research focused on underlying methodological issues, such as risk adjustment, sample size, weighting, and models of shared accountability.
> - Design and testing of reporting formats for consumer usability.
> - Evaluation of the performance measurement and reporting system.

The NQCB should receive funding adequate to enable it to oversee and ensure the implementation of a robust research agenda. The committee recommends that the NQCB work closely with AHRQ, which has an established track record in funding evidence-based health services research, and other groups that can provide linkages at the local level between foundations and community collaborations, such as Grantmakers in Health, to align investment strategies for carrying out this agenda.

> Recommendation 6: Congress should provide the financial resources needed to carry out the research agenda developed by the NQCB. The Agency for Healthcare Research and Quality should collaborate with Grantmakers in Health and others that have ties to local foundations to convene public- and private-sector stakeholders currently investing in various aspects of this research agenda for the purpose of identifying complementary investment strategies.

The stakeholders convened should include private foundations, government research and development programs, and health systems with internal research capacity.

CONSEQUENCES OF INACTION

Failure to establish a well-functioning national performance measurement and reporting system would severely compromise our ability to achieve the essential quality improvements called for in the *Quality Chasm* report. Because payment incentives, public reporting, and quality improvement initiatives all require the existence of meaningful and valid performance measures, their potential impact would be limited by a constrained, fragmented, and ineffective measurement system. Yet without strong, central leadership, individual stakeholders will have great difficulty in acting together voluntarily to create the kind of system that is needed.

Improving performance measurement will vastly improve the nation's ability to provide better health care services, and will catalyze action to provide high-quality, patient-centered care consistently and efficiently to all Americans. Providers will face less frustration from having to respond to multiple requests for reports on often conflicting measures; performance measurement will become less of a burden and more of a resource for internal quality improvement to enhance care processes of care. Improved reporting formats will facilitate better access to information that is understandable, meaningful, and important to patients, families, and communities. Public trust will grow as a greater balance between the information available to health care system and its consumers is achieved. Current participants in measurement initiatives who are suspicious of national leadership may find themselves better off in the long run as a consistent national approach to measurement allows them to add greater value and compete more on execution in contributing to an industrywide endeavor. In sum, the committee believes that, in the absence of a centralized organizing structure such as the NQCB to set clear goals, coordinate measurement efforts, and ensure stable funding for organizations involved in performance measurement, a robust and well-functioning system to support fair comparisons of cost and quality is unlikely to emerge on its own.

REFERENCES

Baicker K, Chandra A. 2004. Medicare spending, the physician workforce, and beneficiaries' quality of care. *Health Affairs*. Jan-June Suppl Web Exclusive: W4:184–197.

CMS (Centers for Medicare and Medicaid Services). 2004. *2004 CMS Statistics*. Washington, DC: CMS.

Fisher ES, Wennberg DE, Stukel TA, Gottlieb DJ, Lucas FL, Pinder EL. 2003a. The implications of regional variations in Medicare spending. Part 2: Health outcomes and satisfaction with care. *Annals of Internal Medicine* 138(4):288–298.

Fisher ES, Wennberg DE, Stukel TA, Gottlieb DJ, Lucas FL, Pinder EL. 2003b. The implications of regional variations in Medicare spending. Part 1: The content, quality, and accessibility of care. *Annals of Internal Medicine* 138(4):273–287.

Hussey PS, Anderson GF, Osborn R, Feek C, McLaughlin V, Millar J, Epstein A. 2004. How does the quality of care compare in five countries? *Health Affairs* 23(3):89–99.

IOM (Institute of Medicine). 1990. *Medicare: A Strategy for Quality Assurance. Volume 1.* Washington, DC: National Academy Press.

IOM. 2000. *To Err Is Human: Building a Safer Health System.* Kohn LT, Corrigan JM, Donaldson MS, eds. Washington, DC: National Academy Press.

IOM. 2001. *Crossing the Quality Chasm: A New Health System for the 21st Century.* Washington, DC: National Academy Press.

IOM. 2002. *Unequal Treatment: Confronting Racial and Ethnic Disparities in Health Care.* Smedley BS, Stith AY, Nelson BD, eds. Washington, DC: The National Academies Press.

IOM. 2004. *Insuring Health—Insuring America's Health: Principles and Recommendations.* Washington, DC: The National Academies Press.

Jencks SF, Cuerdon T, Burwen DR, Fleming B, Houck PM, Kussmaul AE, Nilasena DS, Ordin DL, Arday DR. 2000. Quality of medical care delivered to Medicare beneficiaries: A profile at state and national levels. *Journal of the American Medical Association* 284(13):1670–1676.

Leatherman S, McCarthy D. 2002. *Quality of Health Care in the United States: A Chartbook.* New York: Commonwealth Fund.

Leatherman S, McCarthy D. 2004. *Quality of Care for Children and Adolescents: A Chartbook.* New York: Commonwealth Fund.

Leatherman S, McCarthy D. 2005. *Quality of Health Care for Medicare Beneficiaries: A Chartbook.* New York: Commonwealth Fund.

McGlynn EA, Asch SM, Adams J, Keesey J, Hicks J, DeCristofaro A, Kerr EA. 2003. The quality of health care delivered to adults in the United States. *New England Journal of Medicine* 348(26):2635–2645.

President's Advisory Commission on Consumer Protection and Quality in the Health Care Industry. 1998. *Quality First: Better Health Care for All Americans—Final Report to the President of the United States.* Washington, DC: U.S. Government Printing Office.

Reinhardt UE, Hussey PS, Anderson GF. 2004. U.S. health care spending in an international context. *Health Affairs* 23(3):10–25.

1

Introduction

CHAPTER SUMMARY

This report is a product of the Redesigning Health Insurance Performance Measures, Payment, and Performance Improvement Programs project, established by the Institute of Medicine in 2004. This 3-year project is producing a series of reports on various aspects of health insurance, including performance measurement, performance improvement activities, and payment policies. This introductory chapter provides an overview of the entire series of reports, as well as background on the rationale for the project.

In 2001, the Institute of Medicine (IOM) released the report *Crossing the Quality Chasm: A New Health System for the 21st Century* (IOM, 2001). That report identified six aims for the health care system—health care should be safe, effective, patient-centered, timely, efficient, and equitable—and challenged the health care sector to achieve substantial improvements in each of these dimensions of quality over the coming decade. The report acknowledged that achieving significant improvement in quality across all six dimensions would necessitate behavioral and structural change at many levels, including patient–clinician relationships, small practice settings, health care organizations (e.g., hospitals and health plans), and the environment of care (e.g., regulatory processes and payment policies) (Berwick, 2002).

The IOM project Redesigning Health Insurance Performance Measures, Payment, and Performance Improvement Programs, initiated in 2004, is focused at the environmental level. It addresses the redesign of public and private health insurance programs, with an initial emphasis on the Medicare system. The committee impaneled by the IOM to carry out the project is producing a series of three reports (see Table 1-1):

• *Performance measurement report.* This first report lays the groundwork for the subsequent two reports on payment incentives and Quality Im-

TABLE 1-1 Mapping of IOM Reports of the Committee on Redesigning Health Insurance to Congressional Mandates

P.L. 108-173 Section 238

EVALUATION-

(1) IN GENERAL-Not later than the date that is 2 months after the date of the enactment of this Act, the Secretary shall enter into an arrangement under which the Institute of Medicine of the National Academy of Sciences (in this section referred to as the 'Institute') shall conduct an evaluation of leading health care performance measures in the public and private sectors and options to implement policies that align performance with payment under the Medicare program under title XVIII of the Social Security Act (42 U.S.C. 1395 et seq.).

(2) SPECIFIC MATTERS EVALUATED-In conducting the evaluation under paragraph (1), the Institute shall—

(A) catalogue, review, and evaluate the validity of leading health care performance measures;

(B) catalogue and evaluate the success and utility of alternative performance incentive programs in public or private sector settings; and

(C) identify and prioritize options to implement policies that align performance with payment under the medicare program that indicate—

(i) the performance measurement set to be used and how that measurement set will be updated;

(ii) the payment policy that will reward performance; and

(iii) the key implementation issues (such as data and information technology requirements) that must be addressed.

(3) SCOPE OF HEALTH CARE PERFORMANCE MEASURES-The health care performance measures described in paragraph (2)(A) shall encompass a variety of perspectives, including physicians, hospitals, other health care providers, health plans, purchasers, and patients.

P.L. 108-173 Section 109

IOM STUDY OF QIOs-

(1) IN GENERAL-The Secretary shall request the Institute of Medicine of the National Academy of Sciences to conduct an evaluation of the program under part B of title XI of the Social Security Act. The study shall include a review of the following:

(A) An overview of the program under such part.

(B) The duties of organizations with contracts with the Secretary under such part.

(C) The extent to which quality improvement organizations improve the quality of care for Medicare beneficiaries.

(D) The extent to which other entities could perform such quality improvement functions as well as, or better than, quality improvement organizations.

(E) The effectiveness of reviews and other actions conducted by such organizations in carrying out those duties.

(F) The source and amount of funding for such organizations.

(G) The conduct of oversight of such organizations.

Performance Measurement Report

This report will address issues related to the promulgation and use of standardized performance measures for payment, public reporting, and performance improvement. Specifically, it will do the following:

- Catalogue, review, and evaluate the validity of leading health care performance measures.
- Recommend a process for the ongoing promulgation and maintenance of performance measures, the submission of data by providers, and public reporting of performance information.

Payment Incentives Report

This report will identify and analyze options for aligning Medicare payment policies with provider performance in the original fee-for-service program (under parts A and B of Title XVIII of the Social Security Act), the new Medicare Advantage program (under Part C), and other programs (under Title XVIII). Specifically, it will do the following:

- Select and weight of health care performance measures for use in payment programs.
- Catalogue and evaluate the success and utility of alternative performance incentive programs in public- and private-sector settings.
- Identify and prioritize options for implementing policies that align performance with payment under the Medicare program, indicating:
  - The performance measurement set to be used and how that measurement set will be updated.
  - The payment policy that will reward performance.
  - The key implementation issues (such as data and information technology requirements) that must be addressed.

Performance Improvement Report

This report will provide an evaluation of Medicare's quality improvement program (under Part B of Title XI of the Social Security Act). Specifically, it will provide the following:

- An overview of the quality improvement program, including a description of the duties of private-sector organizations (known as quality improvement organizations, or QIOs) that have contracts with the Secretary under this program, and the source and amount of funding for QIOs.
- An assessment of the effectiveness of reviews and other actions conducted by QIOs, and the extent to which QIOs improve the quality of care for Medicare beneficiaries.
- An assessment of the extent to which other entities could perform such quality improvement functions as well as, or better than, QIOs.
- An assessment of the conduct of CMS oversight of QIOs.

provement Organizations (QIOs). It analyzes leading health care performance measures and the current measurement landscape. In addition to meeting the minimum requirements of its charge, as outlined in Table 1-1, the committee recommends how to develop a system from current fragmented efforts that builds upon existing assets, is responsive to key stakeholder groups, but is also more capable of aligning performance measures with national health care goals and serving the needs of Medicare beneficiaries.

• *Payment incentives report.* Building upon the first report, the payment incentives report will articulate design principles for better linking payment incentives within Medicare, identify a subset of measures to be used for payment incentives, and propose a strategy for implementation.

• *Performance improvement report.* This report will provide an evaluation of the QIO program, including a review of its previous efforts and recommendations for its future roles.

This first report and the subsequent payment incentives report are responsive to a congressional request for an IOM study on how to link payment to performance under Medicare (Public Law 108-173, Section 238). The study of Medicare's QIOs was mandated under that same legislation (section 109) and will be addressed primarily by the performance improvement report. The production of all three reports is sponsored by the Centers for Medicare and Medicaid Services (CMS).

The series of reports is intended to provide guidance to public and private purchasers on how changes in insurance programs can lead to improvements in the quality of health care and increase the value derived from health care investments. Before proceeding, however, the committee notes that while much of the interest in enhancing the quality of health care is driven by a desire to reduce the costs associated with unnecessary or wasteful practices, the rate of increase in health care costs cannot be slowed by enhancements to health insurance programs alone. Many other factors contribute to rapidly rising health care costs, most notably advances in medical knowledge and technology, as well as an aging population eager to take advantage of these advances to extend and improve the quality of life. Moreover, savings that accrue through some quality improvements, such as elimination of unnecessary or risky services that potentially expose patients to more harm than good, may be offset by the cost of others, such as that associated with the institution of provider reminder systems to ensure that patients receive recommended services. And even if significant savings were produced by redesigning health insurance and effecting other quality enhancements, these savings might be applied to other national health goals, such as coverage of the uninsured.

With these caveats in mind, we provide in the remainder of this chapter the context and rationale for the development of the national performance measurement and reporting system proposed in this report as an essential element of the redesign of health insurance programs to enhance health care quality. We emphasize here, as throughout the report, the importance of preserving and building on the many strengths of the existing system while striving to address its shortcomings.

THE CURRENT HEALTH CARE LANDSCAPE

The U.S. health care system provides some of the most scientifically advanced care in the world. Sizable public- and private-sector investments in clinical research have led to tremendous growth in knowledge, technology, and pharmaceuticals. In fiscal year 2005, for example, $27.9 billion was provided through congressional appropriations to fund the National Institutes of Health, while $49.9 billion was invested by the pharmaceutical and biotechnology industries (Cutler and McClellan, 2001; U.S. DHHS, 2005; U.S. FDA, 2004b). Recent medical advances in the areas of cancer treatment, organ transplantation, and joint replacement continue to improve survival and dramatically increase the quality of life. The number of survivors from all cancers combined increased from 3 million Americans living with cancer in 1971 (1.5 percent of the U.S. population) to an estimated 9.8 million in 2001 (3.5 percent of the population) (CDC, 2004). The 336,359 organ transplants performed to date (National Organ Procurement and Transplantation Network, 2005) have enabled survival and productivity for many patients for whom no other treatment was available. And total joint replacement now allows hundreds of thousands of people to live fuller, more active lives (U.S. FDA, 2004a). Numerous other advances have been achieved as well. Advances in cell restoration, prosthetic devices, and rehabilitation, for example, have improved the health and functioning of many people with disabilities, while genomics and other new technologies on the horizon hold great promise for improving health and longevity and alleviating pain and suffering (U.S. DOE Office of Science, 2004). The application of these medical advances would not be feasible without sustained investments in biomedical research, as well as the formal education and training of the health care workforce (U.S. DOL, 2004).

Despite these remarkable achievements, however, the health care system does not consistently provide safe and effective care. A large body of evidence substantiates shortcomings in the safety and effectiveness of health care in the United States (Commonwealth Fund, 2002; IOM, 2000, 2001; Leape and Berwick, 2005; Leatherman and McCarthy, 2004, 2005; McGlynn et al., 2003). The typical American adult receives only 54.9 percent of recommended care; many people do not receive the services they need, while others receive services that expose them to more potential harm than good (McGlynn et al., 2003). Safety problems have been documented in all health care settings, including hospitals, nursing homes, and care in the community (Gurwitz et al., 2000, 2003; IOM, 2000). Fortunately, some progress has been made toward reducing these gaps in safety and quality. The Agency for Healthcare Research and Quality (AHRQ), which maintains a national health care quality tracking system, reported improvement in performance between 2003 and 2004 for most of the system's 98 quality measures (AHRQ, 2004a). Yet the quality chasm in health care persists.

The U.S. health care system is also very costly, and many Americans may not receive good value for the dollars invested in their health care services. Per capita health spending in the United States exceeds that of other industrialized countries by huge margins. The United States spent $4,887 per person on health care in 2001, compared with $2,792 in neighboring Canada, $1,992 in the United Kingdom, and $2,131 in Japan (Reinhardt et al., 2004). Nonetheless, while the United States performs on par with other industrialized countries across a range of quality indicators (e.g., cervical cancer screening rate, influenza vaccination rate, suicide, asthma mortality, smoking rates, survival rates for kidney and liver transplants), it does not exhibit superior performance overall (Hussey et al., 2004). Cross-national surveys of patients' reports on care experiences and ratings of various dimensions of care indicate that, except for a few ratings of access, the U.S. health care system often performs relatively poorly from the patient perspective (Davis et al., 2004). The United States also ranks in the bottom quartile of industrialized countries in terms of life expectancy at birth and infant mortality (Reinhardt et al., 2002).

Across geographic regions within the United States, moreover, higher spending is not consistently associated with higher quality of care and better patient outcomes (Wennberg, 2005). Population-based studies of Medicare beneficiaries residing in communities with nearly two-fold differences in per capita health spending have found that the additional spending was associated with the use of "supply-sensitive" services (i.e., increased use of specialists and hospitals), but no improvement on measures of quality and access (Fisher et al., 2003a). In addition, large regional differences in end-of-life spending are not associated with better health outcomes (i.e., 5-year mortality and change in functional status) or satisfaction with care (Fisher et al., 2003b). And a study assessing patients treated in academic health centers for acute myocardial infarction, colorectal cancer, and hip fracture found that the centers differed in intensity of services delivered by up to 60 percent, but that higher-intensity practice was associated with either no difference or, for some conditions, a small decrement in care quality and patient outcomes (Fisher et al., 2004). These findings suggest that multiple opportunities exist to reduce per capita spending through the elimination of services that do not improve health. Moreover, process reengineering has the potential to deliver health-improving services at a lower cost per unit.

In addition to geographic variations, racial and ethnic disparities in health care are pervasive (IOM, 2002c). An extensive body of research documents that racial and ethnic minorities receive lower-quality care—both routine and specialty—than nonminorities, and these variations persist after accounting for the patient's insurance status and income level (Ayanian et al., 1993, 1999; Barker-Cummings et al., 1995; Epstein et al., 2000; Gaylin et al., 1993; Hannan et al., 1999; Herholz et al., 1996; Johnson et al., 1993; Petersen et al., 2002; Williams et al., 1995).

The escalating cost of health insurance not only consumes a sizable proportion of gross national product, but also contributes to rising numbers of uninsured—nearly 45 million people in 2003, or about one in seven Americans (Fronstin, 2004; Kaiser Family Foundation, 2004c). Many other Americans have only minimal insurance coverage and a limited ability to pay for services out of pocket (Collins et al., 2004; Kaiser Family Foundation, 2004a,b). Some of the uninsured and underinsured receive services through safety net providers, such as public and critical access hospitals, community health centers, and rural health clinics, and some providers, such as academic health centers, provide a sizable share of uncompensated services to the uninsured (Moy et al., 1996; Reuter and Gaskin, 1998). But a large gap remains between the services that are available and those that are needed by the uninsured. On the whole, the uninsured are less likely than those with insurance to receive services from which they would likely benefit, and the services that are provided are less timely (IOM, 2002a). This is also the case for insured individuals with high deductibles and copayments and modest financial resources (Rice and Matsuoka, 2004). The lack of insurance for so many Americans results in serious health consequences and economic costs not only for the uninsured, but also for their families, the communities in which they live, and the entire nation (IOM, 2004b). Most families with one or more uninsured members have lower incomes and are more likely to spend a high proportion of family income on health relative to insured families (IOM, 2002b). In communities with high uninsurance rates, even those with insurance may encounter reduced access to clinic-based primary care, specialty services, and hospital-based care, particularly emergency medical services and trauma care (IOM, 2003b). Society as a whole incurs other costs for gaps in health insurance, including lost health and longevity and lost workforce productivity (IOM, 2003c).

The United States is among the few industrialized countries in the world that does not guarantee access to health care and health insurance coverage for its population (IOM, 2004b). Although many factors likely contribute to the nation's high rates of uninsurance, there is little doubt that rapidly rising health care costs, driven in part by waste in the current health system, hamper efforts to expand coverage.

Among those populations with limited access to high-quality care are those living in rural communities, representing approximately 20 percent of the American population (IOM, 2005). Associated with rural as compared with urban communities are single providers, lower rates of health insurance, poorer health behaviors, higher infant mortality, and greater incidence of chronic diseases (Kaiser Family Foundation, 2004c). The unique factors surrounding discrepancies in rural health perpetuate the inequalities of the health care system.

Americans are concerned about the state of health care. Their primary concern is health care costs: a 2002 survey indicated that 38 percent of respondents were worried about overall costs, and 31 percent were particularly troubled by prescription drug costs (Kaiser Family Foundation, 2002). At the same time, however, concerns regarding quality and safety within the health care sector are attracting increasing attention. Between 2000 and 2004, the proportion of respondents to another survey who were dissatisfied with the quality of their health care grew from 44 to 55 percent (Kaiser Family Foundation et al., 2004); 40 percent of the respondents to this survey also reported that the quality of care had deteriorated during this period.

NEED TO ACCELERATE THE PACE OF IMPROVEMENT

The primary purpose of the IOM project on Redesigning Health Insurance is to accelerate the pace of change in the health system. In the 5 years since the publication of the *Quality Chasm* report (IOM, 2001), virtually every stakeholder group has taken important steps to improve quality in a range of areas (Leape and Berwick, 2005):

• *Information technology*—The federal government has assumed a leadership role in the development of the National Health Information Network with the appointment of a National Coordinator for Health Information Technology (The White House, 2004) and the promulgation of an initial set of national data standards to facilitate the meaningful exchange of data among authorized users (U.S. DHHS, 2003a,b). In October 2004, AHRQ awarded $139 million in contracts and grants to communities and health systems to enhance information technology capabilities (AHRQ, 2004b).

• *Knowledge and tools*—AHRQ has sponsored applied research projects aimed at enhancing and transferring knowledge and tools to improve quality; however, funding levels for health services research remain very low compared with those for clinical research (AHRQ, 2005; U.S. DHHS, 2005). Six states (Florida, Maryland, Massachusetts, New York, Oregon, and Pennsylvania) have established patient safety research centers whose activities include educational programs for providers and patients, reporting systems, and clearinghouses for best practices in safety (Rosenthal and Booth, 2004).

• *Education and technical assistance*—The Institute for Healthcare Improvement has developed many quality improvement programs, including breakthrough series collaboratives, IMPACT networks, forums, and Calls to Action, along with the recently launched 100,000 Lives Campaign. These efforts now reach tens of thousands of people in 50 countries (IHI, 2004). Between 2000 and 2003, the Medicare Quality Improvement Organization Program supported quality improvement projects in all states, often reaching all hospitals, nursing homes, home health agencies, and outpatient physicians in the state, with varying degrees of involvement (AMA, 2000; U.S. DHHS, 2003c).

• *Informed purchasing*—Private and public purchasers have launched national initiatives to drive quality through purchasing decisions. The Leapfrog Group and Bridges to Excellence are two large national efforts aimed at encouraging and rewarding quality improvement in both hospital and ambulatory settings (DeBrantes et al., 2003; Galvin and Milstein, 2002). The Consumer-Purchaser Disclosure Project is an alliance of more than 25 consumer, employer, and labor organizations working to ensure that comparative performance data are available in all geographic areas and to all population groups (Consumer-Purchaser Disclosure Project, 2005). Many other purchaser-driven efforts exist at the local and regional levels (Rosenthal et al., 2004).

• *Quality oversight*—Major accreditation organizations have strengthened requirements and programs, especially in the area of patient safety (JCAHO, 2004; NCQA, 2000; Wachter, 2004). Professional certification programs, such as those of the Accreditation Council for Graduate Medical Education and the American Board of Medical Specialties, have adopted new standards requiring health professionals to demonstrate quality-related competencies (ACGME, 2002; American Board of Medical Specialties, 2005).

Despite these many worthwhile efforts, major changes in the health care delivery system are difficult to discern. Investment in information technology has expanded, but the pace of penetration and modernization in the overall health care system has been slow. Of the nearly 70 percent of physicians who operate in small practice settings, only 8 percent use electronic prescribing, and fewer than one in four providers use some form of computer-generated treatment reminders (Reed and Grossman, 2004). Pockets of innovation have emerged, with some health systems making sizable investments in electronic health records (EHRs) (Garrido et al., 2005; Health Data Management, 2003; HealthPartners, 2004; NYC Health and

Hospitals Corporation, 2003; Sutter Health, 2004; U.S. VA, 2003). But the United States continues to rank in the bottom quartile of industrialized countries in the use of EHRs in ambulatory settings: only about 18 percent of U.S. physicians use EHRs, compared with nearly 90 percent in Sweden and the Netherlands (Harris Interactive Health News, 2002). Other countries, such as the United Kingdom, are making far greater investments in the expansion of electronic supports to practice settings (Audet et al., 2004; Virtual Medical Worlds Monthly, 2001).

The pace of modernization has been impeded by financial barriers, as well as cultural and technical barriers to the adoption of information technology (IOM, 2003d). Disruptions in practice and loss of practice revenue are frequently associated with the initial implementation of such reforms. Moreover, while the introduction of new technology can reduce many medical errors, it can also introduce new types of errors (Leape and Berwick, 2005; Werner and Asch, 2005). Yet despite the complexity, fragmentation, and individualism that characterize the health care system and the field of medicine, health professionals must adapt to changes in care processes and in methods of communication between patients and clinicians and among clinicians (Leape and Berwick, 2005).

The lack of organizational supports in so many ambulatory practice settings has major implications for patient care. Large, tightly organized multispecialty groups are significantly more likely to use evidence-based management processes, such as disease registries, reminder systems, guidelines, and case management systems (Audet et al., 2005), than are more loosely organized practice settings (Shortell and Schmittdiel, 2004). A recent comparison of the quality of care provided to patients served by the Veterans Health Administration through a highly integrated health system found that adherence to science-based processes of care typically exceeded that received by a comparable national sample of patients in 12 communities (Asch et al., 2004). In a survey of California physicians, those affiliated with Kaiser Permanente, which consists of large prepaid group practices, were much more likely to report the enrollment of their patients in disease management programs than were other physicians in the state (Rittenhouse et al., 2004).

Many factors undoubtedly contribute to the slow pace of change at the delivery system level, but a growing consensus has emerged among both the public and private sectors that the environment in which care is provided impedes efforts to improve quality (IOM, 2004a). This environment, which is shaped to a great extent by the design of public and private health insurance programs, fails to produce incentives or structures that encourage and reward high-quality care (Nichols et al., 2004).

THE HEALTH CARE ENTERPRISE

The health care enterprise can be viewed as a complex but decentralized system in which multiple providers, consumers, and purchasers are connected by services, information systems, and financial transactions. Much of the data that emerges from the enterprise is related to documentation of specific health conditions, services, and financial reimbursements. Chart review and administrative data are coded as part of individual transactions, and their use is constrained by issues of privacy and confidentiality; information about the overall performance of the health care enterprise is difficult to obtain or develop. In theory, a marketplace achieves desired performance levels by appealing to consumer choice and fostering competition among providers. In both areas, the U.S. health care marketplace faces fundamental challenges.

Health care consumers make several types of decisions: the selection of a health plan, the selection of providers (e.g., primary care providers, specialists, and hospitals), choices among different treatment programs, and the pursuit of health-related behaviors (e.g., diet, exercise, and smoking). Although health care consumers have these choices in theory, the reality is different. The options from which they can choose are often limited; the information available to inform their decision making is usually constrained; some are not well equipped, cognitively or emotionally, to make such decisions; and the health system provides few useful decision supports to assist them.

In most communities, some degree of competition exists among health plans, but such considerations as price and proximity of services and familiarity with a particular provider are more likely to drive decision making than is the quality of care or the value of services. Most Medicare beneficiaries are able to choose between a Medicare Advantage Plan(s) or traditional, fee-for-service Medicare. CMS does make comparative data for clinical quality available to Medicare Advantage Plans (CMS, 2005c), but no such data are provided under traditional Medicare, which accounts for almost 90 percent of beneficiaries (National Health Policy Forum and California Healthcare Foundation, 2004). For most of the working population, the selection of a health plan is a decision made jointly by the employer and the employee, with the employee choosing from a plan or plans offered by the employer. The availability of information on the quality of commercial or self-insured health plans is variable.

Many health plans report performance information on a set of standardized quality measures. For example, Health Plan Employer Data and Information Set measures are reported to the National Committee for Quality Assurance or directly to large employers or employer coalitions (NCQA, 2005). But as the provider networks of health insurance plans have expanded in response to consumer demand for greater choice, it has become difficult to determine differences in provider quality when comparing plans. Differences at the provider level within a plan are particularly difficult to discern, as health plans in a community often contract with most of the same physicians and hospitals and each plan represents only a small fraction of a provider's practice. State Medicaid programs also vary widely in choice of plans and the information provided to beneficiaries to inform their decision making (Center on Budget and Policy Priorities, 2003; CMS, 2004). In addition to being very limited, the information on providers that is available to consumers is often difficult to use (Hibbard et al., 2002). It may not be pertinent to their decisions or "packaged and disseminated so they can easily obtain, trust, understand, and apply it" (Shaller et al., 2003).

CMS has played a leadership role in establishing public reporting systems for nursing homes, home health agencies, dialysis centers, and, most recently, hospitals (CMS, 2005a). Yet in the majority of communities, solo practices do not frequently provide publicly available information on the quality of ambulatory care. Solo practices and other low-volume providers often do not see enough patients to yield statistically significant data for performance measurement. Small sample sizes pose problems such as the need for risk adjustment, producing biased data, and there is currently no mechanism in place for pooling data across purchasers. Individually, moreover, private purchasers (covering both self-insured and commercial populations) and insurers generally do not account for a large enough share of a physician's practice for meaningful measures of performance to be constructed (Milstein, 2004). Meaningful reporting at the physician practice level is thus a challenge, and will require national leadership to foster collaboration across public and private purchasers.

Along with these data limitations, some consumers have a very limited choice of providers. This is particularly true for the uninsured and those living in sparsely populated areas or poorer neighborhoods of metropolitan areas (Blumenthal and Kagen, 2002; National Rural Health Association, 1995).

Finally, in addition to the lack of comparative quality data to support decisions by consumers and purchasers, certain design characteristics of most health insurance programs work against the provision of high-quality care:

- *Lack of coverage for key benefits*—Benefit packages often do not include services that are important to the effective management of chronic conditions, such as care coordination, non-visit-based communications (e.g., e-mail and telephone calls), and patient education and support services (Berenson and Horvath, 2003).
- *Lack of performance incentives*—Historically, the health care marketplace has failed to reward those providers that deliver the highest-quality care.

In recent years, this situation has started to change. In July 2003, CMS announced a demonstration project to provide bonuses to hospitals in the Premier, Inc. system based on performance in five clinical areas (CMS, 2005b). Many private purchasers and health plans are also implementing pay for performance programs that generally link a modest amount of provider payments to performance across a number of measures (Rosenthal et al., 2004).

• *Piecemeal payment*—Many insurance programs employ piecemeal provider payment systems that compensate individual physicians for face-to-face visits and procedures according to a fee schedule and hospitals for patient episodes by diagnosis-related group. This type of microlevel payment system offers little incentive for investment in information technology (e.g., chronic care registries and EHRs), organizational supports (e.g., quality measurement and improvement programs), population health (e.g., healthy lifestyle programs aimed at tobacco cessation and weight loss), or multidisciplinary team-based approaches to care delivery, all of which have been shown to improve health care quality and patient outcomes (Batalden et al., 2003; Coffield et al., 2001; Ellerbeck et al., 2000; Fitzmaurice et al., 2002; IOM, 2003a,e; Jencks et al., 2000; Robert Wood Johnson Foundation, 2001). These types of health system changes, which require collective decision making and investment on the part of many providers, are difficult to accomplish in a highly decentralized delivery system where revenues flow directly to the component parts. These types of investments also generally do not yield a positive financial return at the individual provider level under current payment systems (Leatherman et al., 2003), and may even reduce revenues for certain components of the system. Thus piecemeal payment does not support efficiency in the health care system and may promote overuse of unnecessary services and underuse of services that can improve health outcomes.

• *Accountability void*—Individual providers, whether physicians or hospitals, frequently focus on providing quality care within their own setting. For most chronically ill patients, whose outcomes depend on the receipt of services from many different providers over an extended period of time, no health care professional or organization assumes responsibility for ensuring that all appropriate services (and only those services) are received. This accountability void is particularly evident at the community level, since no provider or group of providers accepts responsibility for ensuring that the entire population of the community has access to appropriate care.

These characteristics are not independent of each other, but rather tightly interwoven. For example, the lack of care coordination as a benefit can be attributed to the piecemeal payment system, which does not reward integrating a patient's care across multiple providers. However, a system devoid of accountability for all the care delivered to a patient, as well as incentives to provide better care, perpetuates the piecemeal payment approach. Efforts addressing all these integrated characteristics are necessary to promote better quality of care.

Many proposals have been offered to improve and reform the functioning of the health care marketplace. Some of these proposals rely on an inherent ability of markets to transform the health care system, some on social planning or government regulatory approaches, some on stronger self-regulation by the health professions, and some on consumer-driven approaches. While each of these proposals is based on a different set of assumptions and values with regard to the fundamental processes and interactions that would best foster the common good, all would require performance measures to achieve their goals.

This IOM report proposes a set of measures, derived from an evidentiary base, that the committee believes can be used for multiple purposes: data collection and analysis, public reporting, development of professional standards, payment and benefit design, governmental oversight, and purchasing benchmarks. Implementation of this measure set must be carefully considered, however, since the measures will leverage each other when initially used to improve and reform health care services. Additionally, the value of current measures is limited because they cannot always attribute responsibility for improvements to those being measured. Therefore, the report also proposes a coordinating entity to guide and inform the judgments required to align standards and measures with the appropriate purposes within the complex health care enterprise.

After reviewing the research literature, the committee did not take a position on which types of health care reform strategies offer the most promise for achieving quality improvement and better health outcomes. Market-based incentives are one approach to enhancing quality, but they are far from perfect. Government regulation may be necessary in some situations, but this option also has inherent limitations. Vigorous efforts on the part of the health professions or consumer advocates to improve quality through professional and public education, self-monitoring, and robust public planning and regulatory processes also merit consideration. As noted, however, all approaches—market incentives, regulation, professional education and monitoring, and consumer advocacy—will benefit from a well-designed and operational performance measurement and reporting system. Thus, the committee is united in issuing a strong call for improvements in performance measurement and transparency of its results.

THE NEED FOR A NATIONAL SYSTEM FOR PERFORMANCE MEASUREMENT AND REPORTING

Public and private purchasers have powerful levers at their disposal to facilitate change in the health care delivery system. Three overall approaches—public disclosure of performance data, payment policies, and performance improvement processes—can all provide strong incentives for change to providers (both clinicians and institutions), purchasers, and beneficiaries. Yet to do so, all three approaches depend upon the availability of accurate, reliable, and valid performance measures. These measures can serve as the foundation for public reporting programs intended to promote accountability among providers and aid consumers in making informed choices. They can also provide the basis for initiatives that create incentives for providers to deliver more effective and efficient care. Public disclosure and payment policies are then presumed to work in tandem to motivate quality improvement efforts that affect the actual processes of care delivery. However, such synchronicity is not always achieved, and as a result, potential improvements are not fully realized.

Taken together, these three approaches offer a continuum of options for influencing provider and patient behaviors in ways that can produce improvements in health and health care. For example, diabetic patients who receive care from multiple providers in numerous settings often fail to receive services from which they would likely benefit, such as testing for hemoglobin A_1c and cholesterol levels. Measuring these processes can reveal such shortcomings and thereby result in better-quality care and improved health outcomes (Harris Interactive, 2001). Potential options for addressing such failures and ensuring they are not continued include (1) bonus payments to primary care providers whose performance profiles indicate high levels of compliance with practice guidelines (a payment policy option); (2) disclosure of comparative performance reports on providers to assist consumers in selecting the highest-quality providers (a public disclosure option); (3) reduced levels of regulatory burden for primary care providers with exemplary performance (a performance improvement option); and (4) the establishment of communitywide diabetes registries by Medicare's QIOs to assist all providers in monitoring beneficiaries' receipt of effective services (a performance improvement option).

To drive change in the status quo of measurement, all such levers should reinforce achievement of the six aims of the *Quality Chasm* report cited earlier—safe, effective, patient-centered, timely, efficient, and equitable care. Together, the effects of multiple changes at different levels of the health care system—patient and community, microsystem, organizational context, and environmental context—must be sufficient to encourage and enable payers, providers, and patients to close the quality gap (IOM, 2001).

Although performance data are integral to the success of efforts targeting public disclosure of performance data, payment policies, and performance improvement processes, currently available performance data on many types of providers are quite limited. Most performance measurement projects to date have relied on a small set of technical quality measures (i.e., medical care process measures) derived from administrative data produced by particular types of provider settings and patient surveys. These measure sets do not answer key questions, such as whether patients received the full set of services, and only those services, from which they would likely benefit; whether services were provided in a timely and efficient manner; and whether patients achieved the desired short- and long-term outcomes.

A common performance measurement infrastructure is necessary to support the efforts of public and private insurance plans to realign incentives. Developing this infrastructure involves such tasks as specifying the criteria or rules that performance measure sets should satisfy, identifying and specifying the measures to be included in standardized measure sets, and implementing the information technologies (e.g., EHRs and secure platforms for interconnectivity) required to monitor and improve performance. The absence of a carefully crafted, comprehensive approach to performance measurement and realignment of incentives across all purchasers and all three approaches to change (public disclosure of performance data, payment policies, and performance improvement processes) results in an excessive burden on providers and weakens the impact of incentives for quality improvement.

In sum, a national strategy for the measurement and reporting of provider performance is a fundamental building block in the efforts of all stakeholders to improve health care quality through public reporting, ongoing quality improvement, pay for performance programs, quality-based benefit design, and health insurance purchasing benchmarks. Through the identification of improvement goals and the selection of specific measures, this national strategy should focus provider attention on areas and activities that will lead to a fundamental redesign of the health care delivery system.

SCOPE AND ORGANIZATION OF THIS REPORT

This first report in the Redesigning Health Insurance series addresses requirements for a common performance measurement infrastructure:

- Chapter 2 provides an overview of the accomplishments to date of many stakeholder groups that have advanced the field of performance measurement. It also reviews the limitations of current efforts and argues for a national system for performance measurement and reporting.
- Chapter 3 presents the committee's recommendations for an entity—working collaboratively with existing stakeholders groups—to oversee and coordinate the key functions of a national system for performance measurement and reporting.
- Chapter 4 describes the analytic framework used by the committee to aid in the selection of a starter set of performance measures and the

identification of gaps in existing measures. Approaches to address these gaps are also proposed.

• Chapter 5 recommends a multifaceted research agenda to address four areas: development of new measures to address the performance measurement gaps articulated in Chapter 4, methodological barriers, usability of public reports, and evaluation of the performance measurement and reporting system.

REFERENCES

ACGME (Accreditation Council for Graduate Medical Education). 2002. *Report of the ACGME Work Group on Resident Duty Hours.* [Online]. Available: *http://www.acgme.org/new/wkgreport602.pdf* [accessed March 22, 2005].

AHRQ (Agency for Healthcare Research and Quality). 2004a. *National Healthcare Quality Report.* Rockville, MD: AHRQ.

AHRQ. 2004b. *HHS Awards $139 Million to Drive Adoption of Health Information Technology.* [Online]. Available: *http://www.ahrq.gov/news/press/pr2004/hhshitpr.htm* [accessed October 19, 2004].

AHRQ. 2005. *Fiscal Year 2006.* [Online]. Available: *http://www.ahrq.gov/about/cj2006/cj2006.pdf* [accessed March 22, 2005].

AMA (American Medical Association). 2000. *A Study of the Quality of Care Beneficiaries Get in Traditional Medicare Shows Wide Performance Variation among the States.* [Online]. Available: *http://www.ama-assn.org/amednews/2000/10/23/gvsb1023.htm* [accessed March 23, 2005].

American Board of Medical Specialties. 2005. *Medical Specialty Board Certification.* [Online]. Available: *http://www.abpm.org/about/news/board_certification.html* [accessed March 22, 2005].

Asch SM, McGlynn EA, Hogan MM, Hayward RA, Shekelle P, Rubenstein L, Keesey J, Adams J, Kerr EA. 2004. Comparison of quality of care for patients in the Veterans Health Administration and patients in a national sample. *Annals of Internal Medicine* 141(12):938–945.

Audet AM, Doty MM, Peugh J, Shamasdin J, Zapert K, Schoenbaum S. 2004. *Information Technologies: When Will They Make It into Physicians' Black Bags?* [Online]. Available: *http://www.cmwf.org/publications/publications_show.htm?doc_id=251984* [accessed March 28, 2005].

Audet AM, Doty MM, Shamasdin J, Schoenbaum S. 2005. Measure, learn, and improve: Have physicians begun to engage in the quality improvement cycle? *Health Affairs* 24(3):843–853.

Ayanian JZ, Udvarhelyi IS, Gatsonis CA, Pashos CL, Epstein AM. 1993. Racial differences in the use of revascularization procedures after coronary angiography. *Journal of the American Medical Association* 269(20):2642–2646.

Ayanian JZ, Weissman JS, Chasan-Taber S, Epstein AM. 1999. Quality of care by race and gender for congestive heart failure and pneumonia. *Medical Care* 37(12):1260–1269.

Barker-Cummings C, McClellan W, Soucie JM, Krisher J. 1995. Ethnic differences in the use of peritoneal dialysis as initial treatment for end-stage renal disease. *Journal of the American Medical Association* 274(23):1858–1862.

Batalden PB, Nelson EC, Edwards WH, Godfrey MM, Mohr JJ. 2003. Microsystems in health care: Part 9. Developing small clinical units to attain peak performance. *Joint Commission Journal on Quality and Safety* 29(11):575–585.

Berenson RA, Horvath J. 2003. Confronting the barriers to chronic care management in Medicare. *Health Affairs* Suppl. Web Exclusives:W3-37-53.

Berwick DM. 2002. Public performance reports and the will for change. *Journal of the American Medical Association* 288(12):1523–1524.

Blumenthal S, Kagen J. 2002. The effects of socioeconomic status on health in rural and urban America. *Journal of the American Medical Association* 287(1):109.

CDC (Centers for Disease Control and Prevention). 2004. *Cancer Survivorship in the United States: 1971-2001.* [Online]. Available: *http://www.cdc.gov/mmwr/preview/mmwrhtml/mm5324a3.htm* [accessed March 28, 2005].

Center on Budget and Policy Priorities. 2003. *Medicaid-Medicare Link: State Medicaid Programs Are Shouldering a Greater Share of the Costs of Care for Seniors and People with Disabilities.* [Online]. Available: *http://www.house.gov/commerce_democrats/medicaidblockgrant/cbpp.fact.1.pdf* [accessed March 22, 2005].

CMS (Centers for Medicare and Medicaid Services). 2004. *CMS Encourages States to Give Medicaid Beneficiaries More Control over the Long-Term Care Services They Receive.* [Online]. Available: *http://www.cms.hhs.gov/media/press/release.asp?Counter=1167* [accessed March 22, 2005].

CMS. 2005a. *Medicare Compare Series: Nursing Home Compare, Home Health Compare, Dialysis Compare, and Hospital Compare.* [Online] Available: http://www.Medicare.gov [accessed January 24, 2005].

CMS. 2005b. *Premier Hospital Quality Incentives Demonstration.* [Online]. Available: *http://www.cms.hhs.gov/researchers/demos/phqi/default.asp* [accessed January 24, 2005].

CMS. 2005c. *Medicare Personal Plan Finder.* [Online]. Available: *http://www.medicare.gov/default.asp* [accessed March 30, 2005].

Coffield AB, Maciosek MV, McGinnis JM, Harris JR, Caldwell MB, Teutsch SM, Atkins D, Richland JH, Haddix A. 2001. Priorities among recommended clinical preventive services. *American Journal of Preventive Medicine* 21(1):1–9.

Collins SR, Doty MM, Davis K, Schoen C, Holmgren AL, Ho A. 2004. *The Affordability Crisis in U.S. Health Care: Findings from The Commonwealth Fund Biennial Health Insurance Survey.* New York: Commonwealth Fund.

Commonwealth Fund. 2002. *Quality of Health Care in the United States: A Chartbook.* New York: Commonwealth Fund.

Consumer-Purchaser Disclosure Project. 2005. *Consumer-Purchaser Disclosure Project.* [Online]. Available: *http://healthcaredisclosure.org/* [accessed May 12, 2005].

Cutler DM, McClellan M. 2001. Is technological change in medicine worth it? *Health Affairs* 20(5):11–29.

Davis K, Schoen SC, Schoenbaum AJ, Doty MM, Tenney K. 2004. *Mirror, Mirror on the Wall: Looking at the Quality of American Health Care through the Patient's Lens.* New York: Commonwealth Fund.

DeBrantes F, Galvin RS, Lee TH. 2003. Bridges to excellence: Building a business case for quality care. *Journal of Clinical Outcomes Management* 10(8):439–446.

Ellerbeck EF, Kresowik TF, Hemann RA, Mason P, Wiblin RT, Marciniak TA. 2000. Impact of quality improvement activities on care for acute myocardial infarction. *International Journal of Quality Health Care* 12(4):305–310.

Epstein AM, Ayanian JZ, Keogh JH, Noonan SJ, Armistead N, Cleary PD, Weissman JS, David-Kasdan JA, Carlson D, Fuller J, Marsh D, Conti RM. 2000. Racial disparities in access to renal transplantation: Clinically appropriate or due to underuse or overuse? *New England Journal of Medicine* 343 (21):1537–1544.

Fisher ES, Wennberg DE, Stukel TA, Gottlieb DJ, Lucas FL, Pinder EL. 2003a. The implications of regional variations in Medicare spending. Part 1: The content, quality, and accessibility of care. *Annals of Internal Medicine* 138(4):273–287.

Fisher ES, Wennberg DE, Stukel TA, Gottlieb DJ, Lucas FL, Pinder EL. 2003b. The implications of regional variations in Medicare spending. Part 2: Health outcomes and satisfaction with care. *Annals of Internal Medicine* 138(4):288–298.

Fisher ES, Wennberg DE, Stukel TA, Gottlieb DJ. 2004. Variations in the longitudinal efficiency of academic medical centers. *Health Affairs* Suppl. Web Exclusive:VAR19-32.

Fitzmaurice JM, Adams K, Eisenberg JM. 2002. Three decades of research on computer applications in health care: Medical informatics support at the Agency for Healthcare Research and Quality. *Journal of the American Medical Informatics Association* 9(2):144–160.

Fronstin P. 2004. Sources of health insurance and characteristics of the uninsured: Analysis of the March 2004 current population survey. *EBRI Issue Brief* 276:1–31.

Galvin R, Milstein A. 2002. Large employers' new strategies in health care. *New England Journal of Medicine* 347(12):939–942.

Garrido T, Jamieson L, Zhou Y, Wiesenthal A, Liang L. 2005. Effect of electronic health records in ambulatory care: Retrospective, serial, cross sectional study. *British Medical Journal* 330(7491):581.

Gaylin DS, Held PJ, Port FK, Hunsicker LG, Wolfe RA, Kahan BD, Jones CA, Agodoa LY. 1993. The impact of comorbid and sociodemographic factors on access to renal transplantation. *Journal of the American Medical Association* 269(5):603–608.

Gurwitz JH, Field TS, Avorn J, McCormick D, Jain S, Eckler M, Benser M, Edmondson AC, Bates DW. 2000. Incidence and preventability of adverse drug events in nursing homes. *American Journal of Medicine* 109(2):87–94.

Gurwitz JH, Field TS, Harrold LR, Rothschild J, Debellis K, Seger AC, Cadoret C, Fish LS, Garber L, Kelleher M, Bates DW. 2003. Incidence and preventability of adverse drug events among older persons in the ambulatory setting. *Journal of the American Medical Association* 289(9):1107–1116.

Hannan EL, van Ryn M, Burke J, Stone D, Kumar D, Arani D, Pierce W, Rafii S, Sanborn TA, Sharma S, Slater J, DeBuono BA. 1999. Access to coronary artery bypass surgery by race/ethnicity and gender among patients who are appropriate for surgery. *Medical Care* 37(1):68–77.

Harris Interactive. 2001. *Survey on Chronic Illness and Caregiving.* New York: Harris Interactive.

Harris Interactive Health News. 2002. *European Physicians Especially in Sweden, Netherlands, and Denmark, Lead U.S. in Use of Electronic Medical Records.* [Online]. Available: *http://www.harrisinteractive.com* [accessed May 6, 2005].

Health Data Management. 2003. *Around Cleveland Clinic in 100 Days.* [Online]. Available: *http://www.healthdatamanagement.com/html/supplements/himss2003/HimssNewsStory.cfm?DID=9735* [accessed March 22, 2005].

HealthPartners. 2004. *Essential EMR Functions: A Perspective from the Front Lines.* [Online]. Available: *http://www.healthmgttech.com/archives/1104/1104beyond_clinical.htm* [accessed March 28, 2005].

Herholz H, Goff DC Jr, Ramsey DJ, Chan FA, Ortiz C, Labarthe DR, Nichaman MZ. 1996. Women and Mexican Americans receive fewer cardiovascular drugs following myocardial infarction than men and non-Hispanic whites: The Corpus Christi Heart Project, 1988-1990. *Journal of Clinical Epidemiology* 49(3):279–287.

Hibbard JH, Slovic P, Peters E, Finucane ML. 2002. Strategies for reporting health plan performance information to consumers: Evidence from controlled studies. *Health Services Research* 37(2):291–313.

Hussey PS, Anderson GF, Osborn R, Feek C, McLaughlin V, Millar J, Epstein A. 2004. How does the quality of care compare in five countries? *Health Affairs* 23(3):89–99.

IHI (Institute for Healthcare Improvement). 2004. *"The Courage to Act on What If..." Progress Report.* [Online]. Available: *http://www.ihi.org* [accessed November 16, 2004].

IOM (Institute of Medicine). 2000. *To Err Is Human: Building a Safer Health System.* Kohn LT, Corrigan JM, Donaldson MS, eds. Washington, DC: National Academy Press.

IOM. 2001. *Crossing the Quality Chasm: A New Health System for the 21st Century.* Washington, DC: National Academy Press.

IOM. 2002a. *Insuring Health—Care Without Coverage: Too Little, Too Late.* Washington, DC: The National Academies Press.

IOM. 2002b. *Insuring Health—Health Insurance Is a Family Matter.* Washington, DC: The National Academies Press.

IOM. 2002c. *Unequal Treatment: Confronting Racial and Ethnic Disparities in Health Care.* Smedley BS, Stith AY, Nelson BD, eds. Washington, DC: The National Academies Press.

IOM. 2003a. *Health Professions Education: A Bridge to Quality.* Greiner AC, Knebel E, eds. Washington, DC: The National Academies Press.

IOM. 2003b. *Insuring Health—A Shared Destiny: Community Effects of Ununsurance.* Committee on the Consequences of Uninsurance, eds. Washington, DC: The National Academies Press.

IOM. 2003c. *Insuring Health—Hidden Costs, Value Lost: Uninsurance in America.* Committee on the Consequences of Uninsurance, eds. Washington, DC: The National Academies Press.

IOM. 2003d. *Patient Safety: Achieving a New Standard for Care.* Aspden P, Corrigan JM, Wolcott J, Erickson SM, eds. Washington, DC: The National Academies Press.

IOM. 2003e. *Priority Areas for National Action: Transforming Health Care Quality.* Adams K, Corrigan JM, eds. Washington, DC: The National Academies Press.

IOM. 2004a. *1st Annual Crossing the Quality Chasm Summit: A Focus on Communities.* Adams K, Greiner A, Corrigan J, eds. Washington, DC: The National Academies Press.

IOM. 2004b. *Insuring Health—Insuring America's Health: Principles and Recommendation.* Washington, DC: The National Academies Press

IOM. 2005. *Quality through Collaboration: The Future of Rural Health.* Washington, DC: The National Academies Press.

JCAHO (Joint Commission on Accreditation of Healthcare Organizations). 2004. *2004 National Patient Safety Goals.* [Online]. Available: *http://www.jcaho.org/accredited+organizations/patient+safety/04+npsg/* [accessed March 22, 2005].

Jencks SF, Cuerdon T, Burwen DR, Fleming B, Houck PM, Kussmaul AE, Nilasena DS, Ordin DL, Arday DR. 2000. Quality of medical care delivered to Medicare beneficiaries: A profile at state and national levels. *Journal of the American Medical Association* 284(13):1670–1676.

Johnson PA, Lee TH, Cook EF, Rouan GW, Goldman L. 1993. Effect of race on the presentation and management of patients with acute chest pain. *Annals of Internal Medicine* 118(8): 593–601.

Kaiser Family Foundation. 2002. *Kaiser Health Poll Report.* [Online]. Available: *http://www.kff.org/healthpollreport/archive_Aug2003/2.cfm* [accessed May 6, 2005].

Kaiser Family Foundation. 2004a. *Update on Health Insurance.* [Online]. Available: *http://www.kff.org/insurance/loader.cfm?url=/commonspot/security/getfile.cfm&PageID=44678* [accessed March 22, 2005].

Kaiser Family Foundation. 2004b. *Trends and Indicators in the Changing Health Care Marketplace—Section 4: Trends in Health Insurance Benefits.* [Online]. Available: *http://www.kff.org/insurance/7031/print-sec4.cfm* [accessed March 22, 2005].

Kaiser Family Foundation. 2004c. *Health Insurance Coverage in America: 2003 Data Update.* [Online]. Available: *http://www.kff.org/uninsured/loader.cfm?url=/commonspot/security/getfile.cfm&PageID=49550* [accessed March 22, 2005].

Kaiser Family Foundation, Agency for Healthcare Research, Quality Harvard School of Public Health. 2004. *National Survey of Consumers' Experiences with Patient Safety and Quality Information.* [Online]. Available: *http://www.kff.org* [accessed May 6, 2005].

Leape LL, Berwick DM. 2005. Five years after *to err is human:* what have we learned? *Journal of the American Medical Association* 293(19):2384–2390.

Leatherman S, McCarthy D. 2004. *Quality of Care for Children and Adolescents: A Chartbook.* April. New York: Commonwealth Fund.

Leatherman S, McCarthy D. May 2005. *Quality of Health Care for Medicare Beneficiaries: A Chartbook.* New York: Commonwealth Fund.

Leatherman S, Berwick D, Iles D, Lewin LS, Davidoff F, Nolan T, Bisognano M. 2003. The business case for quality: case studies and an analysis. *Health Affairs* 22(2):17–30.

McGlynn EA, Asch SM, Adams J, Keesey J, Hicks J, DeCristofaro A, Kerr EA. 2003. The quality of health care delivered to adults in the United States. *New England Journal of Medicine* 348(26):2635–2645.

Milstein A. 2004. Hot potato endgame. *Health Affairs* 23(6):32–34.

Moy E, Valente E Jr, Levin RJ, Griner PF. 1996. Academic medical centers and the care of underserved populations. *Academic Medicine* 71(12): 1370–1377.

National Health Policy Forum and California Healthcare Foundation. 2004. *Medicare's Chronic Care Improvement Pilot Program: What Is Its Potential?* [Online]. Available: *http://www.chcf.org/documents/chronicdisease/MedicareChronicCareFS.pdf* [accessed March 22, 2005].

National Organ Procurement and Transplantation Network. 2005. *Transplants in the U.S.* [Online]. *Available: http://www.optn.org/latestData/rptData.asp* [accessed March 28, 2005].

National Rural Health Association. 1995. *Managed Care as a Service Delivery Model in Rural Areas.* [Online]. Available: *http://www.nrharural.org/pagefile/issuepapers/ipaper3.html* [accessed March 22, 2005].

NCQA (National Committee for Quality Assurance). 2000. *NCQA to Define Accreditation Program to Focus Attention on Patient Safety.* [Online]. Available: *http://www.ncqa.org/communications/news/patsafrel.htm* [accessed March 22, 2004].

NCQA (National Committee for Quality Assurance). 2005. *Health Plan Report Card.* [Online]. Available: *http://www.ncqa.org/index.asp* [accessed January 24, 2005].

Nichols LM, Ginsburg PB, Berenson RA, Christianson J, Hurley RE. 2004. Are market forces strong enough to deliver efficient health care systems? Confidence is waning. *Health Affairs* 23(2):8–21.

NYC (New York City) Health and Hospitals Corporation. 2003. *Nurses and Physicians in the Implementation of the Electronic Medical Record at NYC Health and Hospitals Corporation.* [Online]. Available: *http://www.ehcca.com/presentations/hitsummit1/6_02_5.pdf* [accessed March 28, 2005].

Petersen LA, Wright SM, Peterson ED, Daley J. 2002. Impact of race on cardiac care and outcomes in veterans with acute myocardial infarction. *Medical Care* 40(Suppl. 1):86–96.

Reed MC, Grossman JM. 2004. Limited information technology for patient care in physician offices. *Issue Brief/Center for Studying Health System Change* (89):1–6.

Reinhardt UE, Hussey PS, Anderson GF. 2002. Cross-national comparisons of health systems using OECD data, 1999. *Health Affairs* 21(3):169–181.

Reinhardt UE, Hussey PS, Anderson GF. 2004. U.S. health care spending in an international context. *Health Affairs* 23(3):10–25.

Reuter J, Gaskin D. 1998. *The Role of Academic Health Centers and Teaching Hospitals in Providing Care for the Poor.* Altman S, Reinhardt U, Shields A. Chicago, IL: Health Administration Press. Pp. 151–165.

Rice T, Matsuoka KY. 2004. The impact of cost-sharing on appropriate utilization and health status: A review of the literature on seniors. *Medical Care Research and Review* 61(4):415–452.

Rittenhouse DR, Grumbach K, O'Neil EH, Dower C, Bindman A. 2004. Physician organization and care management in California: From cottage to Kaiser. *Health Affairs* 23(6):51–62.

Robert Wood Johnson Foundation. 2001. *Substance Abuse: The Nation's Number One Health Problem.* Princeton, NJ: Robert Wood Johnson Foundation.

Rosenthal J, Booth M. 2004. *State Patient Safety Centers: A New Approach to Promote Patient Safety.* [Online]. Available: *http://www.nashp.edu* [accessed November 16, 2004].

Rosenthal MB, Fernandopulle R, Song HR, Landon B. 2004. Paying for quality: Providers' incentives for quality improvement. *Health Affairs* 23(2):127–141.

Shaller D, Sofaer S, Findlay SD, Hibbard JH, Delbanco S. 2003. Perspective: Consumers and quality-driven health care: A call to action. *Health Affairs* 22(2):95–101.

Shortell SM, Schmittdiel J. 2004. Prepaid groups and organized delivery systems: Promise, performance, and potential. In: Enthoven AC, Tollen LA, eds. *Toward a 21st Century Health System: The Contributions and Promise of Prepaid Group Practice* (1st Edition). San Francisco, CA: Jossey-Bass. Pp. 1–21.

Sutter Health. 2004. *Sutter Health Will Implement Nation's Most Advanced Electronic Health Record with Patient Access by 2006.* [Online]. Available: *http://www.sutterhealth.org/about/news/news_emr.html* [accessed March 22, 2005].

U.S. DHHS (U.S. Department of Health and Human Services). 2003a. *HHS Launches New Efforts to Promote Paperless Health Care System.* [Online]. Available: *http://www.hhs.gov/news/press/2003pres/20030701.html* [accessed November 15, 2004].

U.S. DHHS. 2003b. *Federal Government Announces First Federal eGov Health Information Exchange Standards.* [Online]. Available: *http://www.hhs.gov/news/press/2003pres/20030321a.html* [accessed May 6, 2005].

U.S. DHHS. 2003c. *State Nursing Home Quality Improvement Programs: Site Visit and Synthesis Report.* [Online]. Available: *http://aspe.hhs.gov/daltcp/reports/statenh.htm* [accessed March 24, 2005].

U.S. DHHS. 2005. *President Requests 2.6 Percent NIH Budget Increase in 2005.* [Online]. Available: *http://www.nih.gov/news/NIH-Record/03_02_2004/story03.htm* [accessed March 22, 2005].

U.S. DOE Office of Science (U.S. Department of Energy Office of Science). 2004. *Potential Benefits of Human Genome Project Research.* [Online]. Available: *http://www.ornl.gov/sci/techresources/Human_Genome/project/benefits.shtml* [accessed March 22, 2005].

U.S. DOL (U.S. Department of Labor). 2004. *Physicians and Surgeons.* [Online]. Available: *http://stats.bls.gov/oco/ocos074.htm* [accessed March 28, 2005].

U.S. FDA (U.S. Food and Drug Administration). 2004a. *Joint Replacement: An Inside Look.* [Online]. Available: *http://www.fda.gov/fdac/features/2004/204_joints.html* [accessed March 28, 2005].

U.S. FDA. 2004b. *FDA's "Critical Path" Initiative* . [Online]. Available: *http://www.fda.gov/oc/initiatives/criticalpath/woodcock/woodcock.html* [accessed March 22, 2005].

U.S. VA (U.S. Department of Veterans Affairs). 2003. *VA's Electronic Health Records System Pushing National Standards.* [Online]. Available: *http://www1.va.gov/opa/pressrel/PressArtInternet.cfm?id=589* [accessed March 22, 2005].

Virtual Medical Worlds Monthly. 2001. *Electronic Health Record Roll Out Puts Patient at Centre of British National Health Service.* [Online]. Available: *http://www.hoise.com/vmw/01/articles/vmw/LV-VM-03-01-5.html* [accessed March 22, 2005].

Wachter RM. 2004. *The End of the Beginning: Patient Safety Five Years After "To Err is Human."* [Online]. Available: *http://content.healthaffairs.org/cgi/content/abstract/hlthaff.w4.534v1* [accessed March 28, 2005].

Wennberg JE. 2005, *Variation in Use of Medicare Services Among Regions and Selected Academic Medical Centers: Is More Better?* New York: New York Academy of Medicine.

Werner RM, Asch DA. 2005. The unintended consequences of publicly reporting quality information. *Journal of the American Medical Association* 293(10):1239–1244.

The White House. 2004. *Executive Order #13335.* [Online]. Available: *http://www.whitehouse.gov/news/releases/2004/04/20040427-4.html* [accessed April 27, 2004].

Williams JF, Zimmerman JE, Wagner DP, Hawkins M, Knaus WA. 1995. African-American and white patients admitted to the intensive care unit: Is there a difference in therapy and outcome? *Critical Care Medicine* 23(4):626–636.

2

Current and Future State of Performance Measurement and Reporting

CHAPTER SUMMARY

This chapter provides an overview of the current state of health care performance measurement and reporting. To better align and coordinate existing efforts in this area, the committee calls for a national system for performance measurement and reporting and identifies key attributes of a well-functioning system that can meet this need.

In recent years, improving health care quality has become a top priority for all major stakeholders in the health care system—the federal government, group purchasers, health care professionals, health care providers, state governments, oversight organizations, consumer groups, and others. Hundreds of efforts now under way, including public reporting, pay-for-performance, and ongoing quality improvement programs, are aimed at enhancing quality.

Many public- and private-sector health care programs now engage in public reporting of data that allow comparison of the quality of institutional and provider performance. The Centers for Medicare and Medicaid Services (CMS) produces comparative quality reports on many of its participating providers, including health plans, hospitals, nursing homes, home health agencies, and renal dialysis centers (CMS, 2005c). The National Committee for Quality Assurance (NCQA) makes available comparative quality information on health plans (NCQA, 2005c). State governments, private purchasers, coalitions, and others operate additional public reporting programs (AHRQ, 2003; CMS, 2003; Joint Commission Resources, 2005; NBCH, 2004; New York State Department of Health, 2004). A recent review of hospital reporting initiatives found 45 Web sites in the United

States and two in other countries that provide online comparative hospital performance information (Delmarva Foundation, 2005).

Widespread concerns about quality have stimulated quality improvement efforts at all levels of the health care system. Quality monitoring and improvement are critical responsibilities of all types of health care providers, and quality improvement is now regarded as a core competency that all types of health care professionals should possess. Major accreditation and certification bodies have increased requirements for monitoring and demonstrating improvements in quality and safety (ABIM, 2005; JCAHO, 2004; NCQA, 2000). And Medicare, through its Quality Improvement Organization Program, provides about $350 million per year for surveillance functions and technical assistance (U.S. DHHS, 2004a).

In an effort to reward providers for improvements in quality, many private purchasers and health plans have implemented pay-for-performance programs that characteristically link a modest amount of provider payments to performance across a number of measures (Dudley, 2005; Rosenthal and Booth, 2004; Rosenthal et al., 2005). In addition, the public sector has been active in conducting demonstration projects linking performance on a set of standardized measures to bonuses, calling for "value-based purchasing" (U.S. Congress, 2005a,b; U.S. DHHS, 2002, 2004b).

Reflecting the priority accorded to improving quality, many private organizations, such as health plans, hospitals, provider groups, and professional associations, have made considerable progress in developing measures that capture important areas of clinical care and organizational performance. Measures of patients' perceptions or experiences of care have emerged through efforts of consumer advocates. CMS has also demonstrated leadership in encouraging the development of these measures through demonstration projects.

The development of multiple quality measures has been driven by stakeholders eager to see certain features of care recognized and rewarded as part of quality improvement initiatives. These efforts rely greatly upon consensual efforts and private support from key membership organizations. Yet while the private sector has made valuable contributions in moving the quality agenda forward through pioneering and innovative efforts, the emerging quality measures resulting from these efforts are unable to address all six aims for the health care system articulated in the *Quality Chasm* report (IOM, 2001): safety, effectiveness, patient-centeredness, timeliness, efficiency, and equity. The current patchwork of existing measures fluctuates over time and includes many gaps when assessed against the six aims. Few or no measures exist in the areas of efficiency, equity, and patient-centeredness. In addition, the variety of measures that exist in certain areas creates competing demands for data that can be burdensome to providers.

The magnitude of the various quality improvement initiatives has generated high expectations for the use of valid, objective, and reliable performance measures. All of these initiatives—public reporting, quality improvement within providers' offices, and pay for performance—depend upon the availability of an array of measures whose implementation can contribute to realizing the fundamental aims of the nation's health care system. The committee concludes that federal leadership is necessary to ensure that performance measures address all six aims, as well as to balance private-sector initiatives with investments in quality measures for neglected areas that may lack strong constituencies. Federal leadership is also essential to provide stability, coordination, and direction when fluctuations and tensions in the health care system create an unpredictable environment for data collection and reporting. The challenge is multifaceted:

- To identify the national goals that performance measures should serve.
- To clarify data requirements in areas in which multiple measures have been proposed.
- To identify areas in which greater effort is needed.
- To build the capacity to produce, report, and analyze performance data throughout the public and private sectors of the health care system.

PERFORMANCE MEASUREMENT AND REPORTING: WHAT DO WE MEAN?

Quality-related efforts in all of the areas noted above—public reporting, quality improvement initiatives, and pay for performance—rely on some form of performance measurement and reporting. Components of a system that can perform these functions include the following:

- *Standardized performance measures*—Performance measures include measures of the health care process (e.g., periodic blood and urine tests for diabetic patients), patient outcomes (e.g., 60-day survival rate for cardiac bypass patients), patient perceptions of care (e.g., experience with patient–provider communication), and organizational structure and systems associated with the ability to provide high-quality care (e.g., medication order entry systems). Standardized performance measures are those with detailed specifications (e.g., definitions for the numerator and denominator, sampling strategy if appropriate) allowing for "apples-to-apples" comparisons, sometimes requiring effective risk adjustment or stratification of results across key subgroups.
- *Access to patient data*—Calculation of many performance measures requires access to patient-level data from administrative files and chart

reviews. Other measures require asking patients to complete surveys that allow assessment of their perceptions of their care, their quality of life, or their functional status.

• *Data verification and auditing*—A key element of a quality measurement and reporting system is ensuring that data for performance measures are reported accurately. For many measures that are submitted by individual providers (i.e., self-reported), an external auditing function is often desirable and, for some regulators, mandatory.

• *Comparative analysis and reporting capability*—A performance measurement system that produces information to support the decisions of consumers, purchasers, referring physicians, and other stakeholders in choosing plans, providers, or treatment options requires some form of effective comparative reporting capability. Similarly, improvement efforts that draw on knowledge of best practices benefit from comparative data.

While the current proliferation of measure sets and related reporting activities provides important building blocks for a performance measurement and reporting system, it may have unintended consequences. The above components frequently draw upon different data sets. Excessive attention and energy may be required of providers to comply with externally imposed reporting requirements and quality improvement priorities. These resources may be diverted from patient care and internally generated quality improvement efforts. External reporting requirements that fail to yield readily understandable, pertinent, and reliable information may result in frustrated consumers and angry providers. It is not surprising, then, that numerous expert panels have identified the need for greater standardization of performance measures and reporting requirements (IOM, 2002; President's Advisory Commission on Consumer Protection and Quality in the Health Care Industry, 1998).

This chapter includes three sections. The first provides an overview of recent efforts to promote standardized quality measurement and reporting. The second lays out a rationale for a national system for performance measurement and reporting. The final section draws on this analysis and the work of other groups to define the key attributes of an effective national system, including 10 design principles the committee believes should guide the system's development.

RECENT EFFORTS TO PROMOTE STANDARDIZED PERFORMANCE MEASUREMENT

Efforts to standardize quality measurement and reporting in the health care system have been under way for more than 15 years. Of particular significance are the early pioneering efforts of NCQA, the Agency for

Healthcare Research and Quality (AHRQ), the Joint Commission on Accreditation of Healthcare Organizations (JCAHO), and CMS. In recent years, recognition of the need to coordinate and harmonize quality measurement has led to increased collaboration. Widespread participation in standardized measurement and reporting activities has occurred among private purchasers (such as those in the Pacific Business Group on Health, the Leapfrog Group, and Bridges to Excellence), public purchasers (especially CMS, the largest purchaser), private-sector organizations (such as the National Quality Forum [NQF]), and health plans (such as PacifiCare and Aetna).

Pioneering Programs

One of the oldest and perhaps most successful quality measurement efforts is the Health Plan Employer Data and Information Set (HEDIS), first released in 1989 by a coalition of health plans (members of The HMO Group) and large employers. The initial set of measures was subsequently adapted and refined by NCQA (NCQA, 2005b). Health plans seeking accreditation by NCQA are required to report on HEDIS measures, and their performance scores on these measures are factored into the accreditation process.

Originally spearheaded by private purchasers, HEDIS was adapted in the mid-1990s for use by public purchasers (NCQA, 2005b). CMS now requires health plans participating in the Medicare program to submit data on HEDIS-developed measures of health care quality, many of which are incorporated in comparative quality reports available on the CMS Web site (CMS, 2005d). Many state governments also require plans participating in Medicaid to report HEDIS data (New York State Department of Health, 2002; Texas Health and Human Services Commission, 2004; Washington State Department of Health and Human Services, 2005). Additionally, HEDIS measures are frequently used in the nearly 90 pay for performance programs sponsored by private purchasers (Rosenthal et al., 2004).

Most though not all health plans produce HEDIS reports for their privately insured populations. Those plans that choose not to participate in HEDIS reporting are likely to be the very lowest performers (McCormick et al., 2002). NCQA's Quality COMPASS data repository includes comparative HEDIS reports for more than 300 commercial managed care products (NCQA, 2005c). However, as only health maintenance organizations (HMOs) report on HEDIS measures, recent declines in HMO relative to preferred provider organization enrollment have resulted in a decrease in the total population included in the reporting pool. CMS is attempting to address this problem, at least within the Medicare program, and a few employers are beginning to look at HEDIS measures for the commercial sector.

An important complement to HEDIS has been a 10-year program to develop a family of patient survey instruments under the leadership of AHRQ (AHRQ, 1998). Working with a consortium of private-sector research organizations (including Harvard Medical School, Research Triangle Institute, RAND, and, more recently, the American Institutes for Research), AHRQ released the Consumer Assessment of Health Plans Survey (CAHPS) instrument in 1997 to capture consumer assessments of care received. The original CAHPS survey is now required by NCQA for health plan accreditation, and is used by many public and private purchasers (e.g., CMS's Medicare program, many state Medicaid programs, the Federal Employees Health Benefit Plan, and many private employers and business coalitions), as well as quality oversight organizations. The CAHPS family has expanded to include a survey of behavioral health services, recently developed with support from AHRQ and the MacArthur Foundation (CAHPS Survey Users Network, 2005; Shaul et al., 2001). The CAHPS program has also evolved to to include various settings of care, and the acronym now stands for the Consumer Assessment of Healthcare Providers and Systems. A version of CAHPS for hospitalized patients has recently been completed (AHRQ, 2004). Other survey instruments are in various stages of development. These include both a health plan survey and a clinician and group survey (developed through the Ambulatory CAHPS process) and two versions of a nursing home survey—one for residents and the other for family members and others who visit residents regularly (CAHPS Survey Users Network, 2005). Also under development is a survey for patients receiving in-center hemodialysis treatment (CAHPS Survey Users Network, 2005).

In the area of hospital care, both the Department of Health and Human Services (DHHS) and JCAHO have played important roles. The development of standardized performance measurement and public reporting programs for hospitals dates back to 1986, when the DHHS Health Care Financing Administration (now known as CMS) released comparative reports on hospital mortality (HCFA, 1987). Also in the mid-1980s, JCAHO developed and field tested six sets of standardized performance measures (perioperative care, obstetrical care, trauma care, oncology care, infection control, and medication use) and announced its intent to require accredited hospitals to collect and submit data on these measures (JCAHO, 2005d). Both of these early efforts were abandoned in the face of strong objections from the hospital sector and others.

In the late 1990s, JCAHO embarked on a second effort to implement performance measures as a condition of accreditation for hospitals, long-term care organizations, networks, home health agencies, and behavioral health care organizations. Health care organizations were allowed great discretion in selecting measures from a large menu, and the measure specifications were not standardized (JCAHO, 2005d). In 2002, JCAHO introduced a set of standardized core measures into its performance requirements for hospitals (JCAHO, 2005c). Hospitals seeking accreditation (approximately 95 percent of acute care hospitals) are currently required to submit data on three of five standardized measure sets (acute myocardial infarction, heart failure, pneumonia, pregnancy and related conditions, and surgical infection prevention) (JCAHO, 2005a). During the next 5 years, JCAHO plans to introduce standardized measures for other types of organizations and clinical conditions (JCAHO, 2005b). In 2004 CMS, working collaboratively with the American Hospital Association and other partners, announced a voluntary hospital reporting initiative linking a hospital's payment update under Medicare to the submission of data for a set of standardized measures from the JCAHO ORYX system (CMS, 2004). In April 2005, CMS began publicly reporting hospital comparative data based on these measures via its Web-based tool, Hospital Compare (CMS, 2005b).

In the area of long-term care, CMS has played a pivotal role in the development of standardized performance measures. Starting in the mid-1980s, CMS supported the development of patient assessment instruments used by organ transplant centers, nursing homes, and home health agencies. The Minimum Data Set (MDS), the assessment instrument for nursing home patients, was first implemented by CMS in 1990 (Manard, 2002). By 1999, a set of 24 quality indicators based on MDS data had become part of a routinely administered nursing home survey; in 2002, CMS also established a Web-based reporting mechanism, Nursing Home Compare, to provide the public and other stakeholders with comparative quality data on nursing homes (CMS, 2005c; Manard, 2002). In 1999, CMS furthered its efforts by requiring home health agencies to submit patient assessment data using the Outcome and Assessment Information Set (AHRQ, 2002); CMS started making comparative quality data for home health agencies available in 2003 on its Home Health Compare Web site (CMS, 2005c).

In summary, these pioneering performance measurement initiatives have provided a foundation for the identification of standardized measures; laid the groundwork for collaboration; and built a broad base of stakeholder support for public reporting, pay for performance, and quality oversight programs.

Widespread Collaborative Efforts

As the twenty-first century approached, the need to coordinate the national bodies involved in the promulgation of standardized performance measures became increasingly apparent. In addition to the efforts of the major national players, dozens of more narrowly focused or local efforts were aimed at establishing new standardized measure sets. Concern arose that the absence of a national infrastructure for performance measurement would impose an enormous burden on providers, institutions, and health care professionals. More important, the time and resources available to providers to support quality improvement efforts would increasingly be consumed by data collection across a wide range of measures, resulting in less time and fewer resources available for the redesign of care processes.

It also became clear that many stakeholders would use standardized measures and data for a variety of purposes, including public reporting, pay for performance, quality improvement, and professional certification. The existing patchwork of measurement and reporting efforts could not be relied upon to respond to the diverse information needs of consumers, purchasers, providers, and other stakeholders. Publicly available performance information varied greatly in terms of availability by geographic area, participation of various types of providers, comprehensiveness and relevance of quality measures, validity and reliability of data, and usefulness of public reporting formats. Health care leaders recognized the need for a national infrastructure and process for setting goals and priorities for performance measurement and improvement, promulgating standardized measure sets for use by all stakeholders, and streamlining data collection and reporting.

In 1998, the President's Advisory Commission on Consumer Protection and Quality in the Health Care Industry identified key components of a national quality strategy and infrastructure, including (1) the promulgation of a set of aims for improvement, accompanied by specific, measurable objectives; and (2) a measurement and reporting system consisting of standardized measures and data collection and reporting capabilities. The commission also recommended creating two public–private partnership entities (President's Advisory Commission on Consumer Protection and Quality in the Health Care Industry, 1998):

- *Advisory Council for Health Care Quality*—The expert advisory council would identify national aims and specific objectives for improvement, establish goals and objectives for measurement, and track and report on the nation's progress. The council would be located in the public sector and publicly financed.
- *Forum for Health Care Quality Measurement and Reporting*—The forum would define a plan for implementing quality measurement, data collection, and reporting standards, and identify and update core sets of quality measures and standardized reporting methods. The forum would be a private-sector membership organization, financed by member dues.

In 1999, the private-sector component, NQF, was established by a Forum Planning Committee convened under the auspices of the office of the Vice President of the United States. However, the public-sector component (the Advisory Council for Health Care Quality) was not established by

Congress. At the time, other important initiatives, such as the Patient's Bill of Rights, were competing for the President's and Congress' attention and resources. Furthermore, the importance of establishing a public entity that would be responsible for identifying aims for quality improvement, setting national goals for measurement and reporting, and tracking progress was not fully recognized or supported by political will. In hindsight, this omission can be viewed as a missed opportunity.

Once operational, NQF created a Strategic Framework Board (SFB) to provide advice and counsel as it began to pursue its mission. Operating independently from NQF, the SFB consisted of nine experts with a broad spectrum of research and managerial experience. The board's purpose was to (1) design a strategy for national performance measurement and reporting, (2) articulate the guiding principles and priorities for a national system, and (3) identify potential barriers to successful implementation and propose possible solutions (McGlynn, 2003). The SFB was also conceived as a means to fulfill one of the intended roles of the proposed Advisory Council for Health Care Quality: to create and sustain a "dynamic tension" designed to bring an aspirational dimension to the forum's work.

NQF continues today as a not-for-profit membership organization whose governing board includes representatives of consumers, public and private purchasers, employers, health care professionals, provider organizations, health plans, accrediting bodies, labor unions, and other stakeholders. Financial support for the organization comes from two major sources: member dues and project-specific contracts and grants.

The mission of NQF is "to improve American healthcare through endorsement of consensus-based national standards for measurement and public reporting of healthcare performance data that provide meaningful information about whether care is safe, timely, beneficial, patient-centered, equitable and efficient" (NQF, 2005a). The accomplishments of NQF include the following:

- Establishment of a well-described process for endorsing voluntary consensus standards that satisfies the requirements of the National Technology Transfer and Advancement Act of 1995 (NQF, 2004b).
- Review and endorsement of measure sets applicable to numerous health care settings and clinical areas and services, for example, hospital care, diabetes care, and nursing sensitive care (NQF, 2002b, 2003b, 2004a).
- Conduct of educational and convening activities that address key health care challenges, such as patient safety, health care disparities, and the implementation of information technology (NQF, 2002a, 2003a,c).

Despite these noteworthy achievements, the vision for the NQF articulated by the President's Advisory Commission has not yet been fully realized. Indeed, the forum's experience offers valuable lessons learned with regard to the essential components of an effective and sustainable national performance measurement and reporting strategy. The absence of a public arm (the Advisory Council for Health Care Quality) has created a national leadership vacuum and led to insufficient funding for quality improvement initiatives. Consequently, NQF—whose structure is based on a private-sector business model—has few alternatives to depending on outside sources to support its work. Thus, its projects tend to reflect the priorities of available funding sources rather than addressing a discrete set of national goals. As a result, a comprehensive strategy for the development and implementation of health care performance measures does not yet exist. While many collaborative efforts are under way, they are not coordinated; they do not include all the key organizations; and they are not taking place in the context of a comprehensive and ongoing plan specifying aims for improvement, measure development, and implementation.

Although a complete national infrastructure for standardized performance measurement and reporting has not emerged, major national standards-setting bodies, in concert with key public and private purchasers, have taken important actions to focus and harmonize measurement efforts. Much of this collaborative work has focused on performance measurement for physician practices—a particularly challenging problem for several reasons. First, public and private purchaser data must be pooled to obtain meaningful information on small practice settings. Individual insurers do not account for a large enough share of a provider's practice to yield meaningful measures of performance. Second, some aspects of performance are difficult or impossible to assess. At the disease-specific level, for example, individual doctors may simply not see enough patients, and therefore their individual practices cannot yield enough data to support reliable or valid characterizations of their performance (Hofer et al., 1999). Third, growing awareness of the systemic nature of both excellence and defects in quality has increased support for the concept that all providers involved in a patient's care share responsibility for the quality of the care process and for patient outcomes. Designing and implementing shared incentives and reward processes that fairly reflect the degree of influence and responsibility of each individual provider is a new challenge.

In 1998, the American Medical Association (AMA), JCAHO, and NCQA established a Performance Measurement Coordinating Council to integrate the development of performance measures and to "speak with a common private-sector voice on critical public policy issues related to quality and performance measurement" (AMA et al., 2001a). In 2001, the council released pain management assessment and management standards and a standardized measure set for diabetes (AMA et al., 2001a,b; American Pain Society, 2000).

In 2002, the AMA established the Physician Consortium for Performance Improvement, building on prior efforts including the AMA Physician Office Assessment program (AMA, 2002). The consortium, which includes representatives from more than 50 national medical specialty societies, AHRQ, and CMS, has developed measure sets in the following areas: asthma, coronary artery disease, diabetes, heart failure, hypertension, depression, osteoarthritis of the knee, prenatal testing, and preventive care and screening (AMA, 2005). Working collaboratively with JCAHO and NCQA, the consortium recently released a set of Principles for Performance Measurement in Health Care (Physician Consortium for Performance Improvement, 2004).

In 2004, the Physician Consortium for Performance Improvement, CMS, and NCQA released a set of ambulatory care clinical performance measures relevant mainly to primary care (AMA, 2005). This ambulatory measure set includes measures from HEDIS, the various measure sets of the Physician Consortium for Performance Improvement, and measures developed by the federal government (i.e., CMS and the Veterans Health Administration). Most of the measures require use of the costly chart review abstraction method and are therefore expensive to administer.

To build more consensus around a set of standardized measures for physician practices for use in public reporting and pay for performance, the Ambulatory care Quality Alliance[1] (AQA) was launched in the fall of 2004. The alliance has endorsed a standardized set of 26 measures for physician practices that draws heavily on the 2004 ambulatory care clinical performance measure set released by the Physician Consortium for Performance Improvement, CMS, and NCQA, thereby eliminating duplication (ACP, 2005). Concurrently with the work of AQA, NQF conducted an expedited review of ambulatory care clinical performance measures; a set of these measures was endorsed in August 2005 (NQF, 2005b). The administrator of CMS has hailed this initial ambulatory measure set as a "milestone" and pledged CMS's support for the alliance's continued efforts (McClellan, 2005). All of the ambulatory measures endorsed by NQF[2] and the subset of those measures adopted by AQA are "owned" by the Physician Consortium for Performance Improvement or NCQA. The NCQA measures in that set are adaptations of HEDIS measures (used at the health plan level) that have been respecified for use at the physician office level in situations where there is no enrolled population.

---

[1]This collaborative effort involves AHRQ, the American Academy of Family Physicians, the American College of Physicians, the AMA, and America's Health Insurance Plans.

[2]NQF endorsed an initial set of 36 ambulatory measures in August 2005 and an additional 6 measures following the second round of voting and the appeal process.

In addition to public reporting and pay for performance programs, performance measurement systems are now used to support several provider recognition and certification programs. Working in partnership with the American Diabetes Association and the American Heart Association/American Stroke Association, NCQA has established the Diabetes Physician Recognition Program and the Heart/Stroke Physician Recognition Program to identify physicians who demonstrate high-quality care in these clinical areas (NCQA, 2005d). A third physician recognition program, Physician Practice Connections, was developed by NCQA and then adapted to a pay-for-performance application in collaboration with several physician bonus programs, such as Bridges to Excellence and the pay-for-performance program of California's Integrated Healthcare Association. Physician Practice Connections recognizes physician practices that use up-to-date information systems, as well as achievements in such areas as delivery system design, patient self-management support, and decision support that enhance patient care. In February 2005, NCQA and the American Board of Internal Medicine (ABIM) announced an agreement to harmonize their measure systems and activities pertaining to physicians so that internists can submit performance data to NCQA, which in turn will share results with ABIM (NCQA, 2005a). NCQA will use the performance data in its physician recognition programs, while ABIM will use the data in its maintenance-of-certification processes.

In yet another collaborative effort, CMS has furthered its commitment to advancing measure development by awarding a contract for specialty and subspecialty measure development to Mathematica Policy, in collaboration with the Physician Consortium for Performance Improvement and NCQA, starting October 1, 2005. This represents what could be a new level of collaboration around measure development between private-sector entities and CMS (CMS, 2005a).

In summary, the pioneering efforts of a number of organizations have altered the performance measurement landscape (see Appendix B for a synopsis of the contributions of these organizations). Although current national measure sets constitute the major accomplishments, dozens of "niche" measurement sets have emerged as well. The committee reviewed this array of measures (discussed further in Chapter 4) and identified many areas of duplication, inconsistency in specifications, and serious gaps in the assessment of important components of quality care. To overcome these limitations, some key players are collaborating on the development of measure sets that standardize specifications for multiple uses. Beyond harmonization, however, more leadership is necessary to shift the mounting array of efforts from one that is driven principally by individual stakeholder interests to one that is focused on a set of national goals developed through a deliberative process that reflects both public and private concerns.

PERFORMANCE MEASUREMENT EFFORTS
IN OTHER COUNTRIES

The United States is not alone in its efforts to improve performance measurement in health care. Many other nations, for similar reasons, have developed research agendas and public policy initiatives in reporting, assessment, regulation, and improvement of care that depend upon standardized performance measures. Although performance measurement and reporting systems are tailored to each country's political, social, and economic context, much can be learned from those experiences. For one thing, performance measurement in other countries demonstrates the potential value of centralized leadership and a streamlined, coordinated approach. The United States would therefore benefit from a careful assessment of the efforts of the United Kingdom, Australia, and other nations.

Perhaps the strongest such example in the past decade has been the Modernisation Program of the English National Health Service (NHS Modernisation Agency, 2003). In 1998, the Labor government in the United Kingdom, under Prime Minister Tony Blair, launched a massive effort to increase investment in health services from the then-current level of about 6.5 percent of gross domestic product to the European average of about 8.5 percent over 5 years (New Statesman, 2000). A series of carefully developed National Service Frameworks was created to guide this massive new investment and to ensure the value of the Modernisation Program. The frameworks specified hundreds of goals, benchmarks, and associated measures for targeted clinical areas, such as heart disease, cancer care, orthopedics, and primary care. Various agencies and departments within the government were charged to measure, track, and report on progress. That effort continues today. (Note that although the National Health Service has counterparts in Scotland, Wales, and Northern Ireland, the Modernisation Program described here is that in England, rather than throughout the United Kingdom.)

The new government contract with general practitioners constituted a second major advance in measurement and public reporting in the National Health Service (Roland, 2004; Smith and York, 2004; Stevens, 2004). That contract included a bold and innovative measurement system, in which general practitioners are assessed on a 1,050-point system with respect to several dozen performance measures encompassing both structural and process variables in their practices. Substantial financial incentives are linked to point scores at the practice level. The effects of this new contract on care are now under active assessment through several government-sponsored research projects.

Australia established a Council for Safety and Quality in Health Care in January 2000, led by Australian health ministers, to guide national efforts to improve safety and quality throughout the country's health care system. The council reports annually to all health ministers, is supported by all state and territorial jurisdictions, and works closely with other national bodies to complement the efforts of others working to improve care (Australian Council for Safety and Quality in Healthcare, 2004). In January 2005, the council awarded $1 million in grants for 50 innovative projects across Australia to address specific patient safety and quality issues (Australian Council for Quality and Safety in Healthcare, 2005). These efforts have also led to a groundswell of companies implementing multiple ways of measuring and reporting on performance, thus becoming truly transparent and accountable (Australian Government, 2002).

LIMITATIONS OF CURRENT PERFORMANCE MEASUREMENT EFFORTS

The above discussion highlights the scope of performance measurement activities currently under way and the high expectations for these efforts. It also underscores the deep commitment of many key stakeholders to performance measurement and the remarkable progress that has been achieved through their collective efforts. At the same time, the committee believes the current approach to quality measurement in the United States falls short of constituting an effective national system for performance measurement and reporting for the following reasons:

• The current approach fails to set goals and aims consistent with the vision of the *Quality Chasm* report. The focus of the measures presently available is too narrow and does not move the health care system toward that bold vision.
• The current approach produces measures that are inconsistent, complex, and unstable, imposing on providers of care uncertainty and the burden of conflicting measures.
• The current approach faces a continually uncertain future because of inadequate and unstable funding and persistent conflicts among stakeholders, relying on fragile consensus-driven procedures.
• The current approach learns too little and too late from successes and failures. The evidence base for quality improvement, public reporting, and pay for performance is thin, and will remain so without cogent and well-supported evaluation.

Creating a coherent national system that can help stakeholder groups work more effectively, respond to their various needs, and address gaps in leading measure sets is a major challenge. To create such a system, strong, independent leadership is needed to coordinate current efforts. Sustained, adequate funding will be essential to support a structure capable of encouraging multiple initiatives while also withstanding the pressures of narrow stakeholder interests, as well as keeping patients' interests in the foreground. An investment in learning how measurement can best accelerate improvement is imperative as well.

In light of the long history of multiple, sometimes competing efforts to promulgate and report on performance measures, it appears unlikely that the current activities of key stakeholders will lead to the national system that the IOM committee believes to be crucial to quality improvement. To overcome the limitations delineated above and to ensure the emergence of a viable national system for performance measurement and reporting, performance measurement will need to be embraced as a public good requiring leadership—though not a takeover—from the federal government. In the next section, the committee sets forth the attributes of such a national system and proposes a conceptual framework to guide its development.

ATTRIBUTES OF A WELL-FUNCTIONING SYSTEM FOR PERFORMANCE MEASUREMENT AND REPORTING

The major limitations of current performance measurement and reporting capabilities are briefly summarized in Table 2-1. The table also suggests how each of these limitations can be reframed as key attributes of a well-coordinated national system for performance measurement and reporting.

In developing the concept of a national system, the committee drew heavily on the earlier work of the Strategic Framework Board.[3] The committee also conducted a systematic examination of several physician practices that illuminated potential success factors and barriers to the implementation of performance measurement (see Appendix C for details). The committee's analysis led to the conclusion that a national system should possess the following attributes (see Figure 2-1):

- Specify a purpose and aims for the health care system.
- Set national goals.
- Establish and implement a plan for the development and promulgation of performance measures.
- Ensure data collection, data validation, and aggregation processes.
- Develop and promulgate public performance reports to support the decisions of many stakeholders.
- Establish and fund necessary research.
- Continually evaluate, through an impact assessment, the effectiveness of performance measurement, payment reform, and quality improvement initiatives.

---

[3]The board's final report consisted of a series of papers published in *Medical Care Supplement*, Volume 41, No. 1, January 2003.

TABLE 2-1 Major Limitations of Efforts to Measure the Performance of the U.S. Health Care System and Corresponding Attributes of a National System for Performance Measurement and Reporting

Limitations of Current System	Corresponding Attributes of a National System for Performance Measurement and Reporting
Purpose/aims—No coherent approach to specifying purposes and aims of measurement.	Specify a clear national purpose for the health care system and explicit aims for improvement.
Measures—Limited scope of measurement (failure to measure in many domains) and a multiplicity of competing measures in some domains. Lack of clarity and uniformity prevents information technology vendors from planning to include measures.	Establish a national system of standardized performance measures that are linked to aims, comprehensive in scope, and aligned with current and expected capabilities for reporting.
Data aggregation/reporting—Lack of standardization, multiple conflicting stakeholders collecting data independently, unjustifiable reporting burden on providers, and reporting that often confuses consumers.	Ensure well-developed data collection and aggregation processes to minimize the burden on providers while ensuring efficient measurement across payers and providers. Develop public reports that are valid, understandable, and actionable.
Funding—Inadequate and unstable funding for performance measurement activities and research.	Sustain adequate funding for a structure able to withstand pressures of stakeholder interests and keep patients' needs in the foreground.
Capacity to learn—Efforts to improve quality constrained by a lack of evidence on the effectiveness of alternative improvement strategies, potential adverse effects of measurement, best ways to communicate quality information to providers and consumers, and effectiveness of pay-for-performance initiatives.	Evaluate the effectiveness of performance measurement, public reporting, and payment systems and quality improvement initiatives to minimize potential adverse effects, detect unintended consequences, and maximize the eventual benefits of performance measurement.

Additionally, the committee concluded that a national system should support the needs of stakeholders within the public and private health care sectors along three dimensions:

• *Accountability*—Many stakeholders make important decisions that motivate or influence care delivery. Purchasers and consumers make decisions about the selection of health plans, providers, and treatment options;

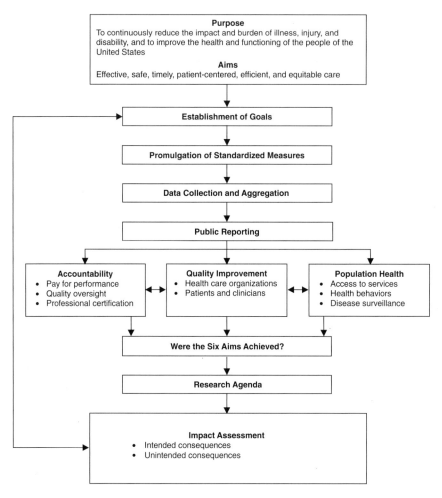

FIGURE 2-1   A national system for performance measurement and reporting.
SOURCE: Adapted from Strategic Framework Board (McGlynn, 2003).

clinicians about the referral of patients to specialists, hospitals, and other providers; public- and private-sector oversight organizations about licensure, accreditation, board certification, and recognition awards; and health plans about which providers to include in their networks.

• *Quality improvement*—Stakeholders engaged in the delivery of health care services need information they can act upon to improve the quality of those services. Clinicians need performance data to support ongoing quality improvement. Health care administrators and managers and the members of their governing boards need performance data to support efforts directed at the redesign of care processes and the operation of systems to support care delivery. Health care providers need both performance data and evidence on those interventions provided by physicians, nurses, and other clinicians that are most likely to yield desired outcomes.

• *Population health*—The health care delivery system is one of many factors that can influence the health of a population. A well-functioning performance measurement and reporting system should provide information to support the broad range of public policy decisions that influence population health and ultimately the need for health care services. The system should be designed to complement and support traditional public health reporting systems. It might include, for example, measures of access to health care services by various populations, including the uninsured and racial/ethnic minorities, the use of preventive services and health behaviors, and disease surveillance. Such a system would be an important asset in such areas as emergency preparedness, disease surveillance, and health protection.

Through its deliberations and its examination of existing measure sets (described more fully in Chapter 4), the committee formulated 10 design principles for a progressively improving national performance measurement and reporting system. Table 2-2 summarizes these design principles (see Appendix D for a complete description). These same principles can guide the future development of measures, as discussed in subsequent chapters.

NEXT STEPS

This committee recognizes that it will take a number of years to fully implement a national system for performanace measurement and reporting. There is a great variation in the degree of knowledge and experience pertaining to the various components of the system. As discussed above, there has been nearly two decades of experience with standardized measurement, but much less experience with public reporting. While data repositories for some measures already exist at the state or national level, no clear consensus has emerged on the proper structure of such registries, and many issues of data ownership and privacy protection must be resolved. It is clear, therefore, that some components of the system can be established immediately; for others, additional work will be needed to identify the best approach. The next chapter analyzes alternatives for achieving a national system that embodies the design principles described in Table 2-2 and presents the committee's recommended strategy.

TABLE 2-2 Design Principles for a National System for Peformance Measurement and Reporting

Principle	Description
Principle 1: Comprehensive Measurement	A performance measurement system should advance the core purpose of the health care system and foster improvements in all six quality aims identified in the *Quality Chasm* report (IOM, 2001): safety, effectiveness, patient-centeredness, timeliness, efficiency, and equity.
Principle 2: Evidence-Based Goals and Measures	A performance measurement system should be guided by a comprehensive set of evidence-based goals for improvement.
Principle 3: Longitudinal Measurement	Standardized performance measures should characterize health and health care both within and across settings and over time.
Principle 4: Supportive of Multiple Uses and Stakeholders	A performance measurement system should provide information for multiple uses, including provider-led improvement efforts, public reporting, payment and benefit design, and population health initiatives.
Principle 5: Measurement Intrinsic to Care	Performance measurement should be intrinsic to the care process.
Principle 6: A Central Role for the Patient's Voice	A performance measurement system should include direct reports and ratings from patients and family caregivers.
Principle 7: Patient-Level, Population-Based, and Systems-Level Measurement	Measurement and measures should assess the health and health care of both individuals and populations and the many systems within which care is provided.
Principle 8: Shared Accountability	Measurement should not be constrained by the absence of a current, identifiable, single responsible agent.
Principle 9: A Learning System	A performance measurement system should be a learning system, continually evaluating its own performance and advancing knowledge regarding performance measurement.
Principle 10: Independent and Sustainable	A performance measurement system should be continually enhanced and financed in a way that ensures its independence and sustainability.

REFERENCES

ABIM (American Board of Internal Medicine). 2005. *About Maintenance of Certification.* [Online]. Available: *http://www.abim.org/moc/index.shtm* [accessed March 30, 2005].

ACP (American College of Physicians). 2005. ACP Online—The Revitalization of Internal Medicine Initiative. *Ambulatory Care Quality Alliance Approves Uniform Starter Set of Performance Measures.* [Online]. Available: *http://www.acponline.org/revitalization/ am_care.htm?hp* [accessed May 3, 2005].

AHRQ (Agency for Healthcare Research and Quality). 1998. *Consumer Assessment of Health Plans (CAHPS[R]): Overview.* [Online]. Available: *http://www.ahcpr.gov/qual/cahps/ dept1.htm* [accessed February 25, 2005].

AHRQ. 2002. *AHRQ Report on Home Health Quality Measures for CMS Public Reporting: Results of Technical Expert Panel Meeting and AHRQ Recommendations.* Rockville, MD: AHRQ.

AHRQ. 2003. *National Healthcare Quality Report.* [Online]. Available: *http:// www.qualitytools.ahrq.gov/qualityreport/archive/2003/browse/browse.aspx* [accessed November 16, 2005].

AHRQ. 2004. *Fact Sheet: Hospital CAHPS(R) (HCAHPS[R]).* [Online]. Available: *http:// www.ahcpr.gov/qual/cahps/hcahpfact.htm* [accessed February 25, 2005].

AMA (American Medical Association). 2002. *Physician Consortium for Performance Improvement: Taking the Lead Together.* Chicago, IL: AMA.

AMA. 2005. *AMA (CQI) Measurement Sets: Clinical Performance Measurement Tools to Support Physicians in Their Efforts to Enhance the Quality of Patient Care.* [Online]. Available: *http://www.ama-assn.org/ama/pub/category/4837.html* [accessed February 23, 2005].

AMA, JCAHO, NCQA (American Medical Association, Joint Commission on Accreditation of Healthcare Organizations, National Committee for Quality Assurance). 2001a. *AMA, JCAHO and NCQA Release Common Measures for Diabetes Care.* Press release. April 25, 2001. Chicago, IL.

AMA, JCAHO, NCQA. 2001b. *AMA, JCAHO and NCQA to Focus on Measuring Effectiveness of Appropriate Pain Management.* Press Release. December 17, 2001. Chicago, IL.

American Pain Society. 2000. *New JCAHO Standards for Pain Management.* [Online]. Available: *http://www.ampainsoc.org/pub/bulletin/jul00/pres1.htm* [accessed March 30, 2005].

Australian Council for Quality and Safety in Healthcare. 2005. *One Million Dollars to Improve Patient Safety.* [Online]. Available: *http://www.safetyandquality.org/index.cfm* [accessed March 31, 2005].

Australian Council for Safety and Quality in Healthcare. 2004. *Safety and Quality Council.* [Online]. Available: *http://www.safetyandquality.org/index.cfm* [accessed March 31, 2005].

Australian Government. 2002. *Triple Bottom Line Measurement and Reporting in Australia: Making it Tangible.* [Online]. Available: *http://www.deh.gov.au/industry/finance/publications/triple-bottom/executive-summary.html* [accessed March 31, 2005].

CAHPS Survey Users Network. 2005. *CAHPS Survey Products.* [Online]. Available: *http:// www.cahps-sun.org/Products/ProductIntro.asp* [accessed February 22, 2005].

CMS (Centers for Medicare and Medicaid Services). 2003. *Nursing Home Compare.* [Online]. Available: *http://www.medicare.gov/NHCompare/Home.asp* [accessed March 29, 2005].

CMS. 2004. Hospital Quality Alliance (HQA): *Improving Care Through Information.* [Online]. Available: *http://www.cms.hhs.gov/quality/hospital/HQAFactSheet.pdf* [accessed March 30, 2005].

CMS. 2005a. *Centers for Medicare and Medicaid Services.* [Online]. Available: *http:// www.cms.hhs.gov/* [accessed October 19, 2005].

CMS. 2005b. *Hospital Quality Initiative.* [Online]. Available: *http://www.cms.hhs.gov/quality/hospital/* [accessed February 21, 2005].

CMS. 2005c. *Medicare Compare for Medicare Advantage Plans, Hospitals, Home Health, Nursing Homes, and End-Stage Renal Dialysis Centers.* [Online]. Available: *http://www.Medicare.gov* [accessed March 1, 2005].

CMS. 2005d. *Medicare Personal Plan Finder.* [Online]. Available: *http://www.medicare.gov/default.asp* [accessed March 30, 2005].

Delmarva Foundation. 2005. *The State of the Art of Online Hospital Public Reporting: A Review of Forty-Seven Websites.* [Online]. Available: *http://www.delmarvafoundation.org/html/public_reporting_summit_052604/WebSummariesFinal9.2.04.pdf* [accessed May 13, 2005].

Dudley RA. 2005. Pay-for-performance research: How to learn what clinicians and policy makers need to know. *Journal of the American Medical Association* 294(14):1821–1823.

HCFA (Health Care Financing Administration). 1987. *Medicare Hospital Mortality Information, 1986.* Washington, DC: U.S. Government Printing Office.

Hofer TP, Hayward RA, Greenfield S, Wagner EH, Kaplan SH, Manning WG. 1999. The unreliability of individual physician "report cards" for assessing the costs and quality of care of a chronic disease. *Journal of the American Medical Association* 281(22):2098–2105.

IOM (Institute of Medicine). 2001. *Crossing the Quality Chasm: A New Health System for the 21st Century.* Washington, DC: National Academy Press.

IOM. 2002. *Leadership by Example: Coordinating Government Roles in Improving Health Care Quality.* Corrigan JM, Eden J, Smith BM, eds. Washington, DC: The National Academies Press.

JCAHO (Joint Commission on Accreditation of Healthcare Organizations). 2004. *Our Commitment to Patient Safety.* [Online]. Available: *http://www.jcaho.org/general+public/patient+safety/index.htm* [accessed March 30, 2005].

JCAHO. 2005a. *Core Measure Information, Specification Manual for National Hospital Quality Measures* [Online]. Available: *http://www.jcaho.org/pms/core+measures/aligned_manual.htm* [accessed February 17, 2005].

JCAHO. 2005b. *Performance Measurement: Future Goals and Objectives.* [Online]. Available: *http://www.jcaho.org/pms/reference+materials/future+goals+and+objectives.htm* [accessed February 17, 2005].

JCAHO. 2005c. *Performance Measurement in Health Care.* [Online]. Available: *http://www.jcaho.org/pms/index.htm* [accessed February 17, 2005].

JCAHO. 2005d. *Performance Measurement: Key Historical Milestones.* [Online]. Available: *http://www.jcaho.org/pms/reference+materials/key+historical+milestones.htm* [accessed February 17, 2005].

Joint Commission Resources. 2005. *Public Information Policy: The Quality Report.* [Online]. Available: *http://www.jcrinc.com/subscribers/perspectives.asp?durki=7712&site=10&return=6062* [accessed March 29, 2005].

Manard B. 2002. *Nursing Home Quality Indicators: Their Uses and Limitations.* Washington, DC: AARP Public Policy Group.

McClellan MB. 2005. Statement of Mark B. McClellan, M.D., Ph.D. Administrator, *CMS on Ambulatory Care Quality Measures.* [Online]. Available: *http://www.cms.hhs.gov/media/press/release.asp?Counter=1443* [accessed May 12, 2005].

McCormick D, Himmelstein DU, Woolhandler S, Wolfe SM, Bor DH. 2002. Relationship between low quality-of-care scores and HMOs' subsequent public disclosure of quality-of-care scores. *Journal of the American Medical Association* 288(12):1484–1490.

McGlynn EAP. 2003. Introduction and overview of the conceptual framework for a national quality measurement and reporting system. *Medical Care* 41(Suppl. 1):I-1–I-7.

NBCH (National Business Coalition on Health). 2004. *Coalition Report Card Weblink Project.* [Online]. Available: *http://www.nbch.org/members/reportcards.cfm* [accessed March 29, 2005].

NCQA (National Committee for Quality Assurance). 2000. *NCQA to Define Accreditation Program to Focus Attention on Patient Safety.* [Online]. Available: *http://www.ncqa.org/communications/news/patsafrel.htm* [accessed March 22, 2004].

NCQA. 2005a. *NCQA, ABIM to Align Requirements, Share Data; Agreement Will Allow Joint Application for Maintaining Board Certification, Recognition.* [Online]. Available: *http://www.ncqa.org/Communications/News/ABIM2-2.htm* [accessed February 23, 2005].

NCQA. 2005b. *NCQA Timeline.* [Online]. Available: *http://www.ncqa.org/about/timeline.htm* [accessed February 21, 2005].

NCQA. 2005c. *Quality Compass 2005: The Most Comprehensive Database of Health Plan Performance Data Anywhere.* [Online]. Available: *http://www.ncqa.org/Info/QualityCompass/index.htm* [accessed February 21, 2005].

NCQA. 2005d. *Recognized Physician Directory.* [Online]. Available: *http://www.ncqa.org/PhysicianQualityReports.htm* [accessed February 21, 2005].

New Statesman. 2000. *Blair has Made a Historic Pledge: Prime Minister Tony Blair Plans to Increase Health Care Spending in the United Kingdom to the European Union Average by the Year 2006.* [Online]. Available: *http://www.findarticles.com/p/articles/mi_m0FQP/is_4470_129/ai_59810465* [accessed March 31, 2005].

New York State Department of Health. 2002. *NYS Managed Care Plan Performance Report.* [Online]. Available: *http://www.health.state.ny.us/nysdoh/mancare/qarrfull/qarr01/qarintro1.htm* [accessed March 30, 2005].

New York State Department of Health. 2004. *Cardiovascular Disease in New York State.* [Online]. Available: *http://www.health.state.ny.us/nysdoh/heart/heart_disease.htm* [accessed March 29, 2004].

NHS Modernisation Agency. 2003. *Real Measurement for Real Improvement Using Statistical Process Control.* [Online]. Available: *http://www.modern.nhs.uk/search/* [accessed March 31, 2005].

NQF (National Quality Forum). 2002a. *Improving Healthcare Quality for Minority Patients: Workshop Summary.* Washington, DC: NQF.

NQF. 2002b. *National Voluntary Consensus Standards for Adult Diabetes Care.* Washington, DC: NQF.

NQF. 2003a. *Information Technology and Healthcare: Proceedings of a Summit.* Washington, DC: NQF.

NQF. 2003b. *National Voluntary Consensus Standards for Hospital Care: An Initial Performance Measure Set.* Washington, DC: NQF.

NQF. 2003c. *Safe Practices for Better Healthcare.* Washington, DC: NQF.

NQF. 2004a. *National Voluntary Consensus Standards for Nursing-Sensitive Care: An Initial Performance Measure Set.* Washington, DC: NQF.

NQF. 2004b. *The National Quality Forum's Consensus Development Process.* Version 1.7. Washington, DC: NQF.

NQF. 2005a. NQF: *Mission Statement.* [Online]. Available: *http://www.qualityforum.org/mission/home.htm* [accessed February 25, 2005].

NQF. 2005b. *NQF-Endorsed National Voluntary Consensus Standards for Ambulatory Care.* [Online]. Available: *http://www.qualityforum.org/docs/ambulatory_care/tbambphase2diabTABLE09-13-05hww.pdf* [accessed October 17, 2005].

Physician Consortium for Performance Improvement. 2004. *Clinical Performance Measurement Tools to Support Physicians in Their Efforts to Enhance the Quality of Patient Care: A Consensus Statement from The American Medical Association and The Joint Commission on Accreditation of Healthcare Organizations and The National Committee for Quality Assurance.* [Online]. Available: *http://www.ama-assn.org/ama1/pub/upload/mm/370/principlesperfmeas.pdf* [accessed May 18, 2005].

President's Advisory Commission on Consumer Protection and Quality in the Health Care Industry. 1998. *Quality First: Better Health Care for All Americans—Final Report to the President of the United States.* Washington, DC: U.S. Government Printing Office.

Roland M. 2004. Linking Physicians' Pay to the Quality of Care: A Major Experiment in the United Kingdom. *New England Journal of Medicine* 351(14):1448–1454.

Rosenthal J, Booth M. 2004. *State Patient Safety Centers: A New Approach to Promote Patient Safety.* [Online]. Available: *http://www.nashp.edu* [accessed November 16, 2004].

Rosenthal MB, Fernandopulle R, Song HR, Landon B. 2004. Paying for quality: Providers' incentives for quality improvement. *Health Affairs* 23(2):127–141.

Rosenthal MB, Frank RG, Li Z, Epstein AM. 2005. Early experience with pay-for-performance: From concept to practice. *Journal of the American Medical Association* 294(14):1788–1793.

Shaul JA, Eisen SV, Stringfellow VL, Clarridge BR, Hermann RC, Nelson D, Anderson E, Kubrin AI, Leff HS, Cleary PD. 2001. Use of consumer ratings for quality improvement in behavioral health insurance plans. *Joint Commission Journal on Quality Improvement* 27(4):216–229.

Smith PC, York N. 2004. Quality incentives: The case of U.K. general practitioners. *Health Affairs* 23(3):112–118.

Stevens S. 2004. Reform strategies for the English NHS. *Health Affairs* 23(3):37–44.

Texas Health and Human Services Commission. 2004. *Behavioral Health Measures across Medicaid Managed Care Plans and Models.* [Online]. Available: *http://www.hhsc.state.tx.us/medicaid/reports/082004_BHDR.html* [accessed March 30, 2005].

U.S. Congress. 2005a. Medicare Value Purchasing Act of 2005. S. 1356.

U.S. Congress. 2005b. Medicare Value-Based Purchasing for Physicians' Services Act of 2005. H.R. 3617.

U.S. DHHS (U.S. Department of Health and Human Services). 2002. *Physician Group Practice Demonstration.* [Online]. Available: *http://www.cms.hhs.gov/researchers/demos/PGP.asp* [accessed March 1, 2005].

U.S. DHHS. 2004a. *FY 2005 Budget in Brief.* [Online]. Available: *http://www.hhs.gov/budget/05budget/centersformed.html* [accessed March 30, 2005].

U.S. DHHS. 2004b. *Rewarding Superior Quality Care: The Premier Hospital Quality Incentive Demonstration Fact Sheet.* [Online]. Available: *http://www.cms.hhs.gov/quality/hospital/PremierFactSheet.pdf* [accessed March 1, 2005].

Washington State Department of Health and Human Services. 2005. *Washington Medicaid Program Compiles New HEDIS Performance Ratings.* [Online]. Available: *http://www1.dshs.wa.gov/mediareleases/2005/pr05021.shtml* [accessed March 30, 2005].

3

Achieving a National System for Performance Measurement and Reporting

CHAPTER SUMMARY

This chapter presents the committee's recommendation for the establishment of an independent board to oversee and coordinate the functions of a national system for performance measurement and reporting. Guidelines for the design and operation of the board to ensure its authority and sustainability are discussed. The chapter closes with a discussion of potential concerns about this newly proposed entity and the committee's responses to those concerns.

ALTERNATIVES TO ACHIEVING A NATIONAL SYSTEM FOR PERFORMANCE MEASURMENT AND REPORTING

A strong evidence base does not yet exist to support the value of a well-coordinated national system for performance measurement and reporting relative to the status quo described in Chapter 2. However, some promising examples of how performance measurement and public reporting have been linked to improved quality helped shape the committee's decision making. For example, the Veterans Health Administration (VHA) has implemented several system changes targeted at improving the quality of care, including measuring and tracking performance on a comprehensive set of indicators. In a cross-sectional comparison of 12 VHA health care systems versus a representative national sample, VHA patients were found to receive higher-quality care than their counterparts in the areas of overall quality, chronic disease care, and preventive care. The greatest differences were seen in areas in which the VHA had well-established performance measures in place and was aggressively monitoring performance and providing feedback (Asch et al., 2004). With regard to public reporting, a recent study comparing hospitals that reported data publicly and those that shared data only privately found that the former hospitals significantly improved their performance in the clinical area studied relative to those that did not use public reports. The results of this study appear to suggest that public reports stimulate quality improvement interventions (Hibbard et al., 2005). In the absence of a strong evidence base, the committee considered three factors in developing its recommendations: (1) the scope of efforts currently under way in public reporting, payment incentives, and quality improvement that are dependent on performance measures; (2) the consequences of inaction; and (3) the merits of alternative approaches to the development of an effective national system for performance measurement and reporting.

The scope of current efforts and expectations for performance measurement are high. The Centers for Medicare and Medicaid Services (CMS), the private sector, and Congress are all committing substantial resources to performance measurement, public reporting, and quality improvement initiatives, and are now embarking on pay for performance initiatives. All of these efforts are being undertaken with the strong expectation of improving the quality of care. Indeed, it was this expectation that led Congress to request that the Institute of Medicine (IOM) provide guidance to CMS to support these efforts.

After reviewing current efforts (see Chapter 2), the committee concluded that extensive resources exist on which to build a national system, including those of national organizations such as the National Committee for Quality Assurance (NCQA), the National Quality Forum (NQF), and the Joint Commission on Accreditation of Healthcare Organizations (JCAHO), as well as numerous state and regional entities. Notwithstanding these considerable accomplishments, however, the nation does not yet have a coherent, integrated system for establishing, measuring, and tracking the performance of the health care system. In fact, there is growing concern in some quarters that the current fragmented approach could create a confusing, duplicative, yet still incomplete set of activities that would absorb too many resources. As the overall enterprise is still young, it is worth asking whether the current efforts can and will evolve into the system that is needed—one in which performance is tied to national health care goals; is viewed as credible, objective, and grounded in evidence; is comprehensive in covering all of the six aims identified in the *Quality Chasm* report; is coordinated and forward looking; and is transparent and accessible to all stakeholders.

In its deliberations, the committee also discussed the potential consequences of failing to move forward and to capitalize on existing resources in a more systematic way. One such consequence is that the pace of change will remain slow, thus not reflecting the sense of urgency the committee views as essential to reach the point at which consistent delivery of high-quality care will become accelerated and more widespread. Another concern is that without a mechanism in place for continuously evaluating the impact of performance measurement initiatives and guarding against unintended consequences, the much-needed evidence base for identifying effective interventions will be less likely to evolve.

ASSESSMENT OF ALTERNATIVES

In the above context, the committee considered four alternatives for achieving a high-functioning national system for performance measurement and reporting, as illustrated in Figure 2-1 in Chapter 2: (1) establishing a large federal entity, (2) establishing an office within CMS or the Agency for Healthcare Research and Quality (AHRQ), (3) delegating functions to existing stakeholder groups, and (4) establishing a new independent board.

Alternative 1: Large Federal Entity

A new federal entity could be established to assume responsibility for the entire spectrum of activities shown in Figure 2-1 in Chapter 2. The advantage of this option is that all of the resources needed to create a national system for performance measurement and reporting would be housed under one roof and supported by a single stream of funding. However, the committee believes this option is not preferable for several reasons. First, creating such a federal entity would duplicate the work already being performed by a host of reputable stakeholder groups. Incurring the high cost of assuming the tasks currently conducted by those existing groups would be imprudent, particularly in the current fiscal environment. Moreover, the transition to a large federal bureaucracy could disrupt current activities in the private sector, thus having the unintended consequence of setting back progress made to date that has been shown to be of value.

Alternative 2: Office Within the Centers for Medicare and Medicaid Services or the Agency for Healthcare Research and Quality

Current public–private, largely voluntary efforts could be sustained with the addition of a special office within CMS or AHRQ that would be charged with encouraging existing players to align those efforts more directly with a specific set of national health goals. The committee believes this option would be an improvement over the status quo, but lacks the capacity to achieve the vision of a full-fledged national system for performance measurement and reporting. The committee believes such an office would be unlikely to have the authority to establish national goals and aims for improvement, and would lack the clout and the resources to convince stakeholder groups to move beyond the sphere of their own special interests.

Additionally, this type of structure could be susceptible to undue political influences that would threaten its independence.

Alternative 3: Other Stakeholder Groups

The responsibility for a national system could be assigned to one of the existing major stakeholder groups, such as NQF, NCQA, or JCAHO. As described in Chapter 2, current private-sector efforts have made substantial progress in shaping and advancing the field of performance measurement in health care. For example, NQF has a reputable track record in endorsing standardized performance measures, while NCQA and JCAHO have rich histories in the development of standardized measures and the public reporting of comparative quality data.[1] In addition to these competencies, however, the committee identified additional functions of a national system that are unlikely to be realized through private-sector efforts alone, as they are framed from the perspective of a public good. These include (1) specifying a purpose and national aims for the health care system, (2) setting national goals, (3) establishing and funding a national research agenda, and (4) evaluating the effectiveness of the performance measurement system and reporting in its entirety. The committee believes that to achieve a broad-based performance measurement and reporting system that is capable of fulfilling all these requirements, public-sector leadership and oversight are essential.

Alternative 4: Independent Board

The committee concludes that a well-functioning national system for performance measurement and reporting is most likely to arise through creation of an entity built on the accomplishments and ongoing efforts of existing organizations. While not impossible, the committee doubts that such a system would evolve on its own from the vast array of efforts by public, for-profit, and not-for-profit organizations currently under way. This assertion is based on history and a number of realities that characterize the present situation:

• As noted above national goals are unlikely to be set and translated into measures, since existing entities have neither the authority nor the overarching leadership required to formulate such goals.

---

[1]NCQA publicly reports Health Plan Employer Data and Information Set measures for participating health plans; JCAHO's ORYX measures are used by CMS for its Hospital Compare Website.

• Gaps in performance measurement, such as the capacity to measure equity and access, are unlikely to be filled because of the lack of clear ownership of these aspects of the nation's quality improvement agenda.

• Wasteful duplication and inconsistencies among measures will continue, since no single stakeholder group has the standing to require others to use specific, standardized definitions and measurements.

• Measures may not be viewed as authoritative, credible, or objective since the measures developed by most stakeholders are more apt to reflect the interests of their constituencies than those of others.

• Public goods, such as investments in better risk adjustment methodologies and data aggregation methods, are unlikely to be addressed adequately in a competitive market among current developers of measures.

• Making all information fully transparent and available to the public is unlikely, since much of the technology and data on performance measurement is currently held as proprietary.

Table 3-1 provides a synopsis of the four alternatives discussed above. Although a large federal entity could assume all the necessary functions for a national performance measurement and reporting system, the committee

TABLE 3-1 Comparison of Alternatives for Achieving a National System for Performance Measurement and Reporting

Key Functions of a National System	Alternative 1: Large Federal Entity	Alternative 2: Office Within CMS or AHRQ	Alternative 3: Other Stakeholder Groups	Alternative 4: Independent Board
Specify purpose and aims	✓			✓
Prioritize national goals	✓			✓
Promulgate standardized measures	✓	✓	✓	✓
Ensure data collection, validation, and aggregation	✓	✓	✓	✓
Establish public reporting methods responsive to the needs of all stakeholders	✓	✓	✓	✓
Identify a research agenda	✓			✓
Evaluate impact of overall system	✓			✓

endorses the model of an independent board with contracting authority to capitalize on existing resources as the most appropriate and judicious approach. As illustrated, public and private entities are currently performing several key tasks, but have not been able to meet national needs and expectations because of the difficulty of relying on consensual measures, the fluctuating nature of private support for these efforts, and the lack of clear goals.

Therefore, the committee recommends a strategy based on the establishment of a new independent board, the National Quality Coordination Board (NQCB), that would be recognized by all public and private stakeholders as the lead agency responsible for ensuring the creation of a national system for performance measurement and reporting. In addition to carrying out general management and coordinating functions, the board would provide leadership and policy guidance that would support existing efforts, and seek to align those efforts with national health goals through contractual agreements, educational programs, and consensus-building initiatives.

Recommendation 1: Congress should establish a National Quality Coordination Board (NQCB) with seven key functions:

- Specify the purpose and aims for American health care.
- Establish short- and long-term national goals for improving the health care system.
- Designate, or if necessary develop, standardized performance measures for evaluating the performance of current providers, and monitor the nation's progress toward these goals.
- Ensure the creation of data collection, validation, and aggregation processes.
- Establish public reporting methods responsive to the needs of all stakeholders.
- Identify and fund a research agenda for the development of new measures to address gaps in performance measurement.
- Evaluate the impact of performance measurement on pay for performance, quality improvement, public reporting, and other policy levers.

The NQCB should be composed of health care leaders capable of understanding the diverse sectors within the health care system, such as consumers, purchasers, educators, clinicians from all disciplines (medicine, nursing, pharmacy), and agencies and research centers with expertise in performance measurement. Expert staff will be needed to monitor routine data collection, coordinate standards-setting efforts, and assess national progress toward the implementation of measures that reflect the six quality aims for the health care system.

To operate effectively, the NQCB must have the authority to function independently while working in close collaboration with public- and private-sector health agencies and health care providers. The board is intended to supplement and strengthen—but not replace—ongoing data collection, standardization, and reporting activities in both the private and public sectors. Ideally, the board will enable these key players to perform their jobs more effectively by ensuring a unified and coordinated approach to performance measurement within a framework of clearly articulated national goals. Additionally, the committee views the NQCB as a federal entity that will complement and support current efforts to guide the development of health care performance measures among professional societies, trade associations, health plans, consumer groups, and other elements of the health care enterprise.

ESSENTIAL ATTRIBUTES OF THE NQCB

The need for a national system for performance measurement and reporting provides the rationale for creating the NQCB. While the development of a detailed operational plan for the board's implementation was beyond the scope of the committee's work, its functions are clear. This section provides further details on what the committee identified as the essential attributes of the NQCB.

Standardizing performance measurement and establishing a useful, bold, and transparent national system for setting goals and reporting on progress will require a difficult transition for many stakeholders in American health care. Although almost all parties—especially patients—will benefit in the end from better measurement and reporting, many of the current stakeholders can initially be expected to defend the status quo.

The sources of resistance will be many. For example, vendors and consultants now maintaining or developing their own measurement systems will regard a more uniform national approach as a potential threat to their current designs and market niche. Organizations and individuals that provide health care will be concerned that bold and transparent measurement may divert them from their current strategic agendas, reveal hidden defects in their care, pose uncomfortable threats to marketplace competition, add new costs for data collection and reporting, and, if not properly adjusted for case mix, be unfair and misleading. Governmental and nongovernmental agencies now charged with surveying and assessing care may be biased toward their own current formats, data definitions, and reporting schemes, and will be concerned about the changes to their current systems and processes required by standardization. If, as the committee recommends, a national system for performance measurement and reporting begins with bold aims for the improvement of care and efficiency, stakeholders lacking confidence that such improvements are achievable can be expected to resist.

History bears this out. In the past, the threshold effect—the pain of transition—has prevented progress at the scale recommended by the committee. Consensus-driven processes have made progress, but not enough to meet the social need. Despite numerous efforts over several decades to improve the nation's health care performance assessment, no effective system yet exists.

An NQCB that can lead the development of a truly effective system of performance measurement and reporting will have to possess a high level of independence and authority if it is to accomplish its purpose. At the same time, the board will need to collaborate with major stakeholders, building upon their good will and social vision, if this initiative is to be more successful than earlier attempts. This means that the NQCB should not ignore or replicate the existing measurement capability represented by these stakeholders. Indeed, the committee recommends that, at the outset, the board seek to accomplish its aims to the extent possible by convening capable existing entities, encouraging them to achieve new levels of cooperation, creating appropriate contractual relationships, and assigning projects and deliverables. In attempting to make use of existing organizations and resources, the NQCB must insist on levels of cooperation, standardization, and transparency not currently characteristic of this array of actors. The committee is hopeful that such cooperation—which represents the most parsimonious way to meet the nation's needs for measurement and reporting—can and will emerge.

> **Recommendation 2: The NQCB's membership and procedures should be designed to ensure that the board has structural independence, protection from undue special interests, substantive expertise drawn from the public and private sectors (including not-for-profit entities), contract authority, standards-setting authority, financial strength, and external accountability.**

The board proposed by the committee should have the capacity to perform the multiple functions outlined in Recommendation 1. These functions require that the board have sufficient independence to ensure its objectivity and the capacity to develop and rely upon evidence-based knowledge to guide its recommendations. At the same time, the board needs to be located within a constellation of governmental agencies so it can coordinate its work with appropriate organizations having the operational resources necessary to implement recommended measurement standards, data collection and reporting procedures, and research and evaluation efforts.

Given these competing needs, the committee has opted to recommend locating the NQCB as an independent entity within the U.S. Department of Health and Human Services (DHHS), reporting directly to the DHHS Secretary. This arrangement will allow the board to perform its functions while preserving its structural independence from other agency priorities that could impede its activities.

The committee believes that an entity without adequate authority and protection cannot succeed in this endeavor. The chance of succeeding through new relationships with and among existing players will depend on the board's ability to withstand the intense short-term political pressures that without doubt will arise as current stakeholders perceive the threats enumerated above. Change will not be accomplished without discomfort, and the NQCB must be able to ride out that discomfort and adhere to the goals articulated in this report. Therefore, the committee proposes that the NQCB be armed with at least the following forms of authority and protection:

- *Structural independence.* The NQCB should have the capacity to move the health care system beyond the status quo. The committee recommends that the board be housed within the DHHS and report directly to the Secretary.
- *Protection from undue influence.* The membership of the NQCB should be appointed by the President, with terms that are staggered and long enough to protect the board against short-term political influence and major stakeholder interests.
- *Substantive expertise.* As noted above, the committee's intention is not to supplant or duplicate the often outstanding work of the many organizations currently involved in developing, evaluating, vetting, and implementing performance measures in health care. Rather, the goal is to accelerate progress through coordination and direct financial support for these current activities. Thus the membership of the NQCB should encompass the technical competence needed to assess and guide that work.
- *Contract authority.* In the event that the major organizations currently engaged in measurement development, implementation, and reporting prove unwilling or unable to undertake the activities outlined by NQCB or to deliver under contract the required levels of standardization, analysis, and reporting, the board should have the backup authority and sufficient funding to broaden the array of contractors through which it can execute its key functions.
- *Standards-setting authority.* The Secretary of DHHS should direct CMS (including Medicare, Medicaid, and the State Children's Health Insurance Program), the Health Resources and Services Administration, and AHRQ to focus on the achievement of all applicable national goals established by the NQCB through public reporting, payment reform and other

incentives, health care improvement programs, health professions education, and organizational and systems capacity building. The Secretary should also direct CMS to require that providers submit to the NQCB (or its designee) performance data that can be used by Medicare for public reporting and quality improvement activities or as a basis for payment. In addition, Congress should activate an interagency task force to explore mechanisms for aligning other government health care programs with these efforts—including the Department of Defense (DoD) TRICARE program and DoD-operated clinical facilities, the Federal Employees Health Benefits Program, and the programs of the Veterans Health Administration and the Indian Health Service.

• *Financial strength.* The NQCB should have sufficient, stable funding to contract for services with outside groups and organizations so it can perform its designated functions effectively. The board should be funded directly from the Medicare Trust Fund and have bypass authority to request an appropriation directly from Congress. This bypass authority would free the NQCB from the unpredictable budgetary cycles commonly associated with preparing discretionary budgets that are subject to review and modification on the basis of other departmental, executive, and legislative priorities. Congress should authorize and appropriate funds to support the work of the NQCB and to implement its recommendations in Medicare and other government programs by the end of fiscal year 2007. More specifically, Congress should authorize an annual allocation from the Medicare Trust Fund, initially in the range of $100–200 million (see the discussion in the next section). This level of investment is based on an analysis of resources that currently support related but more limited activities led by NQF, NCQA and JCAHO (as described below). This figure constitutes approximately 0.1 percent of the Medicare annual budget,[2] a relatively small investment with great potential to enhance value and improve efficiency throughout the health care delivery system. The committee envisions substantial staff requirements to support the functions of the board delineated in Recommendation 1 and substantial costs related to contracts with existing entities to carry out tasks pursuant to the mission of the board. Although the federal government should provide up front the funding needed for the NQCB to become fully operational, particularly with regard to its public-good functions, public–private partnerships could be formed over time to support this ongoing work (see Chapter 5).

• *External accountability.* The NQCB should be required to provide an annual report to Congress on its progress toward implementing an effective system for performance measurement and reporting. In addition, the

---

[2]$278 billion in 2003 (CMS, 2004).

board should undergo periodic independent assessments performed by an external organization such as the Medicare Payment Advisory Commission, the IOM, or the Government Accountability Office.

FUNDING FOR THE NQCB

To estimate the level of resources that may be required to support the work of the NQCB, the board's functions were compared with those of other organizations focused on quality improvement, as previously summarized in Table 3-1. As discussed earlier in the chapter, the primary role of NQF, as now structured, is to endorse standardized performance measures—an important function for a national system. NQF has relatively small revenues ($4 million annually), more than half of which are derived from external sources (Guidestar, 2004c). As the scope of the committee's proposed functions for the NQCB is much broader (see Figure 2-1 in Chapter 2), far greater resources would be needed for its operational and oversight functions.

A better model from which to draw inferences about the funding required for the NQCB is NCQA, as it currently performs three key functions of a national system for performance measurement and reporting: (1) development of performance measures; (2) data collection, validation, and aggregation; and (3) public reporting of performance patterns in various regions and across the country. NCQA's revenues totaled $24 million in 2003 (Guidestar, 2004b). Given the administrative tasks and responsibilities of the NQCB beyond NCQA's existing activities—specifying a purpose and aims for the health care system, setting national goals, establishing and funding a national research agenda, and monitoring the impacts of the overall system—a funding estimate of $100–200 million annually is reasonable.

As described in detail in Chapter 2, JCAHO has been extensively involved in performance measure development and reporting activities. JCAHO's revenues for 2003 totaled $85 million (Guidestar, 2004a). Although a large portion of those revenues is associated with accreditation-related activities, the much broader functions of the NQCB argue for funding within the recommended range.

GUIDELINES FOR THE DESIGN AND OPERATION OF THE NQCB

Establishing the NQCB will be a complex and challenging task that will evolve over time. As noted earlier, preparing a detailed blueprint for the operation of such a system was beyond the scope of this study; however, the committee has developed an overall framework and guidance for the initial steps.

The careful design, operationalization, and management of the NQCB will be critical to its success. The Strategic Framework Board focused special attention on three areas that are applicable to the NQCB (Kizer, 2003).

First, the NQCB decision-making process should be evidence based and continually updated to reflect changes in knowledge. Second, the Board should reinforce local improvement efforts, not superimpose new structures on local communities. Third, the NQCB process should be responsive to the challenges and concerns of health care providers, health plans, consumers, and purchasers alike.

Grounded in Evidence

The decision-making processes of the NQCB will benefit greatly from a strong evidence base and access to specialized expertise (McGlynn, 2003). The board should be a learning system that is supported by and contributes to the generation of evidence relevant to (1) making key decisions, such as setting national goals and specifying performance measures; and (2) evaluating the selected measures and understanding their impact on various types of stakeholders.

A great deal of evidence, much of which is currently unavailable, will be needed to support the work of the NQCB. In setting national goals, the board will need epidemiological evidence (e.g., leading causes of death and disability), clinical evidence (e.g., efficacy or effectiveness of various interventions in curing or slowing the progression of a particular disease), and health services research evidence (e.g., feasibility of successful implementation and cost-effectiveness of various interventions) (McGlynn, 2003). In promulgating standardized performance measures, the NQCB will need evidence on the scientific soundness of the various measures under consideration (e.g., whether claims data can be used to assess whether a particular clinical process was performed on those patients who would likely benefit from it or was performed properly). The NQCB will also need evidence on what measures are most important to patients with various types of preferences and needs (see Chapter 5).

Evidence to support both the setting of goals and the promulgation of measures will have to come from a variety of sources. The Centers for Disease Control and Prevention plays a central role in generating epidemiological evidence. Clinical evidence is produced by both the public sector (e.g., National Institutes of Health) and the private sector (e.g., academic health centers, pharmaceutical companies). Specialty societies and others synthesize this evidence into practice guidelines. Health services research, funded by AHRQ, private foundations, and many health care organizations, is often conducted by researchers located in academic settings or research institutes or within health care delivery systems.

The NQCB should be designed to support the decision making of many different stakeholders and to generate evidence on the impacts of measurement and reporting. The board is intended to generate information that will influence health and health care through three pathways: accountability, quality improvement, and population health. Ultimately, the efforts of the many stakeholders involved in these three areas should result in achievement of the six quality aims of the *Quality Chasm* report (IOM, 2001). Data and analyses required to assess impact will be necessary for determining whether the NQCB and the many other quality-related activities now under way are having their intended effect. Specifically, the NQCB should provide the information necessary to evaluate:

- Changes in the environment of care (e.g., consumer and purchaser selection of providers, pay for performance incentives, use of performance data for public reporting and in accreditation and credentialing decisions).
- Changes in the capacity of the delivery system to provide high-quality care (e.g., changes in care coordination mechanisms, use of multidisciplinary teams, implementation of systematic processes to increase adherence to practice guidelines).

In other words, the NQCB should generate information on areas of progress as well as factors that contribute to or impede the rate of change.

A carefully crafted research agenda will be needed to ensure the availability of the evidence necessary for the NQCB to function as a learning system that incorporates new advances. The development and maintenance of this research agenda will require collaboration among the epidemiological, clinical, consumer, purchaser, and health services research communities. Adequate and ongoing funding will require commitments on the part of public- and private-sector funding agencies.

Supportive of Local Improvement Efforts

Although many important aspects of the U.S. health care system are national in scope (e.g., Medicare payment policies, accreditation and certification programs), the delivery of health care services is for the most part a local enterprise. Where applicable, the design and operation of the NQCB should respond to local goals and improvement priorities. Whenever possible, the board should specify the use of standardized measures and reporting requirements that will yield useful information for the purposes of accountability, quality improvement, and population health at the community, regional, and state levels.

In setting national goals, the NQCB should provide opportunities for local input into the agenda-setting process by giving communities an opportunity to comment (McGlynn et al., 2003). Local communities might also be encouraged to undertake locally driven quality improvement initiatives in addition to pursuing national goals.

Recommendation 3: Local innovation in pursuit of national goals for improving health care quality should be encouraged. Performance measurement, improvement, and reporting activities—including those of public and private purchasers; accreditation and certification entities; and federal, state, and local government programs—should be substantially aligned with the national goals and standardized measures established by the NQCB, but local communities should also be encouraged to identify and pursue local priorities, in addition to helping to achieve national goals.

Improvement efforts will likely be more successful and the reporting burden on providers far less onerous if the performance measures and data requirements specified by the NQCB produce information that is useful at all levels of the care system—from the individual provider (whose efforts to improve require performance measures) to the national level (James, 2001). Overall, the committee believes the NQCB will be far more effective in achieving its purpose and aims if standardized performance measure sets are comprehensive enough to support the efforts of many stakeholders—both those external to health care organizations (i.e., purchasers, planners) and those engaged in health care delivery. The NQCB will also be more efficient and timely if the data used to calculate measures are, to the extent possible, generated in real time as a byproduct of the patient care process, rather than retrospectively.

Responsive to Stakeholder Concerns

The NQCB is a potentially powerful tool intended to support the efforts of all stakeholders to achieve a fundamental redesign of the health care delivery system. As with any powerful tool, it must be used wisely and cautiously, and balance the needs of various stakeholders.

The pace of change and burden of data collection should not overwhelm the provider community, yet it should be rapid enough to address the most important unmet needs of consumers and purchasers. The NQCB should develop a reasonable and prompt schedule for the implementation of various measurement and data submission requirements and for the achievement of its specified goals. Requirements should be phased in and communicated in advance to all stakeholders. The failure to develop a reasonable and prompt plan for implementation (e.g., 1-, 3-, and 5-year requirements) and to communicate this plan to providers, consumers, and purchasers could generate a backlash that would impede progress toward a nationally coherent measurement system.

The stewardship responsibilities of the NQCB should be well defined and carried out with the utmost integrity. To be successful, the board must earn the trust and respect of all stakeholders, but especially the provider and patient communities. As noted above, the board's decision making must be grounded in scientific evidence. Auditing mechanisms must be established to ensure data quality. Adequate data protections must be in place to ensure patient confidentiality. Public reports must provide fair comparisons.

Finally, in any complex system, the change process produces both intended and unintended consequences. An early warning system will be needed to identify unintended consequences of the NQCB and take mitigating action. The unintended consequences of the goal-setting and standardized measurement and reporting processes of the NQCB might include the following:

- *Adverse selection*—In the absence of adequate risk-adjustment techniques, providers who care for some of those patients most in need may appear to be poor performers compared with their peers who treat healthier patients (Werner and Asch, 2005). Some providers may try to improve their performance scores by engaging in adverse selection. As a consequence, patients most likely to experience poor health outcomes, such as those most severely ill or with poor health behaviors, may experience difficulty in gaining access to the health system.

- *Data manipulation*—Providers may engage in data recording and coding practices designed to inflate their performance ratings. For example, if performance measures are adjusted for a patient's complicating and comorbid conditions, providers may inflate the list of secondary diagnoses to include conditions that are inactive or those yet to be confirmed.

- *Stifled innovation*—There is always the potential for innovation to be stifled through the imposition of a more structured process for setting goals and focusing quality improvement efforts. As provider attention becomes focused on the national goals and measurement requirements established by the NQCB, providers may divert resources from other promising quality measurement and improvement activities that could yield even greater returns. Private-sector organizations may reduce investments in the development of new quality measures, survey instruments, and tools, some of which could represent breakthrough technologies.

Recognizing the potential for undesirable consequences such as those described above, the committee included efforts to identify solutions to these problems in the comprehensive research agenda proposed in Chapter 5. That research agenda places particular emphasis on the need to address methodological issues, such as risk adjustment, and to perform an impact assessment to monitor and correct for unintended consequences.

POTENTIAL CONCERNS: THE RATIONALE FOR THE NQCB

While the need for the proposed NQCB is clear and compelling, the committee anticipates understandable concerns regarding the potential repercussions of implementing such a system. However, it is possible to make a strong case for the NQCB that addresses these concerns. The concerns most likely to be raised are summarized in Table 3-2 and discussed below.

The NQCB Will Be Too Bureaucratic

In recommending the NQCB, the committee is not suggesting yet another bureaucratic structure, but a centralized mechanism to promote standardization. The goal of standardization is to ensure a level information

TABLE 3-2 Concerns Regarding the Proposed NQCB and Responses to Those Concerns

Potential Concerns	Responses
The NQCB is too bureaucratic.	The NQCB is a centralized mechanism to promote standardization and a level information playing field.
The NQCB duplicates current functions.	The NQCB is more comprehensive in its proposed measure set, stakeholder groups, and reporting functions than what currently exists.
The NQCB is too costly.	The NQCB is a plausible approach to identifying waste in the health care system and improving efficiency.
The NQCB is too complicated.	The NQCB will simplify performance measurement by providing clear goals, a phased approach to implementation, and alignment of measures.
The NQCB is too burdensome for providers.	The NQCB will decrease the reporting burden by substituting a single data set and reporting format for the multiple data sets and formats currently requested by various stakeholder groups.
The NQCB could result in worse quality.	The NQCB will be responsive to the complexities of good clinical care.
The NQCB is a threat to patient privacy.	The NQCB will ensure appropriate confidentiality protections for patient data in strict compliance with regulations of the Health Insurance Portability and Accountability Act.
The NQCB will stifle local innovation.	The NQCB will serve as a foundation upon which local efforts can build.
The NQCB could pose undue hardship on local providers in underserved areas.	The NQCB will support performance measurement and reporting at the population level. Underserved areas will be carefully monitored for unintended consequences, particularly with regard to access issues related to providers.

playing field for comparison among providers, as well as to promote efficient information collection and transfer analogous to standards setting for transportation and financial systems. Performance measures and quality information represent public goods regardless of one's political perspective or preferred policy approach: a competitive market driven by consumer choice, regulatory approaches based on provider accreditation, or self-motivated efforts by providers to improve. Valid measures of performance are an essential foundation for improving quality and efficiency. Because the unfettered market cannot produce standardized measures, this is a legitimate arena for the government to assume a leadership role. However, the board's focus will be, to the extent possible, on coordinating and building on existing efforts so as to avoid becoming a large bureaucracy.

The NQCB Will Be Too Costly

Some will argue that the NQCB will be too costly. Conversely, the committee argues that not establishing the NQCB will be too costly as the negative consequences of inaction are too great to be ignored. The nation's current health care system is riddled with waste and duplication. A performance measurement system that supports fair comparisons on costs and quality offers a plausible approach to identifying waste and improving efficiency. Present approaches to quality measurement are also wasteful: duplicative, distracting, and sometimes misleading, consuming precious consumer and provider time. The goal of the proposed new measurement system is to provide a common and efficiently collected body of useful and meaningful information for all stakeholders, including providers, payers, and consumers. As stated earlier, the initial investment the committee is recommending is only 0.1 percent of Medicare's annual budget.

The NQCB Will Be Too Complicated

At first blush, the NQCB may appear too complicated. However, current approaches to measurement are both complicated and fragmented. The NQCB, if properly implemented, should provide (1) clear goals for measurement, alleviating the problem of competing measure sets; (2) a phased approach to implementation to ensure that data collection tools and approaches are efficient and supported by electronic health records (EHRs); and (3) alignment of nearly identical measures (similar measures with different data element definitions) that currently require duplicative record collection.

The NQCB Will Impose Too Great a Burden on Providers

A major concern is that the NQCB will be too burdensome for already overtaxed providers. On the contrary, the NQCB will eliminate multiple, often conflicting requests for data from private and public purchasers, accrediting bodies, and others, thus decreasing the burden of data collection. It is anticipated that the NQCB will drive the use of EHRs, enabling data collection to become part of the routine care process rather than an additional task as it is today, with the long-term goal that the data collected will support local quality improvement efforts led by providers. Caution must be exercised, however, with regard to EHRs. Their adoption rate is slow—currently estimated at 27 percent (Bates, 2005)—impeded by costs, privacy issues, lack of national data standards, and physician culture. The NQCB should monitor the adoption rate of EHRs, remaining cognizant of these impediments, and adjust its expectations and timeline accordingly. As the capacity of EHRs to support reporting of performance data is currently uncertain, the NQCB should contribute to the gathering of evidence for evaluating their effectiveness for this purpose (Baron et al., 2005; IOM, 2003; Miller et al., 2005; Sprague, 2004).

The NQCB May Result in Worse Quality

Concern might be raised that a focus on technical process measures may in some cases result in worse rather than better quality. This concern stems from the belief that current technical process measures do not adequately capture the complexity of clinical care, as in the case of frail elderly patients who often have multiple chronic conditions. Good care in this instance requires that physicians prioritize treatment objectives or in some cases choose to focus on functional improvement or quality of life rather than disease treatment. A well-functioning performance measurement and reporting system should be designed to address this concern by (1) ensuring that measures exclude groups or populations of patients for whom the guidelines (and related measures) are inappropriate; (2) allowing evidence-based and verifiable exclusions by practitioners where measures are imperfect; and (3) fostering the development of patient-centered measures of decision quality.

The NQCB Threatens Patient Privacy

Issues concerning the privacy and confidentiality of patient health information warrant heightened attention by the NQCB, particularly with regard to data aggregation. The NQCB will need to be diligent in ensuring that appropriate confidentiality protections are in place for the submission of patient data that are in strict compliance with the regulations of the Health Insurance Portability and Accountability Act. The board will also need to address the potential problem of patients opting not to have their data included in a data repository and the impact this would have on the ability to accurately assess the quality of care both nationally and across communities. These issues are explored further in Chapter 4.

The NQCB Will Stifle Local Quality Improvement Efforts

As with any national compulsory structure, there could be concern that the NQCB will pose a threat to innovative local quality improvement initiatives and programs. Many regions of the country are developing advanced performance measurement systems, and some stakeholders may be concerned that the NQCB will establish a ceiling, thus precluding their own quality improvement targets and local priorities. The NQCB may require local efforts to make some modifications so that common definitions are used by all. However, the board should be flexible enough to serve as a foundation upon which local efforts can build.

The NQCB May Impose Undue Hardship on Local Providers in Underserved Areas

There may be concern that the NQCB will have a negative impact on some communities, particularly those with a shortage of providers, such as in rural and urban areas. The demands of data collection and the impact of public reporting could inadvertently influence providers to leave such underserved areas. This, coupled with emigration of more mobile residents, could force smaller clinics or hospitals to close before they can be competitive on key quality measures. The NQCB will support the collection of data at the population level, as well as the development of public reports appropriate for these communities, and will be flexible in addressing the unique needs of this constituency.

REFERENCES

Asch SM, McGlynn EA, Hogan M, Hayward R, Shekelle P, Rubenstein L, Keesey J, Adams J, Kerr E. 2004. Comparison of quality of care for patients in the Veterans Health Administration and patients in a national sample. *Annals of Internal Medicine* 141(12):938–945.

Baron RJ, Fabens EL, Schiffman M, Wolf E. 2005. Electronic health records: Just around the corner? Or over the cliff? *Annals of Internal Medicine* 143(3):222–226.

Bates DW. 2005. Physicians and ambulatory electronic health records. *Health Affairs* 24(5):1180–1189.

CMS (Centers for Medicare and Medicaid Services). 2004. *2004 CMS Statistics.* Washington, DC: CMS.

Guidestar. 2004a. *2003 Tax Form 990 for JCAHO Surveyor and QHR Consultant Corporation.* [Online]. Available: *http://www.guidestar.org/FinDocuments/2003/363/673/2003-363673595-1-9.pdf* [accessed July 8, 2005].

Guidestar. 2004b. *2003 Tax Form 990 for National Committee for Quality Assurance.* [Online]. Available: *http://www.guidestar.org/FinDocuments/2003/521/191/2003-521191985-1-9.pdf* [accessed July 8, 2005].

Guidestar. 2004c. 2003 *Tax Form 990 for the National Quality Forum.* [Online]. Available: *http://www.guidestar.org/FinDocuments/2003/522/175/2003-522175544-1-9.pdf* [accessed July 8, 2005].

Hibbard JH, Stockard J, Tusler M. 2005. Hospital performance reports: Impact on quality, market, share, and reputation. *Health Affairs* 24(4):1150-1160.

IOM (Institute of Medicine). 2001. *Crossing the Quality Chasm: A New Health System for the 21st Century.* Committee on Quality of Health Care in America. Washington, DC: National Academy Press.

IOM. 2003. *Key Capabilities of an Electronic Health Record System: Letter Report.* Committee on Data Standards for Patient Safety. Washington, DC: The National Academies Press.

James BC. 2001. Making it easy to do it right. *New England Journal of Medicine* 345(13):991–993.

Kizer KW, ed. 2003. Putting the ideas into practice. *Medical Care* 41(Suppl. 1):I-87–I-89.

McGlynn EA. 2003. An evidence-based national quality measurement and reporting system. *Medical Care* 41(Suppl. 1):I-8–I-15.

McGlynn EA, Cassel CK, Leatherman ST, DeCristofaro A, Smits HL. 2003. Establishing national goals for quality improvement. *Medical Care* 41(Suppl. 1):I-16–I-29.

Miller RH, West C, Brown TM, Sim I, Ganchoff C. 2005. The value of electronic health records in solo or small group practices. *Health Affairs* 24(5):1127–1137.

Sprague L. 2004. Electronic health records: How close? How far to go? *National Health Policy Forum Issue Brief* (800):1–17.

Werner RM, Asch DA. 2005. The unintended consequences of publicly reporting quality information. *Journal of the American Medical Association* 293(10):1239–1244.

4

Moving Forward:
What Should Be Measured?

CHAPTER SUMMARY

*This chapter describes the approach used by the committee to se-
lect a starter set of performance measures and identifies significant
gaps in the scope of existing measures. In addition to recommending a starter set of measures drawn from earlier work of stakeholder groups, the committee proposes four approaches to address
identified gaps in existing measures: comprehensive measurement;
longitudinal measurement; patient-level, population-based, and
systems-level measurement; and shared accountability.*

The committee is convinced that performance measurement is a prereq-
uisite for improving both health and health care in the United States, and
that it requires clear stewardship at the federal level. The committee is therefore recommending the establishment of a National Quality Coordination
Board (NQCB) housed within the U.S. Department of Health and Human
Services to perform this guiding function while working collaboratively with
existing stakeholder groups (see Chapter 3).

An important function of the NQCB will be harmonizing current efforts to establish standardized performance measures. Accordingly, this
chapter focuses on how the quality of health care services should be measured. The committee performed a comprehensive review of available standardized performance measures for health care services delivered in
the ambulatory, acute, long-term care, and in-center hemodialysis settings
and evaluated the nature and scope of these measures in light of the
10 design principles articulated in Chapter 2 and Appendix D. Based on
this review, the committee identifies critical gaps in existing measures
and proposes a starter set of measures that are available for immediate
implementation.

APPROACH

The committee approached the challenge of selecting a starter set of performance measures by first identifying the analytic frameworks for quality assessment that have guided the development of measures in the past. The most important of these were the six aims set forth in the *Quality Chasm* report (IOM, 2001) and the Foundation for Accountability's call for assessing care across the lifespan (FACCT, 1997). The committee then identified leading performance measures and measure sets, classifying them within the existing analytic frameworks. A full description of the selection and classification methodology can be found in Appendix E.

The committee recognizes limitations to this approach, as the primary emphasis was on measurement of health care services. This focus constrained the committee's ability to include measures of other important areas that have a profound impact on health outcomes, such as health behaviors and disparities in care. The committee also acknowledges the difficulty of adopting these measures, particularly for certain providers. For example, rural hospitals will face different barriers to implementation from those faced by community-based hospitals or academic health centers. The committee's approach did, however, make it possible to identify the major gaps in current performance measure sets and to specify the 10 design principles for a performance measurement and reporting system set forth in Chapter 2. These 10 design principles, in turn, provided an additional lens for the classification of current measures, as well as a basis for recommending next steps.

GAPS IN CURRENT MEASURES AND IMPLICATIONS FOR THE DESIGN OF A PERFORMANCE MEASUREMENT AND REPORTING SYSTEM

The committee reviewed more than 800 measures within the analytic frameworks noted above. As a result of this effort, the committee identified several major gaps in existing measure sets, summarized in Table 4-1. The following sections highlight those areas in which the committee proposes significant changes in direction or new emphasis in performance measurement, as embodied in the following approaches:

- Comprehensive measurement
- Longitudinal measurement
- Individual patient-level, population-based, and systems-level measurement
- Shared accountability

These approaches represent a change relative to current performance measurement efforts as they provide different frameworks through which

TABLE 4-1 Gaps in Current Performance Measure Sets

Gap	Relevant Design Principles[a]	Description
Limited scope of measurement: Few measures of patient-centered care, equity, or efficiency. Few measures for children or those at the end of life. Many important conditions unrepresented in measures.	*Principle 1:* Comprehensive measurement	A performance measurement system should advance the core purpose of the health care system and foster improvements in all six aims identified in the *Quality Chasm* report (IOM, 2001): safety, effectiveness, patient-centeredness, timeliness, efficiency, and equity.
Narrow time window: Most measures focus on a single point in time and do not assess care across settings.	*Principle 3:* Longitudinal measurement	Standardized performance measures should characterize health and health care both within and across settings and over time.
A provider-centric focus: Current measures focus on existing silos of care (e.g., physician's office, hospital)	*Principle 7:* Individual patient-level, population-based, and systems-level measurement	Measurement and measures should assess the health and health care of both individuals and populations and the many systems within which care is provided.
Narrow focus of accountability: Most measures focus on an individual provider's actions.	*Principle 8:* Shared accountability	Measurement should not be constrained by the absence of a current, identifiable, single responsible agent.

[a]Drawn from Table 2-2 Design Principles for a National System for Performance Measurement and Reporting.

quality can be measured. The committee believes these approaches are essential to achieving higher-quality health care. Box 4-1 illustrates how the above approaches might be implemented to affect the way care is delivered and yield better health and health care.

BOX 4-1   Illustration of How Approaches to Address Gaps in Performance Measures Might Be Implemented

David is a 67-year-old man living with diabetes mellitus. Over the years, his diabetes has contributed to other conditions, such as heart disease, hypertension, and neuropathy. David sees multiple clinicians, including a primary care physician, cardiovascular specialist, podiatrist, and ophthalmologist. He also takes a total of eight prescription drugs to manage his multiple chronic conditions.

Current Health Care Delivery System

During a recent visit, David's primary care physician ordered a battery of tests to monitor his condition, including hemoglobin A_1c and cholesterol testing. His physician also referred him to an ophthalmologist based on David's self-report of blurred vision. In addition, David is seeing a cardiologist, who repeated the blood tests ordered by his primary physician as his medical records were not readily available at the time of his visit. His cardiologist also prescribed a cholesterol-lowering drug and high blood pressure medication, which were called in to the pharmacy. Upon checking David's medication history, the pharmacist noticed that one of the drugs prescribed by the cardiologist was known to have an interaction with another medication he was taking. The pharmacist alerted the cardiologist, who had an incomplete drug history on David, as it was hard for David to remember all the "pills" he was taking and he forgot to bring his prescription bottles to his visit like a friend had recommended. David also had an appointment with a podiatrist as his primary care physician also noted he should have an annual foot exam on his chart. David did not make it to his podiatrist appointment because of transportation issues. Nor did he see the ophthalmologist because he never received the referral paperwork required by his insurance carrier. Upon returning to his primary care physician with complaints of fatigue and "not feeling so good" his physician noticed there were no results in his chart for his eye or foot exam, and the blood work he ordered showed David's hemoglobin A_1c was elevated. His physician makes another referral explaining how important it is for him to get these screenings. He also spoke with David about his diet and monitoring his glucose levels and requested another referral to a dietician.

Under the current health care system, David's care is fragmented. Rarely is David asked what he thinks of his care and how well it accommodates his lifestyle. Most of his providers lack a vehicle, such as an electronic health record, with which they can seamlessly communicate patient health information, including treatment plans and laboratory test results. As a result, tests are repeated, histories are retaken, and in some cases, conflicting medications are prescribed.

Not only is David's care inefficient at the patient level, but it also reflects the waste of resources that characterizes the current health care system. David is not alone, for he serves as an example of how patients are often treated today, augmenting the potential waste created by the many inefficiencies of the health care services system.

Assessing the health care system requires expanding measurement from the individual patient treated by individual physicians to that of the larger community in which David lives. In addition to care delivery services, David's health is also influenced by other environmental factors in his community. Thus it is important to know how well the community as a whole is performing in regards to the overall health of its diabetics. For example, promotion of preventive services and environmental factors such as having walking paths to promote exercise can impact health in the community.

Future Health Care Delivery System

Through the approaches identified by the committee as leading to better health care through a national system for performance measurement and reporting—comprehensive measurement; longitudinal measurement; individual-patient-level, population-based, and systems-level measurement; and shared accountability—many of the problems David encountered in his care can begin to be addressed.

Comprehensive measurement. Effectiveness measures that adequately document David's health, especially with respect to his various complex conditions, should be used to assess the quality of care he has received, including safety issues related to drug interactions. Also important to capture in a more inclusive set of measures is David's perspective on his own care. The array of measures collected by his doctors should make it possible to monitor the course of his disease, as well as all of his health care needs, throughout his lifetime.

Longitudinal measurement. A major barrier to the provision of high-quality care was the lack of communication among David's providers. The inability to transfer records quickly among all of his physicians not only was inefficient because of duplication of effort, but also posed a threat to his care. With proper attention to care transitions, much of this waste could be avoided. Moreover, further complications, such as David's

(continued on next page)

BOX 4-1 continued

blurred vision, could be identified and treated more quickly given assurance that proper follow-up services were available and utilized.

When assessing the quality of the health care delivery system treating David, outcomes and costs should be considered. In a hospital, for example, measurements of the ability of David to perform daily activities and function both physically and mentally at normal levels would be important outcomes. Combined with the costs associated with treating these patients, this information would permit an overall assessment of the longitudinal efficiency of the hospital systems.

Individual-patient-level, population-based, and systems-level measurement. While assessing care at the individual patient level, David's doctors could measure the comprehensiveness of his care through the use of composites. Composite measures of his diabetes testing for a predetermined bundle of routine disease-specific measures, such as checking for hemoglobin levels, blood pressure management, and eye and foot exams, would provide a complete picture of the evidence-based care David should be receiving. They would also allow David to become a more informed patient, aware of what types of treatment he should, at a minimum, be receiving. As an active participant in his care, David could also collaborate with his physician to ensure that he received all recommended treatment protocols.

When measuring care based on a given population, David's care measures could be aggregated with those of others, such as members of his local community, socioeconomic group, and state. These measures of personal health can be evaluated in combination with data reflecting the public and population health systems to better assess the overall health care system. This information would depict how well those in his population were living with their chronic illnesses, as well as provide tangible data for comparison with other populations.

Shared accountability. David's multiple caregivers should take responsibility for ensuring that his care is well coordinated and responsive to his individual needs. This would require his clinicians to embrace a more holistic approach to care, as opposed to practicing in a way that targets a single specialty. For example, David's cardiovascular specialist would also want to ensure that preventive testing, such as foot and eye exams, was performed. If these tests were not performed, she could take corrective action and contact David's other providers. This does not ensure that David's health care will be more coordinated; however, it is important that all the players involved with providing David's care have the opportunity to affect his health without having to worry about being held liable for the actions of others. Finally, just as David is an example of how well an individual patient's physicians interact, care provided to larger patient populations reflects the interactions among the various systems these populations encounter.

Comprehensive Measurement

Current performance measure sets are far too limited in scope. The vast majority of current measures assess the quality of health care in terms of effectiveness and safety. Only a few, limited measures examine timeliness and provide insight into patients' experiences, and hardly any adequately assess the efficiency or equity of care. Nor do measures adequately cover the entire human lifespan, as very few evaluate care for children, adolescents, or those at the end of life. Finally, too few measures exist that address matters particularly salient for the Medicare population, such as chronic obstructive pulmonary disease, stroke, dementia, and Alzheimer's disease.

The committee believes a complete set of measures should offer a far more comprehensive assessment of performance across all of these important dimensions. A measurement system should fully address all six quality aims, in part to help keep providers from focusing on only one area of improvement to the detriment of others. Achieving such comprehensive measurement will require substantial investment in both fine-tuning existing measures and developing new measures where significant gaps exist.

There are a number of reasons for the limited breadth of existing measures, such as the absence of a leader to coordinate and guide existing efforts; a shortage of consensus, evidenced-based guidelines; inadequate financial support for ongoing measurement-related activities; and consensus-driven processes as opposed to goal-driven agendas. The committee recommends that the NQCB assume a leadership role by establishing national goals on which future measure development should focus. In this role, the NQCB should collaborate with stakeholders to produce guidelines that can serve as the foundation for measure development. With this more focused and coordinated effort, private and public funding could be garnered to support innovation and measure development that would aid in achieving national goals.

Longitudinal Measurement

The committee's emphasis on longitudinal measurement is based on two distinct concerns. First, both the U.S. fee-for-service system and the performance measures currently in use reinforce, although not intentionally, the separation of settings of care by design (i.e., ambulatory care, home health care, hospital care, and nursing home care). This emphasis on separate care settings has several adverse effects, including fragmentation, lack of continuity, and poor communication. Second, the effectiveness of a care system should ideally be reflected in its capacity to prolong life, maintain or improve functioning and the quality of life, and achieve these health outcomes with a high degree of patient centeredness and efficiency. Achievement of these results generally involves care that crosses boundaries, rather than the actions of a particular caregiver at a specific point in time. Measurement that focuses only on such fragments of care misses too much of what really matters to patients. Rather, measure sets should focus on measures of continuity and transitional care, as well as on longitudinal assessments of health outcomes and costs (Coleman et al., 2003; Rogers et al., 2004).

The committee recognizes that measuring care across settings, long-term outcomes, and costs for selected conditions will be complex, as it will require a shift away from assessing and reporting how care is delivered at one point in time to a given patient in a given setting. It will also be necessary to acknowledge and incorporate patients' perspectives on their care and health outcomes when evaluating quality. The committee believes, however, that these areas of measurement are integral to a broader understanding of how well health services are provided and can be addressed through organized and focused research efforts.

Measures of Continuity and Transitions

Patient transfers between care settings are common. Issues of care transition affect primarily those living with multiple or complex conditions and are highly relevant to the Medicare population of adults 65 and over, to children with special health care needs, and to the disabled. A study tracking posthospital transitions for 30 days after discharge among a national sample of Medicare beneficiaries found that 61 percent of care episodes resulted in one transition, 18 percent in two transitions, 9 percent in three transitions, and 4 percent in four or more transitions, while 8 percent resulted in death. Transitions in this study were defined as transfers to or from an acute hospital, skilled nursing or rehabilitation facility, or home with or without home health care (Coleman et al., 2004b). No measurement system that ignores the integrity and quality of these transitions can be considered complete.

Attending to transitions implies, among other design principles, listening directly to patients' reports on their own care. Patients and their family caregivers are uniquely positioned to report on their care experiences as they are often the only common thread across disparate health care settings (Coleman et al., 2004a). Therefore, in addition to following patients across multiple settings to assess the care provided instead of focusing on single sites, it is essential to ask patients and their families about their experiences with the care in each setting, the transitions, and overall.

Longitudinal Measures of Outcomes and Costs

Research has documented important differences across providers in the outcomes of care following major surgical procedures (Finlayson and

Birkmeyer, 2002; Hannan et al., 1999; O'Connor et al., 1999) and medical hospitalizations (Barnato et al., 2005; Dudley et al., 2000; Shapiro et al., 1999), as well as in the care of those with chronic diseases (Every et al., 2000). In addition, substantial differences in the longitudinal costs of care for similar populations have been documented at both the community and provider levels, with no evidence that greater costs resulted in higher-quality or better outcomes (Baicker and Chandra, 2004; Fisher and Wennberg, 2003; Fisher et al., 2003, 2004; Wennberg, 1999). The committee believes standardized performance measure sets must incorporate the routine monitoring and reporting of long-term health outcomes (mortality and functional status) and costs for selected conditions to promote the attainment of better outcomes at lower cost.

Individual-Patient-Level, Population-Based, and Systems-Level Measurement

The committee proposes several innovative approaches to collecting and reporting performance measures. The key notion is to collect data on each measure at the level of the individual patient and maintain individual-level records to allow the aggregation of measures along three important dimensions: (1) composite measures of the care provided to the individual, documenting, for example, whether a patient received all of his or her recommended preventive services within a specified time window; (2) reporting of measurement results for strata of the population defined on the basis of socioeconomic status, race, and ethnicity; and (3) reporting of measurement results at multiple levels of the care delivery system—physician, physician group, hospital, and community—to identify gaps in performance and foster accountability at each level. These approaches to aggregation are applicable both to the starter set of measures proposed by the committee and to future measure development. Their implementation is dependent upon adequate data collection, reporting, and aggregation, key functions of a performance measurement and reporting system that the NQCB will ensure. The committee strongly believes that data collection protocols should be planned and implemented to support these functions.

Individual-Patient-Level Perspective

A critical concept that emerged from the committee's deliberations was the use of composite measures. Composites are a relatively new concept in the area of performance measurement, denoting, at minimum, the combining of dichotomous indicators for several specific measures into a single number. The term can also refer, for example, to calculation of a simple mean of rates for several measures, the mean of the fraction of appropriate processes of care received, and the fraction of opportunities to receive all appropriate care for a defined population. The committee has chosen to define composites as the bundling of measures for specific conditions to determine whether all critical aspects of care for a given condition have been achieved for an individual patient, thereby enhancing measurement to extend beyond tracking performance on separate measures.

The committee chose this definition of composite measures for multiple reasons. First, it allows for continuous measurement across providers through aggregation by patient (reinforcing the approach longitudinal measurement) and for an examination of all aspects of required care at the community/population level. On a larger scale, composite measures thus defined can provide a different and potentially deeper view of the reliability of the care system as a whole, encouraging and facilitating systems-level changes by highlighting the need for better care coordination and accountability across multiple providers. They can also serve as a powerful stimulus for the adoption of electronic health records to ensure that patients receive recommended care. The committee believes patients could play a more active role in their care if they were armed with evidence-based information on the complete set of clinical services they should expect and ultimately demand. In addition, the use of composite measures does not require the large sample sizes needed for some other approaches. Thus, the committee proposes that this approach to measurement be taken in addition to measuring performance on discrete indicators.

The committee believes this concept represents a turning point, and a relatively new challenge, for performance measurement. Composite scores centered on individual patients could be calculated for many preventive, acute, and chronic care services, with careful consideration for age and gender appropriateness. The use of composite measures suggests performance goals considerably more stringent than those captured by the usual single-variable measures. Using composites in this manner allows for a patient-centered approach that takes into account the full constellation of health care needs (McGlynn et al., 2003a).

The technical challenges to the construction of accurate, valid, and reliable composite measures and their elements for all conditions are substantial. Among these challenges are the following:

• The rate automatically tends to go down as more process measures are added to the composite, since it is more difficult to provide all the required measures of a large set than of a small one.
• Improvement will not be fully reflected by composites if several processes are measured, some of which are received at a high rate and others at a generally low rate.

• The composite score will be lower if different people receive each of the various processes than if some people receive all and most receive none, for a given rate on each process.

Thus, although the committee's approach to composites readily identifies poor performance, it is not necessarily appropriate for making comparisons or solely summarizing improvement.

The efforts of HealthPartners Inc., the Centers for Medicare and Medicaid Services (CMS), the RAND Corporation, the Foundation for Accountability, and other organizations that have explored this approach, as well as a simple inspection of the scientifically grounded array of current measures, can serve as a good starting point for the development of an initial set of composite measures. One example of how the proposed approach to composites can be implemented is described in Box 4-2.

Despite these efforts, further research is required before this concept of composites can be fully developed and expanded upon. An important issue to be addressed is whether the various components of a composite should be weighted differently, such as according to their level of clinical importance. On the whole, the committee favors a simple yet integrated approach whereby composite measures in the first instance would be "all or none"

**BOX 4-2 Example of the Implementation
of Composite Measures**

A pioneering organization in composite measurement, HealthPartners Inc., a health plan in Minnesota, has been collecting and publicly reporting composite scores for diabetes, coronary artery disease, and preventive care. HealthPartners calculates a composite score for its diabetic population by examining the percentage of its members with Type I and Type 2 diabetes aged 18 through 75 who are optimally managed, not just for each but for all of the following factors: $HbA_1c \leq 8$ percent mg/dl; LDL cholesterol ≤ 130 mg/dl; blood pressure <130/85 mmHg; aspirin use for members >40 years old; and documentation of nonuse of tobacco. A single rate is then reported, indicating the percentage of eligible members who achieved this complete bundle of intermediate outcomes. In the 2004 reporting period, although each separate clinical variable showed performance in the range of 45.5 percent (BP $\leq$130/85) to 82.8 percent (not smoking), the composite score revealed that only 18.4 percent of eligible patients were receiving the complete set of needed interventions (Personal communication, G. Amundson, HealthPartners, December 2004; Amundson et al., 2005).

measures. Accordingly, a composite measure would be designated as "1" only if all the required services or procedures had been performed or all outcomes reached and as "0" if at least one of those services or procedures had not been performed or all outcomes reached; thus weighting would not be an issue. The rationale for this proposal is a recognition that if any of the services required for taking care of an individual (or a population) is absent, care is suboptimal. However, this notion should ultimately be tempered so as to be applied in addition to the proportion of criteria met, as the provider's cost of improvement has many implications for how a weighting system should be structured.

Population-Based Perspective

The Institute of Medicine's (IOM) definition of quality includes population health: "the degree to which health services for individuals and populations increase the likelihood of desired health outcomes and are consistent with current professional knowledge" (IOM, 1990:4). The term "population health" is widely used and often understood to be a product of multiple determinants of health—genetic endowment and physical environment and social environment. The personal health care delivery system, which focuses on the care of individuals, represents an important but limited element of population health, whereas the public health system takes a broader and more inclusive perspective on these determinants. The focus of this report is on the contribution that the personal health care delivery system can make to improving population health—a measure that encompasses not only health but also its distribution among the population. The report does not attempt to speak to the full range of measures one would want in a population health monitoring and reporting system, such as environmental measures, as this would be beyond the committee's charge. The committee does, however, address how the personal health care delivery system can contribute to the public health system in the domains of health promotion, disease prevention, and clinical preventive services.

For example, the nation's public health goals, as articulated by *Healthy People 2010*, include many areas of overlap between the personal health care delivery system and the public health system, such as preventive screenings, immunizations, and tobacco cessation counseling (U.S. DHHS, 2000). Another example of a measure set that intersects both of these systems is the Prevention Quality Indicators developed by the Agency for Healthcare Quality and Research (AHRQ), based on hospital inpatient data that reveal how well care is being delivered by identifying such events as avoidable hospitalizations. The committee recognizes the substantial need to bridge the gap between public and private health care systems and to promote core performance measures that can foster collaborative efforts. Communication among stakeholders in these systems is critical to enhancing performance measurement and achieving the ultimate goal of better health.

The committee calls for a move toward an important method for narrowing the divide between the personal health care and public health systems: the more comprehensive system of individual-patient-level measures, drawn from the population of a community and aggregated by different levels of care providers (individual physician, group practice, hospital, or nursing home), geographic regions (community, state, or national), and demographic groupings (race and ethnicity, socioeconomic status, class, age, sex) when appropriate. This more clinical perspective on health care services is distinct from measuring the determinants of the health of populations and non–health care services.

This approach to gathering performance data allows information to be collected across multiple sites instead of in a site-specific manner, and to be used for multiple purposes, such as internal quality improvement, accountability, and public reporting at the provider, community, and national levels. Moreover, this approach supports an important shift in focus from the care delivered by some part of the health care system (a health practitioner, for example) to the care needs met by the overall system. This change in measurement strategy will support analyses of the extent to which all patients are receiving the right care at the right time for their specific individual needs.

Unfortunately, this concept of measuring care across the continuum of time and space conflicts with how care is currently organized and financed, as the individual patient is usually the only consistent factor across settings of care (and noncare). The way data are managed today tends to render the care continuum opaque, not transparent. Data are often exclusively stored and "owned" by specific care settings and providers, not by patients themselves. This problem of ownership and control compounds the difficulty of sharing and analyzing data across settings in a timely fashion, with or without electronic health records (IOM, 2004; Walker et al., 2005). The committee anticipates that a commitment to a population-based approach to data collection and management will generate the scaling and data management requirements that will eventually drive the use of data warehousing, information technology, and other data management capabilities and strategies, and accelerate the universal adoption of electronic health records as an American standard.

An evolving population-based perspective also is facilitated by patient-level data warehouses that can provide opportunities for testing emerging hypotheses, such as examining the effects of interventions designed for patients with coincident diabetes, heart failure, and depression. The current absence of patient-level data that can be aggregated for populations of evolving interest requires researchers to build a cohort, follow a sample of patients with a designated condition or set of conditions, and respecify and recollect data each time a new hypothesis is formulated. Patient-level data, capable of flexible and varied aggregation to reflect populations of interest, form an "epidemiologic utility" that could be used for knowledge development (Halvorson and Isham, 2003; Wallace, 2005).

A population perspective also addresses the quality aim of equity and the related issue of access by assessing the delivery of the right treatment to the right person at the right time *for everyone who would potentially benefit*. The italicized phrase distinguishes the proposed approach to measuring health care delivery from other perspectives, drawing attention to issues of equity and the existence and impact of disparities among groups. An adequate performance measurement system should illuminate the status of people who do not receive care as much as that of people who do. Especially important from a population perspective are performance measures that target improvement in the health status of different ethnic, racial, and class groups. The heterogeneity of any community offers a strong incentive for organizing the data on its constituents at the patient level. Yet these patient-level data can then be aggregated to any level of granularity, from individual patient reports to the entire community, making it possible, for example, to measure both over- and underuse of interventions within whole populations. Examples of waste and neglect can be obscured if granularity to the patient level is not obtained. Arguably, especially within this perspective, missing or inaccessible data to support the delivery of needed services within a population are defects in quality of care.

Systems-Level Perspective

Few Americans receive their health care from fully integrated delivery systems. Nonetheless, patients and communities often depend upon systems-level performance that requires effective interactions among discrete caregivers and institutions and across time, regardless of whether those providers are in formal, intentional relationships with each other. The committee believes a complete set of performance measures must encompass this type of systems-level performance. As discussed above, measures obtained at the individual patient level could be aggregated to different levels of the system, including physician groups, hospitals, the continuum of care, or communitywide care delivery systems.

At the hospital level, systems-level performance measures could be applied to the hospital as a whole, with its executive and clinical leadership and governing board presumably being responsible for improvement on these measures. At the level of the continuum of care, an accountable entity could be difficult to identify absent an accountable integrated delivery system with responsibility for the care of a defined population over space and time. Nonetheless, patients and families should and do care about outcomes and processes at this level. The committee therefore proposes that such measures be developed, used, and reported to drive shared accountability throughout the health care system. In addition, participation is required from policy makers at all levels if the health care delivery system is to improve. Adoption of systems-level measures should help American communities become more aware of their met and unmet health care needs, and over time could induce innovations and relationships among care providers that could lead to better performance.

The ultimate measures of the performance of American health care would assess the nation's effectiveness in meeting the needs of communities. Few American communities organize their health care as a communitywide system. By measuring and tracking systems-level performance at the community level, however, it may ultimately be possible to assess the national consequences of policy and financing environments as a whole. For assessment of performance at the level of the community as a whole, federal agencies such as the Centers for Disease Control and Prevention can offer guidance. In addition, the state-level reports produced by AHRQ in the context of the National Healthcare Quality and Disparities Reports are good first steps in community-level performance measurement (AHRQ, 2003).

A commitment to systems-level performance measurement will require both scientific innovation and new loci of responsibility for measurement itself, as well as the taking of action in accordance with measurement results. Below the committee proposes a uniform set of hospitalwide measures and measures across the continuum of chronic disease care as the starting point for this effort.

Shared Accountability

Improved performance on many of the measures proposed by the committee can be achieved only through the collaborative efforts of multiple providers and multiple care settings. The committee believes the NQCB should include and report on measures—such as care transitions and longitudinal outcomes and costs—that reflect the performance of multiple providers who should, ideally, collaborate to improve the quality of care. As discussed earlier, the committee also believes that measures should be diffused to different levels of the delivery system, including the community. For example, performance measures for racial, ethnic, or socioeconomic groups (such as the uninsured) should be collected and reported at multiple levels. Analysis of these data would force discussion of the underlying reasons for disparities and the opportunities available to multiple stakeholders for addressing these issues. This notion of shared accountability will have substantial impacts on payment-based incentive policies and will be further addressed by the payment incentives report in this *Pathways* series (see Chapter 1).

In short, the committee concludes that measurement of the health care delivery system should not be impeded by the impossibility of first identifying an accountable actor or the perception that responsibility for care is outside one's realm of control. Indeed, one valuable and intended effect of the integrated measurement system proposed by the committee could be to induce new parties to assume such responsibility. This position represents a significant break from commonly accepted criteria for performance measurement.

SELECTION OF SPECIFIC PERFORMANCE MEASURES

To this point, the discussion has focused primarily on insights that emerged from the committee's review of currently available performance measures and an analysis of the quality of these measures against the goals and aims of health care measurement. The committee's primary charge was to recommend a subset of measures—derived from leading performance measure sets—that could be used to align performance with payment under the Medicare program. The committee addressed this task within a more general framework designed to move the U.S. health care system toward the overarching goals discussed earlier. Its ultimate objective was the creation of a measure set that would be consistent both with the goals and aims for health care improvement set forth earlier in this chapter and with the 10 design principles for performance measurement articulated in Chapter 2. The resulting measures encompass what we need to know about health care quality to guide future payment policies and practices.

Criteria for Selection

In addition to the 10 design principles articulated in Chapter 2, the committee identified criteria to guide the selection of specific measures. The criteria in Box 4-3 apply to individual characteristics of either a specific measure (e.g., validity and reliability) or the collective measure set (e.g., comprehensiveness). Other groups have articulated these criteria: measures should be scientifically sound, feasible, important, aligned with other leading measure sets, and comprehensive. However, it is important to point out the absence of one criterion often used by other groups: *that a measure be within the control of an identifiable actor.* As discussed above, the committee takes the position that improvement across many important domains of care will require action by multiple parties—including patients, providers, and other stakeholders (such as health plans, payers, and public health agencies), and the committee therefore endorses public reporting on measures, such as longitudinal care, that foster shared accountability.

BOX 4-3 Criteria for Measure Selection Considered by the Committee and Other Selected Groups

- **Scientifically Sound:** This criterion concerns the reliability, validity, and explicitness of the evidence base. Reliability means a measure consistently produces the same result when repeated within the same population and setting. Validity addresses the question of whether a measure reflects what it is intended to measure. Finally, the evidence base from which a measure is derived must be explicit—for example, randomized controlled trials, case control studies, observational studies, or formal consensus processes.

- **Feasibility:** To assess feasibility, the data needed for a measure must be in current use, available across the system, and examined for the cost or burden of measurement on providers.

- **Importance:** The health problem addressed by a measure should be a leading cause of death or disability or associated with high resource use. A measure must have an impact on health, be tied to national goals, and be susceptible to being influenced by the health care delivery system. Ideally, a measure should be stratified by race, gender, and age.

- **Alignment:** Optimally, measures should be selected from existing leading measure sets that are calculated with the same technical specifications for both the numerator and denominator to reduce redundancy and the burden of reporting.

- **Comprehensiveness:** Measures selected should be part of a set to reflect quality in a particular area of care or bundled services of necessary care for a given condition. Each measure in the set should meet the criterion of importance to warrant inclusion. To demonstrate comprehensiveness, the set of measures must address the way the care is delivered and the nature of the quality problem involved—underuse, misuse, or overuse.

Note that, as discussed in the text, the committee did not support the criterion that only measures under the control of a specific system of care should be used.
SOURCE: AHRQ, 2001; CMS, 2004a; McGlynn et al., 2003a,b; MedPAC, 2005a; NCQA, 2001.

Methodological Limitations of Existing Measures

The committee recognized that many current measures, while meeting the above criteria, have methodological limitations that may reduce their applicability or utility in certain settings. These limitations include a degree of statistical variability for some measures that may constrain the ability to characterize the performance of individual physicians or small practices, a need for case-mix or risk adjustment in some instances that cannot be met by currently collected data, and requirements for data collection that may impose a substantial burden on providers in the absence of registries or computerized health information systems (Birkmeyer, 2004; Birkmeyer et al., 2004; Hofer et al., 1999; Landon et al., 2003). (A more detailed overview of the methodological limitations of existing structure, process, and outcome measures is provided in Appendix F.) Experience has shown that starting with less-than-perfect publicly reported measures can stimulate the development of improved measures, as illustrated by care safety measurement efforts and by the development of the National Committee for Quality Assurance's Health Plan Employer Data and Information Set (HEDIS) measures of the performance of health maintenance organizations (Personal Communication, Arnold Milstein, October 11, 2004). Thus the committee is confident that aggressive implementation of existing measures would both improve those measures and, assuming that the measures led to action, enhance the quality of care.

Recommended Measures for Implementation

The committee's analysis of existing performance measure sets revealed many measures consistent with one or more of the articulated measurement goals that also meet the criteria shown in Box 4-3. For some of the six quality aims, such as efficiency, equity, and patient-centeredness, however, the committee was unable to identify standardized performance measures already in widespread use. Many measures have been used in research settings or are at various stages of pilot testing and development for use in standardized performance measurement. Therefore, the committee recognized that the creation, promulgation, and reporting of new measures need to be included in a research agenda to achieve the goals of performance measurement set forth above.

The committee recommends the immediate implementation of the starter set of measures derived from leading measure sets shown in Table 4-2 and discussed in detail in the next section. To this end, a data repository system will need to be in place, along with a mechanism for public reporting. In addition, the NQCB will need to identify a strategy for data aggregation. There are two particularly thorny issues to be addressed:

• *National versus local/regional data repositories*—Data could be submitted to a national repository and then transmitted to the local/regional level for reporting purposes. Another alternative is to create local/regional repositories that would transmit data to the national level. Each strategy has implications for data confidentiality and security, operational

TABLE 4-2 Recommended Starter Set of Performance Measures

Ambulatory Care	**Ambulatory care Quality Alliance (26)** Prevention measures[a] (7), coronary artery disease[a] (3), heart failure[a] (2), diabetes[a] (6), asthma[a] (2), depression[a] (2), prenatal care[a] (2), quality measures addressing overuse or misuse (2) **Ambulatory Care Survey** CAHPS Clinician and Group Survey: getting care quickly, getting needed care, how well providers communicate, health promotion and education, shared decision making, knowledge of medical history, how well office staff communicate
Acute Care	**Hospital Quality Alliance (20)** Acute coronary syndrome[a] (7), heart failure[a] (3), pneu-monia[a] (5), smoking cessation[a] (3), surgical infection pre-vention[a] (from the Surgical Care Improvement Project) (2) **Structural Measures** (computerized provider order entry, intensive care unit intensivists, evidence-based hospital referrals) **Hospital CAHPS** Patient communication with physicians, patient communication with nurses, responsiveness of hospital staff, clean-liness/noise level of physical environment, pain control, communications about medicines, discharge information
Health Plans and Accountable Health Organizations	**Health Plan Employer Data and Information Set (HEDIS) (61)** Integrated delivery systems (health maintenance organizations): effectiveness (26), access/availability of care (8), satisfaction with the experience of care (4), health plan stability (2), use of service (15), cost of care, informed health care choices, health plan descriptive information (6) Preferred provider organizations within Medicare Advantage: selected administrative data and hybrid measures **Ambulatory Care Survey** CAHPS Health Plan Survey: getting care quickly, getting needed care, how well providers communicate, health plan paperwork, health plan customer service
Long-Term Care	**Minimum Data Set (15)** Long-term care (12), short-stay care (3) **Outcome and Assessment Information Set (11)** Ambulation/locomotion (1), transferring (1), toileting (1), pain (1), bathing (2), management of oral medications (1), acute care hospitalization (1), emergent care (1), confusion (1)
End-Stage Renal Disease	**National Healthcare Quality Report (5)** Transplant registry and results (2), dialysis effectiveness (2), mortality (1)
Longitudinal Measures of Outcomes and Efficiency	1-year mortality, resource use, and functional status (SF-12) after acute myocardial infarction

[a]The committee recommends the aggregation of individual measures to patient-level composites for these areas.

costs and complexity, ongoing innovation and local access/acceptability, and locus of management. The committee does not endorse one strategy over the other, as these issues require further deliberation by the NQCB. The Ambulatory care Quality Alliance (AQA) is currently developing a model that includes a framework and governing structure for aggregating, sharing, and stewarding data that could provide guidance in this area (AHRQ, 2005).

  • *Comprehensive scope*—Data repositories that included data for all patients (i.e., privately insured patients, Medicare and Medicaid beneficiaries and other publicly insured patients, and the uninsured) would provide a more complete picture of an individual provider's practice if the provider cared for multiple populations. Comprehensive repositories would also provide better population-level information. But legal, regulatory, ownership, and operational issues must be addressed if such repositories are to be established.

Additionally, as learned from the committee's case studies, technical and financial assistance to providers will require greater attention. Providers of all types will need assistance in implementing quality improvement strategies in addition to data collection and reporting. These and many other issues will require careful assessment before the NQCB can move forward.

> **Recommendation 4: The NQCB should promulgate measure sets that build on the work of key public- and private-sector organizations. Specifically, the NQCB should:**
>
> • **As a starting point, endorse as national standards performance measures currently approved through ongoing consensus processes led by major stakeholder groups.**
> • **Ensure that a data repository system[1] and public reporting program capable of data collection at the individual patient level are established and open to participation by all payers and providers.**
> • **Ensure that technical and financial assistance is available to all providers who need help in establishing performance measurement and improvement capabilities.**

The following discussion details the starter set of performance measures proposed by the committee. This starter set of measures represents what can be done now to move toward a national system for performance measurement and reporting.

---

[1]The data repository system would collect, validate, and aggregate provider performance data (see Recommendation 1).

RECOMMENDED STARTER SET OF PERFORMANCE MEASURES

The committee recommends the leveraging of existing efforts, but stands firm that an immediate gearing up of resources must occur to address the shortcomings in current approaches to performance measurement discussed in this chapter.

Starter Set Measures for Ambulatory Care Performance

To accelerate performance measurement in the ambulatory care setting, the committee proposes the immediate adoption of the 26 clinical performance measures recently selected by AQA. The individual measures in this set, detailed in Appendix G-1, cover four domains of care in which quality problems are well documented and continue to persist:

- *Preventive care*—cancer screening, vaccinations, and tobacco use/ counseling
- *Chronic care*—coronary artery disease, heart failure, diabetes, asthma, and depression
- *Prenatal care*—HIV screening and administration of anti-D (Rh) immune globulin
- *Efficiency of care*—appropriate prescribing of antibiotics to children

The committee proposes that patient-level composite scores, as previously described, be collected and reported for measures of asthma, coronary artery disease, depression, diabetes, heart failure, and prenatal care, as well as a preventive care composite consisting of age- and sex- appropriate services.

Preventive Care

The committee devoted considerable attention to preventive care, with the rationale that these services, such as earlier diagnoses for common cancers, would yield benefits in the long run in terms of both improved quality of life and in some cases potentially lower costs. Measures of preventive care provide an opportunity to highlight issues associated with both effective and equitable care. Disparities among racial and ethnic groups in cancer-related deaths and survival rates are well documented. For example, death rates for breast cancer are higher among African Americans than among whites—36 per 100,000 versus 27 per 100,000.[2] In addition, 5-year survival rates for breast cancer (74 percent) among African Americans are

---

[2]Age-adjusted to the 2000 U.S. standard population.

lower than those among whites (88 percent) (American Cancer Society, 2004; IOM, 2003).

Assessing adults for tobacco use and providing tobacco cessation counseling ranks second among the top 30 clinical preventive services recommended by the U.S. Preventive Services Task Force based on the criteria of clinically preventable burden and cost-effectiveness.[3] However, counseling services have one of the lowest national delivery rates (less than 50 percent) (Coffield et al., 2001). More than 440,000 tobacco-related deaths occur annually as a result of cardiovascular diseases, cancers, respiratory diseases, and perinatal conditions. Accordingly, the committee endorses the rapid uptake of these measures (Centers for Disease Control and Prevention, 2002).

Chronic Care

Serious quality problems, particularly underuse of services, have been documented for all of the chronic conditions in the AQA set. For those chronic conditions—diabetes, asthma, depression, heart failure, and coronary artery disease—a national study found that Americans receive only 45–68 percent of recommended care (McGlynn et al., 2003a). Recent data on elderly Medicare beneficiaries also demonstrate serious quality problems. For example, only one-third of the elderly received effective treatment for depression, while only one-quarter of elderly diabetics received an annual dilated eye exam, a recommended screening test for retinopathy (Leatherman and McCarthy, 2005). Since the number of individuals with chronic conditions continues to grow (an estimated 133 million Americans in 2005, expected to rise to 157 million in 2020), and 78 percent of all health care spending in all care settings is attributable to these conditions, performance measurement in this area becomes a top priority (Partnership for Solutions, 2002).

Prenatal Care

In 2002, approximately 4 percent of pregnant women either did not receive prenatal care until the third trimester or received no such care at all (National Center for Health Statistics, 2004). Inadequate prenatal care can lead to infant mortality, as well as complications during pregnancy and childbirth. The United States ranked twenty-second in infant mortality among Organisation for Economic Cooperation and Development countries

---

[3]Clinically preventable burden is defined as the proportion of disease and injury prevented by the clinical preventive service in usual practice if the service were delivered to 100 percent of the target population at recommended intervals. Cost-effectiveness is defined as net cost per quality-adjusted life-years saved.

in 2003, with a rate of 7.0 deaths per 1,000 live births (Organisation for Economic Co-operation and Development, 2005), as compared with Iceland, ranked first with a rate of 2.4 deaths per 1,000 live births. The cost burden over a lifetime for a child born with birth defects is estimated to be $8 billion (U.S. Preventive Services Task Force, 1996). These problems are the outcome of many factors; however, they can begin to be alleviated through better prenatal care.

Two preventive services for prenatal care are included in the AQA measure set and are supported by the United States Preventive Services Task Force: anti-D (Rh) immune globulin and HIV screening. Providing anti-D (Rh) immune globulin to women who are Rh negative promotes prevention of life-threatening outcomes, such as newborn hemolytic disease due to maternal sensitization. HIV screening significantly lowers rates of mother-to-child HIV transmission, an important benefit as between 280 and 370 newborns are diagnosed with HIV in the United States each year (Bulterys et al., 2002). Thus the committee proposes the inclusion of both of these measures in the starter set by the NQCB.

Efficiency of Care

Overuse and misuse of resources are results of poor-quality care. This issue is addressed in the AQA set through measurement of appropriate treatment of viral infections leading to upper respiratory conditions and pharyngitis. Antibiotics are effective only in treating bacterial infections. Therefore, the use of antibiotics for respiratory infections that are viral in nature is not efficacious and leads to the negative consequence of increased microbial antibiotic resistance. While the trend in prescribing antibiotics for children has been declining (from a rate of 838 per 1,000 in 1989 to 503 per 1,000 in 1999), the practice remains unacceptably common (McCaig et al., 2002). To counter these trends in overuse and misuse, the committee proposes inclusion of these measures in the starter set.

Ambulatory Care Surveys

Although the AQA measures are a reasonable starting point for performance measurement in the ambulatory care setting, assessment in this area would be incomplete without a component of patient feedback. To complement the above clinical measures, the committee proposes implementing surveys of ambulatory care in conjunction with those measures upon completion of field testing.[4] The CAHPS program has developed two prod-

---

[4]See Chapter 2 for an overview of the CAHPS family of surveys.

BOX 4-4 Core Domains of Ambulatory Care Surveys

CAHPS Health Plan Survey
Getting care quickly
Getting needed care
How well providers
  communicate
Health plan paperwork
Health plan customer service

CAHPS Clinician and Group Survey
Getting care quickly
Getting needed care
How well providers communicate
Health promotion and education
Shared decision making
Knowledge of medical history
How well office staff communicate

---

ucts specific to ambulatory care: the CAHPS Health Plan Survey and the CAHPS Clinician and Group Survey (AHRQ, 2004). Core domains in each of these surveys are presented in Box 4-4.

Starter Set Measures for Acute Care Performance

Of the $1.5 trillion spent on health care in 2002, 33 percent is attributable to hospital care (American Hospital Association, 2004). Widespread performance measurement in hospitals has built upon past efforts involving collaboration among a multitude of stakeholders, as discussed in Chapter 2. These efforts have culminated in the measures chosen by the Hospital Quality Alliance (HQA), a partnership of 13 public and private sponsors (see Appendix G-2). Measures were selected on the basis of severity of clinical condition and ease of data submission for public reporting. The 20 measures endorsed by the National Quality Forum (NQF) originate from the voluntary starter set of 10 measures that, under the Medicare Prescription Drug, Improvement and Modernization Act of 2003, are linked to a 0.4 percent reduction in Medicare annual payment update if not reported. Currently, an estimated 4,200 hospitals are participating in this public reporting effort. As with the AQA measures, the committee proposes the reporting of these individual measures as patient-level composites for the following areas: acute coronary infarction, heart failure, pneumonia, smoking cessation, and surgical complications.

Structural Measures

In an effort to address patient safety in the hospital setting, the committee proposes assessment of the following structural measures: (1) implementation of computerized provider order entry for prescriptions, (2) staffing of intensive care units with intensivists, and (3) evidence-based hospital referrals. These measures originate from the Leapfrog Group's original "three leaps," which have been widely implemented and are part of the NQF's 30 safe practices (NQF, 2003).

Hospital CAHPS

Hospital CAHPS is currently slated for inclusion in the HQA measure set by 2007. The domains of measurement for this survey are listed in Box 4-5. The committee strongly supports the expedient collection and reporting of these patient-centered measures.

Starter Set Measures for Health Plan Performance

Health plans have a long and credible history of collecting and reporting performance measures, beginning with the adoption of HEDIS measures. The 2005 HEDIS measure set includes 61 measures that are recommended for the starter set. With respect to Medicare, specifically Medicare Advantage, however, the data collected and reported by preferred provider organization (PPO) plans and health maintenance organization plans will need to be reconciled. Currently, PPOs are required initially to report only those HEDIS measures for which administrative data can be used; nonetheless, additional infrastructure necessary to collect data for measures requiring chart abstraction must be in place and fully functional by 2008 to enable reporting of the full set of HEDIS measures by PPOs (see Appendix G-3) (CMS, 2004a).

Starter Set Measures for Long-Term Care Performance

To receive payment, nursing homes and home health settings are required by CMS to collect data on long-term care measures routinely using the Minimum Data Set (MDS) and the Outcome and Assessment Instru-

---

BOX 4-5   Hospital CAHPS Domains

Patient communication with physicians
Patient communication with nurses
Responsiveness of hospital staff

Cleanliness/noise level of physical environment
Pain control
Communications about medicines
Discharge information

ment Set (OASIS), respectively (CMS, 2004b, 2005a). The MDS, collected since 1990, evaluates such areas as cognitive/behavior patterns, quality of life, functional status, and pain. OASIS, implemented in 2000, assesses outcomes for home care patients, with the data intended for use in quality improvement efforts, including evaluations of sociodemographics, environment, support systems, health status, functional status, and health service utilization.

As these measures are already being collected by providers, the committee proposes that the long-term care measures being publicly reported by CMS[5] in both the MDS and OASIS data sets, as listed in Appendix G-4, initially be used for describing performance in these settings. However, the committee recognizes that measures in the MDS need additional research and development before they can be linked to pay for performance mechanisms (MedPAC, 2005b).

Starter Set Measures for End-Stage Renal Disease Performance

End-stage renal disease (ESRD) affected more than 430,000 people in 2002 at a cost of $17 billion to Medicare (U.S. Renal Data System, 2004). Under the Social Security Act, ESRD patients are eligible to obtain all Medicare benefits, including dialysis and renal transplant. As a result, almost all ESRD patients are covered under Medicare, with only a small percentage paying out of pocket or through private insurers. Data have been collected on this special population since 1988 through a partnership among the National Institutes of Health, CMS, and the United States Renal Data System, which documents the incidence and prevalence of ESRD and its patients, and identifies and furthers the research agenda associated with this disease. Five of these measures[6]—targeting transplant registries and overall dialysis effectiveness—are being collected in AHRQ's National Healthcare Quality Report (see Appendix G-5).

Starter Set Measures for Longitudinal Measurement of Outcome and Efficiency Performance

The committee believes the above starter set measures are sector-specific and thus have several serious shortcomings: they do little to foster improved

---

[5]CMS has developed the Web-based resources Nursing Home Compare and Home Health Compare, which publicly report selected quality indictors to help consumers make informed choices when selecting a nursing home or home health agency, respectively; see Appendix G-4 for measures in both of these sets (CMS, 2005b).

[6]The three outcome measures are derived from the University of Michigan; the two process measures are from the United States Renal Data System.

coordination across all care settings; they provide virtually no information on the costs of care, especially for a population over time; and they offer very limited measures of the outcomes of care. To begin to address these shortcomings, the committee proposes longitudinal measures of outcomes and costs, starting with 1-year mortality, resource use, and functional status measures for acute myocardial infarction.

CLOSING COMMENTS

The next step in enhancing current performance measurement and reporting capabilities is to address the gaps identified in this chapter through a research agenda. Chapter 5 provides a strategy for the development of a research agenda to support the aggressive development of the resolution of underlying methodological issues, the improvement of public reporting methods, and the evaluation of the overall progress of the national system for performance measurement and reporting proposed in this report.

REFERENCES

AHRQ (Agency for Healthcare Research and Quality). 2001. *Approach to Performance Measurement.* [Online]. Available: *http://www.ahrq.gov/about/gpra2001/gpra01app1.htm* [accessed September 1, 2004].

AHRQ. 2003. *National Healthcare Disparities Report.* Rockville, MD: AHRQ.

AHRQ. 2004. *CAHPS.* [Online]. Available: *http://www.ahrq.gov/qual/cahpsix.htm* [accessed March 3, 2005].

AHRQ. 2005. *Ambulatory Care Quality Alliance Third Invitational Meeting Summary (continued).* [Online]. Available: *http://www.ahrq.gov/qual/performance3/perfm3d.htm* [accessed October 20, 2005].

American Cancer Society. 2004. *Cancer Facts and Figures 2004.* Atlanta, GA: American Cancer Society.

American Hospital Association. 2004. *Trends Affecting Hospitals and Health Systems.* Washington, DC: American Hospital Association.

Amundson GM, Gentilli S, Wehrle D. 2005. *HealthPartners 2005 Clinical Indicators Report.* 13th ed. Bloomington, MN: HealthPartners, Inc. [Online]. Available: *http://www.healthpartners.com/files/23463.pdf* [accessed December 6, 2005].

Baicker K, Chandra A. 2004. Medicare spending, the physician workforce, and beneficiaries' quality of care. *Health Affairs.* Jan-June Suppl Web Exclusive: W4:184–197.

Barnato AE, Lucas FL, Staiger DP, Wennberg DE, Chandra AP. 2005. Hospital-level racial disparities in acute myocardial infarction treatment and outcomes. *Medical Care* 43(4):308–319.

Birkmeyer J. 2004. *Does Risk Adjustment Always Matter?* Presentation to the IOM Committee on Payment, Performance Measures, and Performance Improvement. December 1–3, 2004. Washington, DC.

Birkmeyer JD, Dimick JB, Birkmeyer NJO. 2004. Measuring the quality of surgical care: Structure, process, or outcomes? *Journal of the American College of Surgeons* 198(4):626–632.

Bulterys M, Nolan ML, Jamieson DJ, Dominguez K, Fowler MG. 2002. Advances in the prevention of mother-to-child HIV-1 transmission: Current issues, future challenges. *AIDScience* 2(4):1–10.

Centers for Disease Control and Prevention. 2002. Annual Smoking-Attributable Mortality, Years of Potential Life Lost, and Economic Costs—United States, 1995–1999. *Morbidity and Mortality Weekly Report* 51:300–303.

CMS (Centers for Medicare and Medicaid Services). 2004a. *Medicare Advantage PPO HEDIS Measurement Feasibility Assessment Report.* Washington DC: CMS.

CMS. 2004b. *OASIS Overview.* [Online]. Available: *http://www.cms.hhs.gov/oasis/ hhoview.asp* [accessed February 25, 2005].

CMS. 2005a. *Minimum Data Set (MDS) 3.0.* [Online]. Available: *http://www.cms.hhs.gov/ quality/mds30/* [accessed March 2005].

CMS. 2005b. *Medicare Compare Series: Nursing Home Compare, Home Health Compare, Dialysis Compare, and Hospital Compare.* [Online]. Available: *http://www.Medicare.gov* [accessed January 24, 2005].

Coffield AB, Maciosek MV, McGinnis JM, Harris JR, Caldwell MB, Teutsch SM, Atkins D, Richland JH, Haddix A. 2001. Priorities among recommended clinical preventive services. *American Journal of Preventive Medicine* 21(1):1–9.

Coleman EA, Boult C, American Geriatrics Society Health Care Systems Committee. 2003. Improving the quality of transitional care for persons with complex care needs. *Journal of the American Geriatrics Society* 51(4):556–557.

Coleman EA, Mahoney E, Parry C. 2004a. Assessing the quality of preparation for post-hospital care from the patient's perspective: The Care Transitions Measures (CTM). *Medical Care* 43(3):246–255.

Coleman EA, Min S, Chomiak A, Kramer AM. 2004b. Post-hospital care transitions: Patterns, complications, and risk identification. *Health Services Research* 39:1449–1465.

Dudley RA, Johansen KL, Brand R, Rennie DJ, Milstein A. 2000. Selective referral to high-volume hospitals: Estimating potentially avoidable deaths. *Journal of the American Medical Association* 283(9):1159–1166.

Every NR, Fihn SD, Sales AE, Keane A, Ritchie JR. 2000. Quality enhancement research initiative in ischemic heart disease: A quality initiative from the Department of Veterans Affairs. QUERI IHD Executive Committee. *Medical Care* 38 (6 Suppl 1):I-49–I-59.

FACCT (Foundation for Accountability). 1997. *The FACCT Consumer Information Framework: Comparative Information for Better Health Care Decisions.* [Online]. Available: *http://www.facct.org/information.html* [accessed June 4, 2002].

Finlayson EV, Birkmeyer JD. 2002. Should consumers trust hospital quality report cards? *Journal of the American Medical Association* 287(24):3206; author reply 3207–3208.

Fisher ES, Wennberg JE. 2003. Health care quality, geographic variations, and the challenge of supply-sensitive care. *Perspectives in Biology and Medicine* 46(1):69–79.

Fisher ES, Wennberg DE, Stukel TA, Gottlieb DJ, Lucas FL, Pinder EL. 2003. The implications of regional variations in Medicare spending. Part 1: The content, quality, and accessibility of care. *Annals of Internal Medicine* 138(4):273–287.

Fisher ES, Wennberg DE, Stukel TA, Gottlieb DJ. 2004. Variations in the longitudinal efficiency of academic medical centers. *Health Affairs* Suppl Web Exclusive: VAR19-32.

Halvorson, G, Isham G. 2003. *Epidemic of Care: A Call for Safer, Better, and More Accountable Health Care.* San Francisco, CA: Jossey-Bass.

Hannan EL, van Ryn M, Burke J, Stone D, Kumar D, Arani D, Pierce W, Rafii S, Sanborn TA, Sharma S, Slater J, DeBuono BA. 1999. Access to coronary artery bypass surgery by race/ ethnicity and gender among patients who are appropriate for surgery. *Medical Care* 37(1):68–77.

Hofer TP, Hayward RA, Greenfield S, Wagner EH, Kaplan SH, Manning WG. 1999. The unreliability of individual physician "report cards" for assessing the costs and quality of care of a chronic disease. *Journal of the American Medical Association* 281(22):2098–2105.

IOM (Institute of Medicine). 1990. *Medicare: A Strategy for Quality Assurance* (Volume 1). Washington, DC: National Academy Press.

IOM. 2001. *Crossing the Quality Chasm: A New Health System for the 21st Century.* Washington, DC: National Academy Press.

IOM. 2003. *Priority Areas for National Action: Transforming Health Care Quality.* Adams K, Corrigan JM, eds. Washington, DC: The National Academies Press.

IOM. 2004. *1st Annual Crossing the Quality Chasm Summit: A Focus on Communities.* Adams K, Greiner A, Corrigan J, eds. Washington, DC: The National Academies Press.

Landon BE, Normand S-LT, Blumenthal D, Daley J. 2003. Physician clinical performance assessment: Prospects and barriers. *Journal of the American Medical Association* 290(9):1183–1189.

Leatherman S, McCarthy D. 2005. *Quality of Health Care for Medicare Beneficiaries: A Chartbook.* New York: Commonwealth Fund.

McCaig LF, Besser RE, Hughes JM. 2002. Trends in antimicrobial prescribing rates for children and adolescents. *Journal of the American Medical Association* 287(23):3096–3102.

McGlynn EA, Asch SM, Adams J, Keesey J, Hicks J, DeCristofaro A, Kerr EA. 2003a. The quality of health care delivered to adults in the United States. *New England Journal of Medicine* 348(26):2635–2645.

McGlynn EA, Cassel CK, Leatherman ST, DeCristofaro A, Smits HL. 2003b. Establishing national goals for quality improvement. *Medical Care* 41(Suppl. 1):I-16–I-29.

MedPAC (Medicare Payment Advisory Commission). 2005a. *Report to the Congress: Medicare Payment Policy.* Washington, DC: MedPAC.

MedPAC. 2005b. *Report to the Congress: Medicare Payment Policy. Section C: Skilled Nursing Facility Services.* Washington, DC: MedPAC.

National Center for Health Statistics. 2004. *Health, United States.* [Online]. Available: *http://www.cdc.gov/nchs/hus.htm* [accessed November 15, 2005].

NCQA (National Committee for Quality Assurance). 2001. *Principles for Performance Measurement in Health Care.* [Online]. Available: *http://www.ncqa.org/communications/news/prinpls.htm* [accessed August 30, 2004].

NQF (National Quality Forum). 2003. *Safe Practices for Better Healthcare.* Washington, DC: NQF.

O'Connor GT, Quinton HB, Traven ND, Ramunno LD, Dodds TA, Marciniak TA, Wennberg JE. 1999. Geographic variation in the treatment of acute myocardial infarction: The Cooperative Cardiovascular Project. *Journal of the American Medical Association* 281(7):627–633.

Organisation for Economic Co-operation and Development. 2005. *Infant Mortality Rate, Deaths per 1000 Live Births.* [Online]. Available: *http://www.oecd.org/dataoecd/35/19/35027658.xls* [accessed August, 2005].

Partnership for Solutions, A Project of The Johns Hopkins University and The Robert Wood Johnson Foundation. 2002. *Chronic Conditions: Making the Case for Ongoing Care.* [Online]. Available: *http://www.partnershipforsolutions.com/DMS/files/chronicbook2002.pdf* [accessed November, 14, 2005].

Rogers WH, Kazis LE, Miller DR, Skinner KM, Clark JA, Spiro III A, Graeme FB. 2004. Comparing the Health Status of VA and Non-VA Ambulatory Patients. *Journal of Ambulatory Care Management* 27(8):1–14.

Shapiro MF, Morton SC, McCaffrey DF, Senterfitt JW, Fleishman JA, Perlman JF, Athey LA, Keesey JW, Goldman DP, Berry SH, Bozzette SA, Additional Authors from the HCSUS Consortium. 1999. Variations in the care of HIV-infected adults in the United States: Results from the HIV cost and services utilization study. *Journal of the American Medical Association* 281(24):2305–2315.

U.S. DHHS (U.S. Department of Health and Human Services). 2000. *Healthy People 2010: Understanding and Improving Health*. Washington, DC: U.S. Government Printing Office.

U.S. Preventive Services Task Force. 1996. *Guide to Clinical Preventive Services*. Baltimore, MD: Williams & Wilkins.

U.S. Renal Data System. 2004. *Annual Data Report*. [Online]. Available: *http://www.usrds.org/* [accessed March 3, 2005].

Walker J, Pan E, Johnston D, Adler-Milstein J, Bates DW, Middleton B. 2005. *The Value of Health Care Information Exchange and Interoperability*. [Online]. Available: *http://content.healthaffairs.org/cgi/content/abstract/hlthaff.w5.10* [accessed January 25, 2005].

Wallace P. 2005. Personal communication to Karen Adams, March 28.

Wennberg JE. 1999. Understanding geographic variations in health care delivery. *New England Journal of Medicine* 340(1):52–53.

5

Research Agenda

CHAPTER SUMMARY

This chapter recommends an aggressive research agenda for the National Quality Coordination Board (NQCB) with four primary components: (1) development, implementation, and evaluation of new performance measures; (2) applied research to address underlying methodological issues; (3) design and testing of reporting formats for consumer usability; and (4) evaluation of a performance measurement and reporting system. A collaborative effort among private and public stakeholder groups led by the NQCB will be necessary to develop and fund this agenda.

In Chapter 4, the committee identifies significant gaps in current performance measurement and reporting capabilities. We argue for an accelerated effort to move beyond the status quo to ensure a broader and deeper understanding of how well the health care system is performing across all six aims of the *Quality Chasm* report (IOM, 2001) and, most important, where the system can be improved. This chapter focuses on the development of a research agenda that can help realize the kind of performance measurement and reporting system proposed by the committee.

One primary component of the necessary research agenda involves the development, implementation, and evaluation of performance measures. Second is applied research to address methodological issues related to data analysis, including how to minimize the effects of confounders and safeguard against misclassification of providers. Third, research is needed to determine the best formats for public reporting of performance data so that the data can be used by consumers as a decision tool in selecting high-quality providers. Finally, on a broader front, the committee has asserted the need for a national system for performance measurement and reporting to improve the quality of care for all Americans. This assertion is based on the committee's expert analysis and lessons learned from past experience, but is not as yet supported by an evidence base. Therefore, research is needed to develop a business case either supporting or refuting the need for the National Quality Coordination Board (NQCB). Moreover, the NQCB as envisioned by the committee will be a learning system. Thus it will be necessary to understand how well the entire system is functioning and to what extent these efforts to improve quality are affecting health and processes of care.

> Recommendation 5: The NQCB should formulate and promptly pursue a research agenda to support the development of a national system for performance measurement and reporting. The board should develop this agenda in collaboration with federal agencies and private-sector stakeholders. The agenda should address the following:
>
> • Development, implementation, and evaluation of new measures to address current gaps in performance measurement.
> • Applied research focused on underlying methodological issues, such as risk adjustment, sample size, weighting, and models of shared accountability.
> • Design and testing of reporting formats for consumer usability.
> • Evaluation of the performance measurement and reporting system.

Advances in the quality of health care delivery will be markedly slower without a performance measurement and reporting system that articulates a focused research agenda. The NQCB should take responsibility for leading efforts to develop such a research agenda and to ensure its timely implementation. In this role the board will need to have contracting and grant-making authority to support external research as well as the internal capacity to perform this function. To provide a base for these efforts, the Agency for Healthcare Research and Quality (AHRQ) and other stakeholders—both public and private—should take steps now to assess and sponsor developmental work addressing current barriers to performance measurement and reporting. The following sections address how action on the four fronts enumerated above can advance a national performance measurement and reporting system designed to enhance the quality of health care delivery.

DEVELOPMENT, IMPLEMENTATION, AND EVALUATION OF NEW MEASURES

Current efforts to develop performance measures to fill some of the gaps identified in Chapter 4 are unlikely to succeed without the more coordinated and effective leadership that the NQCB can provide in prioritizing and adequately funding a targeted research agenda to address those gaps.

TABLE 5-1 Priority Areas for Measure Development

Approach	Research Focus	Areas for Measure Development
Comprehensive measurement	Extend quality domains through the development of new measures.	• Efficiency • Equity • Patient-centeredness
Longitudinal measurement	Expand a longitudinal perspective to encompass other care settings and clinical conditions.	• Longitudinal experiences of care • Outcomes and efficiency of care
Patient-level, population-based, and systems-level measurement	Develop measures and approaches to measurement that support decision making by leaders at the physician group, hospital, and community levels.	• Systems-level measures
Shared accountability	Develop measures and methods that foster shared accountability.	This is a cross-cutting approach that will be fostered by measures in the above six areas.

As recommended in Chapter 3, the research agenda developed by the NQCB should be linked to well-specified goals and aims of the health care delivery system. In Chapter 4, the committee highlights four approaches that could be taken to achieve a high-quality performance system: (1) comprehensive measurement; (2) longitudinal measurement; (3) patient-level, population-based, and systems-level measurement; and (4) shared accountability. Table 5-1 identifies six priority areas for future development of performance measures within these broad approaches. The committee believes measures developed in these areas have the potential for yielding the greatest impact on quality of care within the next 3 years.

The NQCB should identify short- and long-term goals for the development of measures in these six areas by 2008 and beyond. The NQCB should work with public and private stakeholders to support the development and promulgation of measures in these six areas. Additionally, as the identification of measurement gaps is a dynamic process, the priority areas of focus should be updated periodically.

Comprehensive Measurement

In the short term, comprehensive measurement can best be achieved by developing adequate measures that address the all of the six aims identified in the *Quality Chasm* report. The most important gaps identified by the committee are measures of efficiency, equity, and patient-centeredness.

Efficiency

Substantial work is under way on the development of measures of efficiency that can represent the value of medical care. Prior Institute of Medicine (IOM) studies have endorsed the basic concept of avoiding waste: a more efficient care process or delivery system will produce an equal or better outcome at lower cost. The key is to be able to measure both quality and resource use for well-defined episodes of care. The following principles guided the committee's thinking in this area: (1) measures of efficiency should be based on episodes of care of adequate duration so that the quality of care and/or outcomes of treatment can be reliably determined; (2) the scope of services and time window of observation should be broad and long enough to ensure that providers being evaluated cannot improve their apparent efficiency simply by shifting costs to other providers or to periods outside the window of observation; (3) multiple measures of efficiency (i.e., of costs and quality) for a given provider are preferable because performance may vary across the types of service provided (e.g., care for diabetes versus congestive heart failure); and (4) when possible, reliance should be placed on measures that have been reported in the peer-reviewed literature to enhance both affordability and validity.

Two broad types of efficiency measures warrant consideration: longitudinal and episodic. The committee recommends an aggressive research agenda to develop and pilot test efficiency measures of both types.

Longitudinal efficiency An example of measures of longitudinal efficiency for defined populations over relatively prolonged periods is 1-year mortality and resource use for acute conditions. The feasibility of collecting these data has been demonstrated for different types of care delivery systems (Tarlov et al., 1989; Ware et al., 1996), hospitals (Fisher et al., 2004; Guadagnoli et al., 1995), and for regional care systems within the United States (Fisher et al., 2003a,b). Such data have also been used to monitor the impact of the introduction of a prospective payment system on hospitalized patients (Kahn et al., 1990). In addition to the measure of longitudinal efficiency recommended by the committee for the starter set of measures detailed in Chapter 4—1-year mortality, resource use, and functional status after acute myocardial infarction—attention should be paid to collecting long-term follow-up data on additional conditions for which longitudinal outcomes and costs can be reliably assessed. Candidates include hip fracture and colorectal cancer, given their relative frequency, the high rates of hospitalization associated with these conditions (allowing population-based comparisons of outcomes at the community level), and the potential for these data to provide insight into multiple care systems (orthopedics and oncology) and care settings (rehabilitation, ambulatory care, and acute hospital).

Episodic efficiency Measurement of the efficiency of episodic care refers to a unit of analysis that reflects the level of resources used in the care of a specific, relatively brief episode (e.g., acute back pain) as part of the total care received by patients. Examples of such measures are methods for calculating adjusted average payments for all patient refined-diagnosis related groups and episode treatment groups. Many researchers have identified the need for measuring episodic efficiency to address issues ranging from cost containment and attribution to reduction in waste. Issues such as non-standardized use of these measures, validity of and availability of data sources, and risk adjustment hinder progress in this area, however. (For further discussion, refer to Appendix H.)

Equity

Multiple studies have demonstrated marked variations in access to health care (Cassil and Sorian, 2002; IOM, 2002, 2003, 2005; Isaacs and Schroeder, 2004; Sheikh and Bullock, 2001). As equity is a cross-cutting quality aim, it is important that it be measured not only to achieve comprehensive measurement, but also to test how well the health care system is functioning on all other quality aims. The committee was thus concerned by the relatively few measures available for evaluating equity, particularly with regard to issues of access and disparities in care. Greater attention should be focused on these issues, with consideration of the following measures and methods.

Access An important area of disparity in care is health insurance coverage. Ambulatory care measures, which reflect the quality of care for individuals in any ambulatory care setting, are one useful kind of equity measure. Yet they are obtained most easily by sampling only insured populations. Thus greater use should be made of hospital-based measures, which include all patients at a given institution regardless of their payer or insurance status. Other important issues of access include those related to transportation, service hours, and manpower. Rural communities are a particularly critical population to assess, as they often have limited access to high-quality care (IOM, 2005). The committee believes that in the short term, it will be necessary to identify representative samples of patients from all sites where the uninsured may receive care—whether uncompensated care from physicians' office-based practices or emergency rooms, or care provided by established safety net providers.

Disparities The committee strongly advocates the collection of performance measures addressing health care services at the individual level, allowing for aggregation to various levels of providers, geographic regions, and demographics. The critical issue in measuring racial, ethnic, or socioeconomic disparities is the need for data aggregation and reporting systems that can provide this stratification when sample sizes are large enough to yield reliable estimates. These efforts should be coordinated with those of other organizations characterizing the equity of care. The National Healthcare Disparities Report has made significant progress in this area, but much research remains to be done (AHRQ, 2003).

Additionally, equity should be assessed using measures that can capture variations in care by (1) region of the country; (2) type of community (i.e., rural versus urban, as the former tend to comprise sicker and poorer populations); (3) availability of care; and (4) patient race, ethnicity, and class. The committee views such research as a top priority of the NQCB so as to minimize the detrimental impacts of inequity in health care on underserved and disadvantaged populations (AHRQ, 2003; IOM, 2001, 2002, 2004). Although data systems may not be sufficient to support reporting of such measures within the next year, the committee believes such systems can be in place by 2008, and calls for an aggressive effort to that end.

Patient-Centered Care

The committee recommends expanding the current repertoire of patient-centered measures so as to gain insight based on patients' experiences, as patients are a valuable part of the interconnected chain of care delivery. In accordance with design principle 6 for a national system for performance measurement and reporting—a central role for the patient's voice (see Chapter 2)—the committee defines patient-centered care as "providing care that is respectful of and responsive to individual patient preferences, needs, and values and ensuring that patient values guide all clinical decisions" (IOM, 2001:6). Data that capture measures of health care that matter to patients can be a powerful influence on how care is delivered by providers, purchased by payers, and adhered to by patients.

The CAHPS initiative, discussed in Chapter 2, has been a forerunner in systematically capturing patients' perspectives on their care. The committee endorses use of the entire CAHPS family of surveys, which have been developed for a variety of settings—ambulatory care, hospital, health plan, in-center dialysis center, and nursing home—as part of the NQCB's measurement strategy. In addition, three promising dimensions of patient-centeredness that require attention are (1) self-assessment of patients' level of engagement in their care (Hibbard, 2004; Hibbard et al., 2004); (2) patients' input on the quality of the delivery of their chronic disease care

(Bodenheimer et al., 2002; Glasgow et al., 2005; Lorig et al., 2001, 2004); and (3) information on whether patients who faced major treatment choices received accurate information and support in making choices aligned with their values, a parameter termed "decision quality" (Mulley, 1989, 2004; Sepucha et al., 2004). The committee views the incorporation of additional patient-centered measures as a top priority for achieving a more balanced, less provider-centric approach to performance measurement.

Longitudinal Measurement

As suggested earlier, longitudinal measurement will help break down the boundaries created by the current silos of the health care system. Two sets of measures are needed: measures of care transitions, or how well patients' care is coordinated as they enter into and out of different health care settings, and measures of longitudinal efficiency. As the latter was discussed above, this section focuses on measures of care transitions, characterized as both longitudinal experiences of care and outcomes of care. While gains have been made in care transitions within the hospital setting, further emphasis should be placed on patients transferring from ambulatory to other care settings.

Longitudinal Experiences of Care

The assessment of care transitions is critical as it is at these points that breakdowns and errors in care are most likely to occur (Coleman and Berenson, 2004). Evaluation of transitions requires longitudinal measurement to determine whether the health care needs of patients have been met irrespective of where their care is delivered—hospital, nursing home, or home care. Measures in this area should provide the impetus for moving toward care that transcends the various care settings and the fragmentation promoted by disease-specific care.

Four measure sets for care transitions are candidates for implementation within the next 3 years: (1) the California Healthcare Foundation's Patients' Evaluation of Performance in California Survey, (2) the University of Colorado Health Sciences Center's Care Transitions Measure, (3) Hospital Consumer Assessment of Healthcare Providers and Systems, and (4) the Assessing Care of Vulnerable Elders measure. All of these measures reflect the patient's experiences and rely on self-reported responses to items during either a telephone or written survey. (For further discussion of care transitions and these measures, see Appendix I.) The committee proposes that the NQCB evaluate which of these candidate measures would be most appropriate for immediate use.

Outcomes of Care

Patient outcomes are the ultimate indicator of the quality of care received. These important measures reflect the extent to which providers are delivering high- or low-quality care, as well as the functioning of the broader health care system. However, outcomes measures are often difficult to use for quality improvement purposes. Multiple confounders are associated with health outcomes, such as patient adherence, societal factors, and the long time frames required to yield significant results. Health services researchers have wrestled for decades with models for statistical adjustment that can protect against holding providers accountable for such confounding determinants of outcome. Much progress has been made in understanding simple adjustments, such as for age, as well as more difficult ones, such as for comorbidity. In addition, more is now understood about the policy implications of the choices of adjusters. For example, race may correlate with outcome. A mortality measure that adjusts for race in effect excuses the care system from responsibility for race-related factors—a decision with profound policy implications.

The committee believes consideration should be given to measures of two outcomes of care particularly salient to patients: disease-specific mortality and pain control.

Disease-specific mortality The committee proposes the following 30-day and 1-year disease-specific mortality measures for consideration: acute myocardial infarction, coronary artery bypass graft, percutaneous coronary intervention, and end-stage renal disease. Sufficient epidemiologic work has been done on these measures to permit both appropriate adjustments for demographics and comorbidities and widespread practical adoption. As always, consideration must be given to the available sample sizes and to the expression of risks in terms of confidence intervals. It is likely that small hospitals and individual practitioners simply have too few relevant cases to be included in a disease-specific mortality measurement strategy.

Pain control Qualitative studies have demonstrated that recognition and treatment of pain are important priorities for patients receiving palliative care; however, validated measures of pain control are not yet available for widespread use (Lynn, 2000). The committee proposes that the NQCB consider which measures of pain assessment and changes in pain management are the most promising candidates for implementation, with evidence for their reliability and validity. (For more discussion of the evidence base and areas for further research with respect to pain control, see Appendix J.)

Individual-Patient-Level, Population-Based, and Systems-Level Measurement

The importance of individual-patient-level and population-based measures was highlighted above. In addition, systems-level measures are needed to assess the performance of both the smaller entities constituting the overall health care delivery system (such as hospitals and health plans) and the overall system itself. Measures of this type therefore have implications for purchasers and providers wishing to compare the performance of these smaller systems relative both to each other and to larger systems. The committee believes that with targeted attention, systems-level measures could be ready for implementation by 2008.

An example of such measures is mortality measures, which entail some controversy. The primary issue is the classic problem of severity or case-mix adjustment. Hospitals and other care providers facing comparisons of outcome measures, especially those as significant as mortality, understandably become concerned about fairness with respect to severity variables beyond their control. Unmeasured determinants of outcome, unevenly distributed among providers, may masquerade as effects of care itself, thus penalizing providers who simply are dealing with more problematic, higher-risk patients at the outset.

The committee considered two types of mortality measures: (1) disease-specific mortality, such as from cancer or ischemic heart disease, discussed in the previous section, and (2) hospitalwide mortality, summing experience over many diagnoses. The former could, in principle, characterize the quality of specialty care or clinical services, while the latter might reflect systemic and organizational characteristics with broader impact, such as teamwork, supervision, information management, or adequacy of the physical plant.

The committee achieved consensus on disease-specific mortality measures, but was unable to do so with respect to hospitalwide mortality measures. The Hospital Standardised Mortality Rate model has been widely discussed in the peer-reviewed literature and is now in significant use in the United Kingdom and, in earlier stages, in the United States (Jarman et al., 1999). Several committee members suggested that this model should be included in the initial set of performance measures to provide additional experience with its use, as well as information on its correlations with other structural, process, and outcome measures. These members suggested that mortality, as a systemic characteristic, is simply too important to ignore when initiating a consolidated measurement system, and that the use of a recognized approach, even if still developmental, would be prudent. Other committee members expressed skepticism about the technical aspects of the Hospital Standardised Mortality Rate model in particular and about the more general theoretical foundation for attempting to measure mortality as a hospitalwide characteristic, given how hospital-specific variations in end-of-life care can influence such measures (Fisher et al., 1994). The NQCB will need to address these issues as the measurement development effort goes forward.

Shared Accountability

Shared accountability is cross-cutting in that it holds all providers who partake in a patient's care responsible for the outcomes of that care. There is no single method for achieving shared accountability. Assessing care longitudinally across time and space can require the evaluation of care for a patient from the hospital to the nursing home. Composite measures of care reinforce this overall approach by focusing on treatment for all aspects of a patient's condition. Measurement at both the population and systems levels addresses the larger health care system and includes the societal factors that contribute to the health of the general public. The committee therefore believes that development and promulgation of measures in all of these areas foster shared accountability. It will become increasingly necessary to develop models of shared accountability as the focus shifts away from measuring care by setting, as discussed in the next section.

APPLIED RESEARCH TO ADDRESS UNDERLYING METHODOLOGICAL ISSUES

The NQCB should support research aimed at resolving key methodological issues surrounding performance measurement so as to enhance the accuracy and integrity of the data obtained. If measurement methodologies are flawed, data can be misleading, potentially threatening providers' reputations and falsely portraying the quality of care provided. The committee calls particular attention to the following issues:

- *Risk adjustment*—This statistical tool allows data to be modified to control for variations in patient populations. For example, risk adjustment could be used to ensure a fair comparison of the performance of two providers: one whose caseload consists mainly of elderly patients with multiple chronic conditions and another who treats a patient population with a less severe case mix. Risk adjustment makes it possible to take these differences into account when resource use and health outcomes are compared.

- *Sample size*—Small sample sizes may make conclusions statistically invalid, particularly when used for ranking individual providers. For instance, depictions of a physician's performance may be inaccurate if she has treated only five patients for congestive heart failure, because if a random event has occurred, her performance rating will be skewed.

• *Weighting of elements for composite measures*—The issue here is whether to place more emphasis on any particular component of a composite measure, as discussed in Chapter 4. For example, weighting of components of the prevention composite measure would address whether a physician treating a woman with a history indicating an increased risk of breast cancer should be scored higher for providing this screening as opposed to giving smoking cessation advice.

• *Shared accountability*—As noted, the committee espouses the concept of shared accountability as a way to encourage better care coordination and to shift away from measuring and rewarding care by setting. Models are needed for determining how best to hold accountable all providers involved in a patient's care—e.g., a group of providers who prevented hospital readmission for a typical Medicare beneficiary with four chronic conditions—and to reward high-quality care.

Resolution of these methodological issues is critical for accurate data reporting. The NQCB should therefore ensure that these issues, as well as others it deems important, are promptly addressed.

DESIGN AND TESTING OF REPORTING FORMATS FOR CONSUMER USABILITY

If performance measures are to have the intended effects on the way care is provided, as well as on the health outcomes of patients, it is essential that they be reported so as to be clear and meaningful for those who wish to use the data. There is a broad audience for public reports on care, ranging from providers and purchasers to patients. To date, attention has focused mainly on how purchasers and providers respond to public reports and how their responses affect their behaviors; little attention has been focused at the patient level. Additionally, reports often are not tailored to the needs of special populations who may vary widely in their specific health information needs, language, and level of health literacy. The committee believes the usability of public reports of comparative health care performance data needs to be a focus of further research, as these reports currently are not produced in formats that resonate with consumers. Inadequate or inaccurate public reports can undermine the confidence of both consumers and clinicians in the value of public disclosure of performance information. Knowing what measures are meaningful to consumers is also important. Reports need to be produced so they can be understood by consumers and assist those searching for a provider (Farley Short et al., 2002; Hibbard et al., 2002). If these goals are not met, then public reports will have little effect, if any, on consumers and their choice of care. Emphasis in this area of research should be placed on how best to design and test formats for public reporting for consumers of health care (Shaller et al., 2003; Vaiana and McGlynn, 2002).

EVALUATION OF A SYSTEM FOR PERFORMANCE MEASUREMENT AND REPORTING

The NQCB should not be a static entity, but rather a dynamic learning system that continually evaluates itself and advances understanding of the impact of performance measurement. The committee proposes that assessment of the NQCB be carried out at time intervals that allow for continual improvement and midcycle corrections as needed (Deming, 1994; Langley et al., 1996). It is critical to determine whether the NQCB is having the intended consequences—ultimately the attainment of the six quality aims of the *Quality Chasm*—through intermediate outcomes such as better care processes. Just as important, the ongoing monitoring of the NQCB should serve to safeguard against unintended consequences, such as adverse selection. Table 5-2 presents a summary of what should be encompassed by an impact assessment of the NQCB, as discussed in detail below.

Intended Consequences

Performance measurement should yield knowledge and enable inferences about the effects of health system changes in such areas as payment policies, public reporting, benefit design, accreditation/certification, and quality oversight. Assessment of the NQCB should elucidate whether these changes to the health care system are inducing behaviors, particularly among providers, that result in improved patient care. For example, it should be possible to address the following key questions more fully as a result of the performance measurement activities overseen by the NQCB:

- Is performance measurement contributing to a closer evaluation of care processes so that providers are capable and desirous of changing the way they organize and deliver care to achieve improved quality?
- Does performance measurement assist providers in making wiser choices concerning the allocation of resources by addressing efficiency and the overuse of services that have been demonstrated to show no benefit or possibly even harm to patients?
- Does performance measurement encourage more rapid uptake of information technology by physician practices, thus facilitating the exchange of patient information among multiple providers?

TABLE 5-2 Impact Assessment of the NQCB

Intended Consequences	Unintended Consequences
Gain knowledge of important health system changes • Payment policies of public and private purchasers • Pay for performance • Public reporting programs • Benefit design • Accreditation and certification programs • Quality oversight processes	Foster belief that measurement in and of itself can improve care • Investment in measurement without a focus on improving care • Data collection burden • Misclassification
Induce desirable provider behaviors • Better understanding of care processes, leading to actions that improve quality • Wise use of resources • Investment in information technology infrastructure • Enhanced cooperation among providers • Accelerated innovation	Induce undesirable provider behaviors • Gaming • Adverse selection
Close known quality gaps • 22 priority areas • Populations of focus (equity)	Sustain quality gaps • Patient harm • Community harm

• Does performance measurement foster cooperation among providers so that care is better integrated and more patient-centered?

• Does performance measurement spur innovation rather than stifle creativity?

In addition to lessons learned about interventions introduced into the health care system to improve care (e.g., pay for performance) and influence provider behavior, the NQCB needs to be assessed to determine whether it is indeed closing known quality gaps, as well as eliminating disparities in health care. A potential risk of not doing so is that measurement will be done simply for its own sake, without serving the primary purpose of moving closer to achieving the six quality aims.

Unintended Consequences

In addition to assessing whether the NQCB is having the intended consequences or desired outcomes, it will be equally important to identify any unintended consequences of the demands imposed by the system. As noted above, measurement itself must not be viewed as capable of improving care, but as a catalyst for actions that can do so. Other potential consequences that warrant close monitoring include the potential burden of data collection on the health care system, as well as on individual providers; misclassification of providers, particularly if data are publicly reported; gaming of the system; and adverse selection of healthier patients to improve scores. Perhaps the most serious unintended consequence is that quality gaps will persist, resulting in harm to both patients and communities.

FUNDING

Recommendation 6: Congress should provide the financial resources needed to carry out the research agenda developed by the NQCB. The AHRQ should collaborate with Grantmakers in Health and others that have ties to local foundations to convene public- and private-sector stakeholders currently investing in various aspects of this research agenda for the purpose of identifying complementary investment strategies.

Achieving the goal of a comprehensive national system for performance measurement and reporting will require the development and implementation of new measures, methodologies, and reporting formats, as well as thorough evaluation of the system. Accomplishing these tasks will in turn require commitment from both public and private stakeholders. Collaboration among these stakeholders could jumpstart much-needed development of measures to fill the gaps identified in this report, as well as the formulation of evidence-based consensus guidelines to serve as the basis for measure development. The NQCB should receive adequate funding to ensure the implementation of a robust research agenda, such as that proposed in this chapter. The committee recommends that the NQCB work closely with AHRQ, who has an established track record in funding evidence-based health services research, and other groups that can provide linkages between foundations and community collaborations, such as Grantmakers in Health, to align investment strategies for carrying out this agenda.

REFERENCES

AHRQ (Agency for Healthcare Research and Quality). 2003. *National Healthcare Disparities Report*. Rockville, MD: AHRQ.

Bodenheimer T, Lorig K, Holman H, Grumbach K. 2002. Patient self-management of chronic disease in primary care. *Journal of the American Medical Association* 288(19):2469–2475.

Cassil A, Sorian R. 2002. *1 in 4 Uninsured Americans with Chronic Conditions Can't Get Needed Care.* Washington, DC: Center for Studying Health System Change.

Coleman EA, Berenson RA. 2004. Lost in transition: Challenges and opportunities for improving the quality of transitional care. *Annals of Internal Medicine* 141(7):533–536.

Deming WE. 1994. *The New Economics for Industry, Government, and Education* (2nd Edition). Cambridge, MA: Massachusetts Institute of Technology Center for Advanced Engineering Study.

Farley Short P, McCormack L, Hibbard J, Shaul JA, Harris-Kojetin L, Fox MH, Damiano P, Uhrig JD, Cleary PD. 2002. Similarities and differences in choosing health plans. *Medical Care* 40(4):289–302.

Fisher ES, Wennberg JE, Stukel TA, Sharp SM. 1994. Hospital readmission rates for cohorts of Medicare beneficiaries in Boston and New Haven. *New England Journal of Medicine* 331(15):989–995.

Fisher ES, Wennberg DE, Stukel TA, Gottlieb DJ, Lucas FL, Pinder EL. 2003a. The implications of regional variations in Medicare spending. Part 1: The content, quality, and accessibility of care. *Annals of Internal Medicine* 138(4):273–287.

Fisher ES, Wennberg DE, Stukel TA, Gottlieb DJ, Lucas FL, Pinder EL. 2003b. The implications of regional variations in Medicare spending. Part 2: Health outcomes and satisfaction with care. *Annals of Internal Medicine* 138(4):288–298.

Fisher ES, Wennberg DE, Stukel TA, Gottlieb DJ. 2004. Variations in the longitudinal efficiency of academic medical centers. *Health Affairs* Suppl. Web Exclusive: VAR19-32.

Glasgow RE, Wagner EH, Schaefer JM, Mahoney LD, Reid RJ, Greene SM. 2005. Development and validation of the patient assessment of chronic illness care (PACIC). *Medical Care* May 43(5):436–444.

Guadagnoli E, Hauptman PJ, Ayanian JZ, Pashos CL, McNeil BJ, Cleary PD. 1995. Variation in the use of cardiac procedures after acute myocardial infarction. *New England Journal of Medicine* 333(9):573–578.

Hibbard J. 2004. *Measuring Patient Activation.* PowerPoint Slides, Alliance of Community Health Plans Advancing Better Care Conference, February 9–10.

Hibbard JH, Slovic P, Peters E, Finucane ML. 2002. Strategies for reporting health plan performance information to consumers: Evidence from controlled studies. *Health Services Research* 37(2):291–313.

Hibbard JH, Stockard J, Mahoney ER, Tusler M. 2004. Development of the Patient Activation Measure (PAM): Conceptualizing and measuring activation in patients and consumers. *Health Services Research* 39 (4 Pt 1):1005–1026.

IOM (Institute of Medicine). 2001. *Crossing the Quality Chasm: A New Health System for the 21st Century.* Washington, DC: National Academy Press.

IOM. 2002. *Unequal Treatment: Confronting Racial and Ethnic Disparities in Health Care.* Smedley BS, Stith AY, Nelson BD, eds. Washington, DC: The National Academies Press.

IOM. 2003. *Insuring Health—Hidden Costs, Value Lost: Uninsurance in America.* Washington, DC: The National Academies Press.

IOM. 2004. *Insuring Health—Insuring America's Health: Principles and Recommendation.* Committee on the Consequences of Uninsurance, eds. Washington, DC: The National Academies Press

IOM. 2005. *Quality Through Collaboration: The Future of Rural Health.* Washington, DC: The National Academies Press.

Isaacs SL, Schroeder SA. 2004. Class: The ignored determinant of the nation's health. *New England Journal of Medicine* 351(11):1137–1142.

Jarman B, Gault S, Alves B, Hider A, Dolan S, Cook A, Hurwitz B, Iezzoni LI. 1999. Explaining differences in English hospital death rates using routinely collected data. *British Medical Journal* 318(7197):1515–1520.

Kahn KL, Keeler EB, Sherwood MJ, Rogers WH, Draper D, Bentow SS, Reinisch EJ, Rubenstein LV, Kosecoff J, Brook RH. 1990. Comparing outcomes of care before and after implementation of the DRG-based prospective payment system. *Journal of the American Medical Association* 264(15):1984–1988.

Langley G, Nolan KM, Norman CL, Provost LP, Nolan TW, Norman CL. 1996. *The Improvement Guide: A Practical Approach to Enhancing Organizational Performance.* San Francisco, CA: Jossey-Bass.

Lorig KR, Sobel DS, Ritter PL, Laurent D, Hobbs M. 2001. Effect of a self-management program on patients with chronic disease. *Effective Clinical Practice* 4(6):256–262.

Lorig KR, Ritter PL, Laurent DD, Fries JF. 2004. Long-term randomized controlled trials of tailored-print and small-group arthritis self-management interventions. *Medical Care* 42(4):346–354.

Lynn J. 2000. Learning to care for people with chronic illness facing the end of life. *Journal of the American Medical Association* 284(19):2508-2511.

Mulley AG Jr. 1989. Assessing patients' utilities. Can the ends justify the means? *Medical Care* 27(Suppl. 3):S269–S281.

Mulley AG Jr. 2004. *Performance Measurement Workshop: Patient-Centered Measurement of Decision Quality.* Presentation to the IOM Committee on Performance Measures, Payment and Performance Improvement Programs, December 1–3, 2004, Washington, DC.

Sepucha KR, Fowler FJ Jr, Mulley AG Jr. 2004. Policy support for patient-centered care: The need for measurable improvements in decision quality. *Health Affairs* var.54.

Shaller D, Sofaer S, Findlay SD, Hibbard JH, Delbanco S. 2003. Perspective: Consumers and quality-driven health care: A call to action. *Health Affairs* 22(2):95–101.

Sheikh K, Bullock C. 2001. Urban-rural differences in the quality of care for Medicare patients with acute myocardial infarction. *Archives of Internal Medicine* 161(5):737–743.

Tarlov, AR, Ware JE Jr., Greenfield S, Nelson EC, Perrin E, Zubkoff M. 1989. The Medical Outcomes Study. An application of methods for monitoring the results of medical care. *Journal of the American Medical Association* 262(7):925–930.

Vaiana ME, McGlynn EA. 2002. What cognitive science tells us about the design of reports for consumers. *Medical Care Research and Review* 59(1):35–59.

Ware, JE Jr., Bayliss MS, Rogers WH, Kosinski M, Tarlov AR. 1996. Differences in 4-year health outcomes for elderly and poor, chronically ill patients treated in HMO and fee-for-service systems: Results from the Medical Outcomes Study. *Journal of the American Medical Association* 276(13):1039–1047.

Appendix A

Glossary

Care transitions. A set of actions designed to ensure the coordination and continuity of health care as patients transfer between different locations or different levels of care within the same location. Transitional care encompasses both the sending and the receiving of aspects of care (Coleman and Berenson, 2004).

Chronic conditions. A condition that lasts a year or longer, limits what one can do, and may require ongoing care. Examples of chronic conditions are diabetes, cancer, glaucoma, and heart disease (Partnership for Solutions, 2001).

Clinicians. Individual health care providers, such as physicians, nurse practitioners, nurses, physician assistants, and others.

Electronic health record. A repository of electronically maintained information about an individual's health care and corresponding clinical information management tools that provide alerts and reminders, linkages with external health knowledge sources, and tools for data analysis (Shortliffe et al., 2001).

Fee for service. An approach to billing for health services in which providers charge a separate price or fee for each service provided or patient encounter. Under fee for service, the level of expenditures for health care depends on both the levels at which fees are set and the number of types of services provided.

Performance measures. Includes both measures of patient perspectives on care, clinical quality, and patient outcomes.

- Measures of patient perspectives include patient assessment and satisfaction with their access to and interactions with the care delivery system (e.g., waiting times, information received from providers, choice of providers).
- Measures of clinical quality are specific quantitative indicators to identify whether the care provided conforms to established treatment goals and care processes for specific clinical presentations. Clinical quality measures generally consist of a descriptive statement or indicator (e.g., the rate of beta blocker usage after heart attack, the 30-day mortality rate following coronary artery bypass graft surgery), a list of data elements that are necessary to construct and/or report the measure, detailed specifications that direct how the data elements are to be collected (including the source of data), the population on whom the measure is constructed, the timing of data collection and reporting, the analytic models used to construct the measure, and the format in which the results will be presented. Measures may also include thresholds, standards, or other benchmarks of performance (IOM, 2002).
- Measures of patient outcomes include mortality, morbidity, and physical and mental functioning.

Providers. Refers to both institutional providers of health care services (e.g., health plans, HMOs, hospitals, nursing homes) and clinicians (e.g., physicians, nurse practitioners, nurses, physician assistants).

Quality. The degree to which health services for individuals and populations increase the likelihood of desired health outcomes and are consistent with current professional knowledge (IOM, 1990).

Quality aims. Descriptive elements of health care delivery goals, specifically:

1. *Safe*—avoiding injuries to patients from the care that is intended to help them.

2. *Effective*—providing services based on scientific knowledge to all who could benefit and refraining from providing services to those not likely to benefit (avoiding underuse and overuse, respectively).

3. *Patient-centered*—providing care that is respectful of and responsive to individual patient preferences, needs, and values and ensuring that patient values guide all clinical decisions.

4. *Timely*—reducing waits and sometimes harmful delays for both those who receive and those who give care.

5. *Efficient*—avoiding waste, including waste of equipment, supplies, ideas, or energy.

6. *Equitable*—providing care that does not vary in quality because of personal characteristics such as gender, ethnicity, geographic location, and socioeconomic status (IOM, 2001).

Quality improvement. A set of techniques for continuous study and improvement of the processes of delivering health care services and products to meet the needs and expectations of the customers of those services and products. It has three basic elements: customer knowledge, a focus on processes of health care delivery, and statistical approaches that aim to reduce variations in those processes (IOM, 1990).

Risk adjustment. A process that modifies the analysis of performance measurement results by those elements of the patient population that affect results, are out of the control of providers, and are likely to be common and not randomly distributed.

Vulnerable populations. Persons who are at increased risk of poor health outcomes. For example, persons with severe and chronic mental illness, the frail elderly, racial minorities, and the poor.

Acronym List

AAMC	Association of American Medical Colleges
ABIM	American Board of Internal Medicine
ACE	Angiotensin Converting Enzyme
ACGME	Accreditation Council for Graduate Medical Education
ACP	American College of Physicians
AHRQ	Agency for Healthcare Research and Quality
AIR	American Institutes for Research
AMA	American Medical Association
AQA	Ambulatory care Quality Alliance
ASIM	American Society of Internal Medicine
CABG	Coronary Artery Bypass Graft
CAHPS	Consumer Assessment of Healthcare Providers and Systems
CMS	Centers for Medicare and Medicaid Services
DHHS	Department of Health and Human Services
EHR	Electronic Health Record
ESRD	End-Stage Renal Disease
FAACT	Foundation for Accountability
GAO	Government Accountability Office
HCFA	Health Care Financing Administration
HEDIS	Health Plan Employer Data and Information Set

HMO	Health Maintenance Organization
HQA	Hospital Quality Alliance
IHI	Institute for Healthcare Improvement
IOM	Institute of Medicine
JAMA	Journal of the American Medical Association
JCAHO	Joint Commission on Accreditation of Healthcare Organizations
MDS	Minimum Data Set
MedPAC	Medicare Payment Advisory Commission
NCQA	National Committee for Quality Assurance
NHS	National Health Service
NQF	National Quality Forum
NSQIP	National Surgical Quality Improvement Program
OASIS	Outcome and Assessment Information Set
PCI	Percutaneous Coronary Intervention
PCPI	Physician's Consortium for Performance Improvement
PPO	Preferred Provider Organization
QIO	Quality Improvement Organizations
SFB	Strategic Framework Board

REFERENCES

Coleman EA, Berenson RA. 2004. Lost in transition: Challenges and opportunities for improving the quality of transitional care. *Annals of Internal Medicine* 141(7):533–536.

IOM (Institute of Medicine). 1990. *Medicare: A Strategy for Quality Assurance. Volume 1.* Washington, DC: National Academy Press.

IOM. 2001. *Crossing the Quality Chasm: A New Health System for the 21st Century.* Washington, DC: National Academy Press.

IOM. 2002. *Leadership by Example: Coordinating Government Roles in Improving Health Care Quality.* Washington, DC: The National Academies Press.

Partnership for Solutions, A Project of Johns Hopkins University and The Robert Wood Johnson Foundation. 2001. *The Problem: Chronic Conditions.* [Online]. Available: *http://www.partnershipforsolutions.com/problem/index.cfm* [accessed November 14, 2005].

Shortliffe EH, Perreault LE, Wiederhold G, Fagan LM. 2001. *Medical Informatics: Computer Applications in Healthcare and Biomedicine.* New York: Springer-Verlag.

Appendix B

TABLE B-1 National Organizations Involved in Performance Measurement

Name	Primary Role	Governance and Major Participants
Agency for Healthcare Research and Quality (AHRQ)	AHRQ sponsors and conducts research that provides evidence-based information on health care outcomes; quality; and cost, use, and access. The information helps health care decision makers—patients and clinicians, health system leaders, purchasers, and policymakers—make more informed decisions and improve the quality of health care services.	A Public Health Service agency in the U.S. Department of Health and Human Services (DHHS). Reporting to the DHHS Secretary, the Agency was authorized in 1989 as the Agency for Health Care Policy and Research and reauthorized in 1999 as AHRQ.

Major Quality Measurement Activities	Source of Core Funding
• The National Healthcare Quality Report (NHQR) is the first comprehensive national effort to measure the quality of health care in America. It includes a broad set of performance measures that can serve as baseline views of the quality of health care and presents data on services for seven clinical conditions: cancer, diabetes, end-stage renal disease, heart disease, HIV/AIDS, mental health, and respiratory disease. Also included are data on maternal and child health, nursing home and home health care, and patient safety.	Federal.

• The National Healthcare Disparities Report (NHDR), companion to the NHQR, provides measures of differences in access and use of health care services by various populations (cut by race/ethnicity, income, education, and insurance status where applicable) for all areas covered in the NHQR.

• The Consumer Assessment of Healthcare Providers and Systems (CAHPS) family of surveys is used by many public and private purchasers, including the National Committee for Quality Assurance (NCQA), to (1) develop and test questionnaires assessing health plans and services, (2) produce easily understandable reports communicate survey information to consumers, and (3) evaluate the usefulness of these reports for consumers in selecting health care plans and services.

• The National Quality Measures Clearinghouse™ houses the most current evidence-based quality measures and measure sets to evaluate and improve the quality of health care.

• The National Guidelines Clearinghouse™ contains evidence-based clinical practice guidelines that are often linked to measures.

• QualityTools (www.qualitytools.ahrq.gov) house the NHQR and the NHDR.

• The Prevention Quality Indicators* are a set of 16 measures that can be used with hospital inpatient discharge data to identify "ambulatory care sensitive conditions" for which good outpatient care can potentially prevent the need for hospitalization, or for which early intervention can prevent complications or more severe disease. They measure the outcomes of preventive and outpatient care through analysis of inpatient discharge data.

• The Inpatient Quality Indicators* consist of a set of 30 measures that reflect the quality of care inside hospitals and include inpatient mortality; utilization of procedures for which there are questions of overuse, underuse, or misuse; and volume of procedures for which there is evidence that a higher volume of procedures is associated with lower mortality.

(continued on next page)

TABLE B-1   continued

Name	Primary Role	Governance and Major Participants
AHRQ (continued)		
Ambulatory care Quality Alliance (AQA)	AQA is a collaborative effort initially convened by AHRQ, the American Academy of Family Physicians, the American College of Physicians, and America's Health Insurance Plans. The steering group has been expanded to include the American Medical Association, the American Osteopathic Association, the American College of Surgeons, the Society of Thoracic Surgeons, AARP, the National Partnership for Women and Families, and the Pacific Business Group on Health. Their mission is to improve health care quality and patient safety through a collaborative process in which key stakeholders agree on a strategy for measuring performance at the physician level; collecting and aggregating data in the least burdensome way; and reporting meaningful information to consumers, physicians and other stakeholders to inform choices and improve outcomes.	Public–private partnership. The AQA consists of a large body of stakeholders that represents clinicians, consumers, purchasers, health plans, and others. Major participants: **Health care organizations:** ACP, AAFP, AMA, AMA Consortium, American Board of Internal Medicine, American Board of Medical Specialties, ACC, AAP, AAAAI, AOA, ACS, STS, MGMA, AHA, AAMC and state medical societies. **Private participants:** AARP, AFL-CIO, Consumer/Purchaser Disclosure Project, Employer Health Care Alliance Corp., Leapfrog Group, General Motors, National Business Group on Health, National Business Coalition on Health, Pacific Business Group on Health, Medstat, Motorola, UPS, BellSouth, Xerox, and Marriott. **Public purchasers and other government agencies:** CMS, OPM, AHRQ, and Department of Treasury. **Health insurance plans:** Aetna, Anthem, Cigna, Health Net, Health Partners, Humana, Independence BCBS, Kaiser Permanente, Pacificare, Presbyterian Health Plan, Regence BCBS, UnitedHealth Group, Wellchoice, Harvard Pilgrim HealthCare, AHIP, Blue Cross Blue Shield Association. **Accrediting organizations:** NCQA, JCAHO, and URAC.

Major Quality Measurement Activities	Source of Core Funding
• The Patient Safety Indicators* are a set of 29 measures that provide a perspective on patient safety by screening for problems that patients experience as a result of exposure to the health care system and that are likely amenable to prevention by changes at the system or provider level. www.qualityindicators.ahrq.gov *The AHRQ Quality Indicators initially were developed as metrics for quality improvement, however their use has evolved over time to include public reporting, and pay for performance.	
Endorsed key parameters (criteria) for selecting performance measures. For example: evidence-based, clinical importance, scientific validity, feasibility, relevance to physician performance, consumers, and purchasers. Endorsed a standardized set of 26 measures for physician practices that draws heavily on the 2004 ambulatory care clinical performance measure set released by the AMA Consortium, CMS, and NCQA. Expanding the initial "starter" set of measures to include specialty and subspecialty care measures, efficiency measures and patient experience measures. Working with CMS and AHRQ to finalize pilot projects that would utilize the endorsed measurement set and combine public and private payer data.	Combination of federal and private.

(continued on next page)

TABLE B-1   continued

Name	Primary Role	Governance and Major Participants
Centers for Medicare and Medicaid Services (CMS)	The federal agency responsible for administering the Medicare, Medicaid, SCHIP (State Children's Health Insurance Program), HIPAA (Health Insurance Portability and Accountability Act), CLIA (Clinical Laboratory Improvement Amendments), and several other health-related programs. Their mission is to ensure health care security for beneficiaries.	An agency of U.S. DHHS. On July 1, 2001, the Health Care Financing Administration (HCFA) became CMS.
Hospital Quality Alliance (HQA)	The purpose of the HQA initiative is to make information about hospital performance accessible to the public and to inform and invigorate efforts to improve quality. Voluntary reporting is essential to the success of this initiative.	Public–private partnership of hospitals, government agencies, quality experts, purchasers, consumer groups and other health care organizations. These organizations have joined together to develop a shared national strategy for hospital quality measurement and are committed to advancing quality of care. Major participants: • American Hospital Association • Association of American Medical Colleges • Federation of American Hospitals • AARP • AFL-CIO • CMS • AHRQ • JCAHO • AMA • NQF • Consumer-Purchaser Disclosure Project

Major Quality Measurement Activities	Source of Core Funding
• *Technical Assistance*: Under the Quality Improvement Organization (QIO) program, CMS contracts with independent medical organizations to ensure the quality of medical care paid under the Medicare program to Medicare Advantage and fee-for-service beneficiaries. • *Measure Development*: CMS has collaborated with many organizations such as JCAHO, AQA, and HQA to develop measures in nursing homes, home health agencies, hospitals, dialysis facilities, and physician offices. • *Public Reporting*: Web-based tools, such as the Nursing Home Compare, Home Health Compare, and Hospital Compare, allow the public to compare data on the quality of providers were developed by CMS in collaboration with others. • *Financial Incentives Linked to Quality*: CMS is conducting quality incentive demonstrations by awarding bonus payments to providers for high performance, most notably through the Premier Hospital Quality Incentive Demonstration and Physician Group Practice Demonstration. The Medicare Health Support Program is a pilot program under way addressing chronic care disease management for fee-for-service beneficiaries. In addition, hospitals are provided with financial incentive to report on performance measures through MMA 501(b).	Federal.
• Currently has 20 hospital quality measures. • Hospital Compare is a tool patients can use in making care decisions by providing the public with useful information on hospital quality of care in an easily accessible way. • HCAHPS—measuring patient perspectives on hospital care—and anticipated for public reporting in 2007.	Combination of federal and private.

(continued on next page)

TABLE B-1   continued

Name	Primary Role	Governance and Major Participants
Joint Commission on Accreditation of Healthcare Organizations (JCAHO)	JCAHO evaluates and accredits more than 15,000 health care organizations and programs in the United States. Its mission is to continuously improve the safety and quality of care provided to the public.	Private, nonprofit. Governed by a 29-member Board of Commissioners that includes nurses, physicians, consumers, health care executives, purchasers, labor representatives, quality experts, ethicists, and educators. Major participants: Commonwealth Fund, California Endowment, Robert Wood Johnson Foundation, and AHRQ.
Leapfrog Group	The Leapfrog Group is a voluntary initiative to mobilize employer pur-chasing power to improve the safety, quality, and affordability of health care for Americans. Their mission is to trigger leaps forward by supporting informed health care decisions by those who use and pay for and promote high-value health care through incentives.	Private. The Leapfrog Group includes over 170 members from a growing consortium of Fortune 500 companies and other large private and public healthcare purchasers that provide health benefits to more than 34 million Ameri-cans in all 50 states. Major participants: • Business Roundtable • Robert Wood Johnson Foundation
National Committee for Quality Assurance (NCQA)	NCQA is dedicated to improving health care quality through evaluation of health care at various levels of the system from health plans to medical groups and individual doctors. NCQA's mission is to transform health care through measurement, transparency, and account-ability.	Private, nonprofit. Advised by a board of directors. NCQA frequently works with the federal and state governments to advance shared goals. Major participants: • AHRQ • American Diabetes Association • American Heart Association/ American Stroke Association • Bridges to Excellence • California Endowment Foundation • California HealthCare Foundation • Integrated Healthcare Association • Commonwealth Fund • Robert Wood Johnson Foundation • Bristol-Myers Squib • Pfizer

Major Quality Measurement Activities	Source of Core Funding
• In February 1997, the Joint Commission launched its ORYX® initiative, to develop evidence-based performance measures and integrate outcomes and other performance measurement data into the accreditation process. • In July 2002, hospitals began collecting core measure data on four initial core measurement areas: acute myocardial infarction; heart failure; community-acquired pneumonia; and pregnancy and related conditions. In January 2003, hospitals began transmitting their measurement results to the Joint Commission. In 2004, surgical infection prevention measures were added as a data collection and submission option.	Combination of federal and private.
• The Leapfrog Group identified and has since refined four hospital quality and safety practices that are the focus of its health care provider performance comparisons and hospital recognition and reward. All of the practices are endorsed by the National Quality Forum. Based on independent scientific evidence, the quality practices are: computer physician order; entry evidence-based hospital referral; intensive care unit (ICU) staffing by physicians experienced in critical care medicine; and the Leapfrog Safe Practices Score.	Private.
• The Research group engages in collaborative research that explores new approaches to measuring and reporting on the quality and efficiency of health care. • The Analysis group provides both day-to-day analysis of NCQA Accreditation, Health Plan Employer Data and Information Set (HEDIS) and CAHPS databases, and design and analysis of statistical processes used in research projects and measure development and maintenance. • The Measures Development (or Quality Measurement) group is devoted to the development and maintenance of measures in HEDIS. • Working with the American Diabetes Association and the American Heart Association/American Stroke Association, established the Diabetes Physician Recognition Program and the Heart/Stroke Physician Recognition program to identify physicians who demonstrate high quality care in these areas. • Developed Physician Practice Connections, a recognition program based on an evaluation of the presence and use of systems in office practice. All three recognition programs have been adopted for use in pay for performance programs.	Combination of public and private.

(continued on next page)

TABLE B-1 continued

Name	Primary Role	Governance and Major Participants
National Quality Forum (NQF)	Established consequent to a Presidential Commission, the NQF was created primarily to standardize national performance measures, quality indicators, and similar metrics for health care. It was envisioned to be the singular body performing this function. Other functions envisioned for the NQF were to develop and implement a national strategy for health care quality measurement and reporting and to be an "honest-broker" convener for health care quality matters. The mission of the NQF is to improve American health care through endorsement of consensus-based national standards for measurement and public reporting of health care performance data that provide meaningful information about whether care is safe, timely, beneficial, patient-centered, equitable, and efficient.	Not-for-profit membership organization. Unique public–private partnership. About 300 member organizations. NQF is governed by a 29-member Board of Directors representing health care providers, health plans, consumers, purchasers, accreditors, researchers, and quality improvement organizations. Government members of the Board include CMS, AHRQ, VHA, ONCHIT, and NIH. Board also includes JCAHO, NCQA, IOM, AARP, GM, Physician Consortium for Performance Improvement, and elected representatives of the 4 Member Councils. Major participants: • AARP • Leapfrog Group, GM, Ford • 20 largest hospital organizations • CMS • AHRQ • VA • AMA, AAFP, medical specialty societies • National Partnership for Women and Children • Kaiser Permanente • Robert Wood Johnson Foundation
The Physician Consortium for Performance Improvement convened by the American Medical Association (AMA)	The Physician Consortium for Performance Improvement's (the Consortium) mission is to improve patient health and safety by (1) identifying and developing evidence-based clinical performance measures; (2) promoting implementation of effective and relevant clinical performance improvement activities; and (3) advancing the science of clinical performance measurement and improvement.	Professional societies. The Consortium is currently formalizing its governance and structure. The Consortium includes physicians and experts in methodology convened by the AMA. The Consortium includes representatives from more than 70 national medical specialty and state medical societies, the AHRQ, CMS, and others. Representatives from employers, health plans, and consumer groups participate in measure development work groups.

Major Quality Measurement Activities	Source of Core Funding
Over 200 national consensus standards have been endorsed so far for care settings across the continuum of care (e.g., acute care hospitals, ambulatory care, nursing homes, home care, palliative and hospice care, other) as well as for conditions (e.g., cancer, asthma, acute coronary syndrome, diabetes, and deep vein thrombosis) and issues (e.g., patient safety, reportable events, medication use). A variety of workshops have been conducted to address specific issues related to quality.	Membership dues, contracts and grants; combination of federal and private.
• The Consortium selects topics for performance measures development that are actionable, for which established clinical recommendations are available, and for which feasible data sources exist. Work groups review the levels of evidence provided in clinical practice guidelines that demonstrate potential positive impact on health outcomes and propose feasible measures for inclusion in a physician performance measurement set. All specifications for Consortium measures are available at www.physicianconsortium.org, including specifications for electronic health record systems. • As of October 2005, 24 Consortium measures have been NQF-endorsed, and several are included in the AQA starter set.	AMA. In-kind funding, national medical specialty societies. Additional funding for measure development from contracts with CMS.

Appendix C

Case Studies

THEMES FROM CASE STUDIES

The most carefully designed health policy cannot be realized without a reasonable implementation strategy with which to anticipate and prepare to address issues that could impede the envisioned change. In this section, the committee reviews those issues likely to arise in different health care settings, especially small practices, during the implementation of a national system for performance measurement and reporting. Led by the National Quality Coordination Board (NQCB), the call for this national system will require a major shift in the current culture of health care in the United States—a shift away from the traditional provision of care within care settings toward stronger involvement of patients in their care. Along with this redesign of health care delivery, a coordinated system will entail public reporting of performance measures in addition to a greater emphasis on shared accountability among providers and patients for improving the quality of care delivered. Many providers will need assistance as they undertake performance measurement activities. To implement the new processes in their practices and to prepare for participation in a national system, providers may need to invest financial and personal resources in the short run for long-term gain.

Health care organizations will need to be prepared to commit the resources necessary to change their operations to accommodate the measurement tasks called for by the NQCB and retool their internal processes. These tasks will likely strain existing resources, which will need to be redeployed within organizations. A part of the implementation strategy for a national system for measurement and reporting is to have a phase-in period that will allow providers to learn procedures and protocols once the necessary infrastructure is in place, as well as obtain provider support and feedback with regard to performance measurement activities. Economies of scale available to larger organizations may allow them to respond more quickly than smaller organizations with fewer resources to devote to these tasks.

To examine the experience of practices that are currently implementing performance measurement, the committee sought input from a small sample of practices across various regions and communities. Major themes emerged from these case studies to reveal potential issues associated with implementing a national system for performance measurement and reporting. Specifically, the IOM committee sought to address two main questions: (1) What will it take to obtain provider support? and (2) How feasible is it to implement the proposed NQCB? In addition, the committee wished to address the issues associated with implementation of performance measurement, especially those faced by small practices, with particular attention to barriers and successes achieved in overcoming those barriers.

Three main themes emerged from the case studies: (1) the need to obtain physician support, (2) the need to obtain needed resources (human, technical, and financial), and (3) the importance of sustaining change. These themes are discussed below, followed by a review of barriers and successes achieved by the practices studied (see Table C-1).

Obtain Physician Support

The first step in implementing performance measurement within clinical practices is to obtain physicians' agreement to participate. Omitting this important step could delay or undermine the success of the NQCB. The NQCB can obtain physician support in a number of ways, as indicated by the providers contacted in the committee's case studies:

• Support provider participation in federal, state, and local collaborative arrangements for data collection and interpretation of results.
• Encourage those providers who are not already implementing quality improvement to seek help from their colleagues who are doing so or from their professional organizations.
• Promote use of practice guidelines by measure developers to achieve consensus on measures, and include multiple stakeholders in the consensus process.
• Encourage provider innovation in measurement activities that are clinically meaningful and specific to the practice setting, in addition to meeting national requirements.

TABLE C-1 Key Themes for Implementing Performance Measurement

Key Themes	Case Study[a]						
	A	B	C	D	E	F	G
Seek physician support							
• Use of practice guidelines to reach consensus on measures	X	X	X	X	X	X	X
• Provider ownership of data	X	X	X	X	X	X	X
• Prior exposure to performance measurement and quality improvement through professional organizations	X	X			X	X	X
• Participation in federal, state, and local collaboratives	X	X			X	X	X
• Use of pay for performance	X	X	X				
Obtain resources							
➤ **Human (hiring new staff)**							
• Additional clinical staff, such as physician assistants and nurses, for internal quality improvement efforts	X	X	X	X	X	X	
• Outside vendors for system maintenance				X	X	X	
• Full-time technicians for data system management or part-time staff to help with data collection	X			X	X		X
➤ **Technical assistance**							
• Recruiting of staff with prior training in quality improvement, such as a quality assurance coordinator	X	X	X	X			X
• Provider assistance received from an outside organization—e.g., an academic health center helps with data collection and interpretation		X	X		X	X	X
• Provider collaboration with federal, state, and local organizations for assistance with data collection and feedback		X			X	X	
➤ **Information technology**							
• Purchase of hardware and software within the practice	X	X	X	X	X	X	X
• Implementation of EHRs	X	X		X	X	X	X
➤ **Financial**							
• Up-front investments to get the practice ready for performance measurement	X	X	X	X	X	X	X
• Cost sharing through affiliations or partnerships with local collaboratives		X	X		X	X	
• Grants for performance measurement activities						X	

TABLE C-1   continued

Key Themes	Case Study[a]						
	A	B	C	D	E	F	G
Successes							
• Better patient care	X	X	X	X	X	X	X
• Provider and staff satisfaction	X	X	X	X	X	X	X
• Improvement shown by all practices that measure performance	X	X	X	X	X	X	X
• Ability of small practices, even a solo physician, to measure performance successfully				X	X	X	X
• Increased office efficiency	X	X			X		X
• Increased revenue		X		X	X		X
Barriers[b]							
• Provider resistance							
• Difficulty in demonstrating a business case							
• Time required to get EHRs fully operational							
• Requirement of additional resources to redesign practice care teams and ancillary personnel							
Sustain change							
• Review of performance measures annually to adjust criteria and practice goals	X	X	X	X	X	X	X
• Updating of the use of information technology to support quality efforts	X	X	X	X	X	X	X
• Increase in staff as needs dictate to continue internal quality improvement	X	X	X	X			
• Continuation or increase of bonus payments for meeting care targets	X	X	X				
• Creation of internal committees to review performance measurement	X	X	X				
Uses of performance measurement							
• Internal quality improvement	X	X	X	X	X	X	X
• Pay for performance	X	X	X				
• Public reports	X						

[a]Case studies are masked here as the focus is on the synthesis of key themes. This synthesis is based on responses by the 7 case study subjects to a list of questions prepared by the IOM committee.

[b]Barriers were not included in the committee's initial list of questions; however, the practices indicated they had overcome these difficulties over the past 3–5 years, when they began using performance measurement.

• Ensure that providers have ownership of their data. Allow them to check their data before sending it to a repository, and provide a process for them to dispute what they believe to be inaccurate or inappropriate data.

• Encourage the use of pay for performance to help offset some of the personal and financial investments required of participating providers.

Obtain Needed Resources

Many practices examined by the committee indicated that they needed additional human, technical, and financial resources in order to implement performance measurement. The NQCB, in collaboration with other organizations, could help providers locate these resources. The assistance provided might include the following:

• *Human resources*—support additional staff to manage data systems and input data.

• *Technical assistance*

  – Assistance from other organizations at the national and subnational levels in educating practice staff in quality improvement.

  – Help with implementation of electronic health records (EHRs) or practice management systems that link billing and medical records, possibly at the national or subnational level.

  – Help with data interpretation early in the process, especially before public reporting.

  – Adapt data feedback to increase usability by the practice.

• *Financial support*—Offer financial incentives to providers from either private or public funds for implementing performance measurement and achieving higher quality of care, as demonstrated by their data. A common issue is that a focus on performance measurement activities may result in a lower volume of patients because the focus of care is on providing quality, not on increasing office visits.

Sustain Change

Results of the committee's case studies indicated that participation in performance measurement based on temporary support, such as a short-term grant or individual experimentation within a practice, does not lead to successful implementation of performance measurement. The decision to implement quality improvement and performance measurement activities must begin with physician support and the necessary human, technical, and financial resources for the long term, as discussed above. Moreover, initial gains must be translated into long-term success. The small practices examined by the committee provided several examples of ways to sustain quality improvement, such as the following:

- Providers can participate in an annual review process to update performance measures, adjusting criteria and goals to align with the practice's quality improvement efforts.
- Practices need consistency in the levels of reimbursement tied to their performance and established goals, as well as in the associated procedures and policies.
- Several providers mentioned that their reputation in their community for providing high-quality care is important to them and is an important reason for their wanting to continue with performance measurement. They like having quality data that can demonstrate that they provide quality care.
- Public and private financial assistance can be provided for quality improvement and performance measurement activities. As noted above, providing high-quality care is expensive.

Barriers to Implementation

The case studies revealed a number of barriers to the implementation of performance measurement, regardless of practice size: provider resistance, difficulty in demonstrating a business case, time required to get EHRs or paper record systems ready for use, and the need for additional resources (as discussed above) to restructure practice care teams and ancillary personnel.

As noted earlier, since the NQCB tasks include collecting and reporting measures based on both administrative and medical record data, most small practices will need more help in this area than larger organizations. In addition, the small practices in the committee's case studies emphasized both technological and fiscal barriers.

For example, a technological problem that can occur when implementing EHRs was cited by GreenField Health in Oregon (case study 5, described below). GreenField Health noted that the first step for a practice after implementing EHRs is to customize them for its own use and standardize the way clinicians enter the data, facilitating the collection of accurate measures. Thus, it may be useful to have someone in the office familiar with the clinical and database issues to help address these needs. Other major barriers reported by small practices are presented below in Box C-1.

Often it is difficult to collect the data needed by the practice to carry out quality improvement activities. For example, GreenField Health reported that laboratory results, such as hemoglobin A_1c for diabetics or mammogram readings, are not currently retrievable from claims data. This small practice hired a physician with advanced computer skills who streamlined its data sources for performance measurement activities, including database programming when necessary. Likewise, a solo internist in Primer Care Family Practice in Oklahoma (case study 3) hired a part-time college student to scan laboratory results into his EHR system. Another example of practices being required to

---

BOX C-1   Barriers to Performance Measurement in Small Practices

- Large cost of setting up the infrastructure; difficulty of hiring and retaining physicians and other staff who understand the goals of quality improvement.
- Lack of standard software that can collect data for multiple purposes (often gathered using multiple paper forms to respond to different requests).
- Lack of private contracts that reward high performers at low cost to the plan (e.g., high-quality care is not low cost if the guidelines require a certain number of tests and follow-up visits that drive up costs).
- Lack of reimbursement for treating patients via telephone and e-mail (e.g., there is no financial incentive for fewer patient visits).
- Continual costs for maintenance of data systems (in addition to the purchase cost, and usually paid on a monthly basis).

---

report data that are difficult to collect is proof of eye exams for diabetics, which is required by recognition programs for diabetes care. To overcome this difficulty, Community Medicine Associates (case study 6) bought a photo machine to administer eye exams that are interpreted by an ophthalmologist's practice off site and returned for documentation purposes.

GreenField Health also noted that additional technical costs are likely to be incurred once a practice has identified problems with its performance based on the data collected. These costs include the technical assistance and resources required to mine the data from registries or other data sources so as to maximize the information obtained. Moreover, once performance data have been collected voluntarily, there is no source in the market that will pay a small practice for such data; thus a business case or financial incentive for collecting the data does not currently exist.

All of the barriers discussed above were overcome by small practices with perseverance and a commitment to providing the highest-quality care possible for their patients, even when they encountered challenges such as staff turnover, high out-of-pocket expenses, and limitations of technology. Several practices reported that setbacks result in learning that leads to improved internal processes, which eventually make it possible to achieve success.

Successes Achieved

All the practices in the committee's case studies emphasized that they were able to overcome most of the above barriers and gave reasons for continuing to believe and participate in performance measurement and quality improvement. Regardless of the practice size, performance measurement can be implemented successfully given the right cultural environment, resources, and tools. The case study practices reported general such successes as the following: increased office efficiency, provider and staff satisfaction, better patient care, higher quality of life because practitioners could work at home and save time at the office by using EHRs, and in some cases increased revenue after the initial short-term investments.

Specific successes are detailed in the next section. For example, Prime Care Family Practice (case study 3), a small rural practice, was informed by its state Quality Improvement Organization that only 8 percent of its eligible patients had been referred for a mammogram. To address this problem, the practice scheduled times for its patients to receive mammograms at the local hospital every Friday. Within 1 year, 100 percent of eligible patients had been referred for a mammogram, and 76 percent had a mammogram result documented in their patient record. This is a clear example of the improved patient care that can result from access to performance measurement data, without which providers would have been unaware of and thus unable to address the problem.

The case study practices also shared with the committee nonfinancial motivators that attract providers to participate in pay-for-performance arrangements, such as clinician satisfaction, data available for innovative tracking of patients, improvement of one's local reputation, increased billing compliance, and decreased liability. For example, North Texas Medical Group (case study 7) stated it was able to use performance measurement to implement an innovative approach to improving blood test monitoring of patients taking coumadin. By using performance measurement, North Texas Medical Group was able to carefully monitor some of its high-risk patients, which increased its practitioners' satisfaction with their clinical performance. As a result of other performance measurement activities, North Texas Medical Group was also able to develop a local reputation for providing excellent care, and has been able to decrease its liability concerns over the last several years. As an example of how a nonfinancial motivator can be linked to performance measurement, Community Medicine Associates (case study 6) used performance measurement primarily to improve productivity and billing compliance, which rests on billing correctly, and not overbilling, for services. Because of this increased productivity, the organization was able to provide bonuses of up to $5,000 per quarter, or $20,000 per year, to its participating providers.

All practices indicated that neither their financial and personal investments nor any frustrations experienced along the way detract from the value of performance measurement; the effort is worth the time and investment for them and their patients. Thus there is a clear need for a national system for performance measurement and reporting to foster such quality improvement efforts, especially for those small practices that are already struggling with competing market demands.

FULL DESCRIPTIONS OF CASE STUDIES

Case Study 1: HealthPartners, Inc.

HealthPartners, Inc., is a large nonprofit health care organization structured as a mixed-model health plan serving 630,000 members in group practices throughout Minnesota. Organized as a broad network of physicians and hospitals, HealthPartners provides services in practices with 10 to 600 physicians. Among its members, 30 percent receive care from HealthPartners Medical Group and Clinics, a staff-model group, and 70 percent from other contracted medical groups. HealthPartners serves its members across a range of health needs, from preventative to chronic disease services.

In addition to tracking performance on individual measures, HealthPartners calculates a composite score for a set of critical aspects of care received by the patient for a given condition. Data for these composite measures—addressing diabetes, cardiovascular disease, preventive care, and depression—are derived from administrative data and chart abstraction based on either electronic or paper records. Computer-based and paper registries are maintained separately from medical records and are not currently used to report performance. Rigorous validation of measures consists of four functions: drafting technical specifications, testing the measures, applying appropriate sampling methodology, and modifying the measures as needed.

A quality measurement steering committee, including medical group representatives, oversees measurement development and reporting at HealthPartners. The committee develops the composite measures mentioned above to align with provider-developed, evidence-based guidelines of the Institute for Clinical Systems Improvement (ICSI). ICSI is a not-for-profit collaborative in Minnesota consisting of medical groups and hospital systems, and serving as a driving force for improvement in the delivery of health care. The association between ICSI and HealthPartners has facilitated providers' acceptance of and involvement in performance measurement.

The cost to the plan for record review is $12 per review and approximately $0.014 per member per month (PMPM) for all health plan members (see Table C-2). In comparison, the plan's review cost for 2004 Health Plan Employer Data and Information System commercial reporting in 2004 was approximately $0.013 PMPM (see Table C-3). Additional resources needed for data collection activities include staff time for identifying patient samples

TABLE C-2   Total Cost Estimate per Review for Plan Members of
HealthPartners, Inc.

Performance Measure (total members = 631,780)	Sample Size	No. of Groups	No. of Components	No. of Records	Cost[a]
Optimal depression care	60	16	3	960	$11,500
Optimal diabetes care	80	27	5	2,160	$26,000
Optimal cardiovascular disease care	80	26	4	2,080	$25,000
Preventive care up to date (adults)	80	26	7	2,080	$25,000
Preventive care (children and adolescents)	60	27	13	1,620	$19,500
Tobacco assessment[b]	NA[c]	27	1	0	$0
Body mass index[b] assessment	NA[c]	27	1	0	$0
Total	360		34	8,900	$107,000

[a]The actual cost of chart review is under $12 per record.
[b]Tobacco assessment and body mass index measures are collected through chart review on the Preventive Care up to date samples, at minimal incremental costs. For a full list of measures, see the 2004 Clinical Indicators Report, available at http://www.healthpartners.com/files/23463.pdf.
[c]NA = not applicable.

TABLE C-3   Total Cost Estimate per Review for Commercial Plan
Members

Performance Measure (total commercial members = 531,186)	No. of Measures	No. of Records	Cost[a]
Childhood immunization	8	411	$5,000
Adolescent immunization	5	411	$5,000
Colorectal cancer screening	1	411	$5,000
Beta-blocker treatment after a heart attack	1	411	$5,000
Cholesterol screening after an acute event	3	411	$5,000
Comprehensive diabetes care	7	411	$5,000
Timeliness of prenatal and postnatal care	2	411	$5,000
Well-child visits in the first 15 months of life	7	411	$5,000
Well-child visits in the third, fourth, fifth, and sixth years of life	1	411	$5,000
Well-adolescent visits	1	411	$5,000
Total	36	4,110	$50,000

[a]The actual cost of chart review is under $12 per record.

BOX C-2   Key Lessons Learned from HealthPartners, Inc.

- Performance measurement is a powerful tool. It should be focused on what is important, not what is easy to measure.
- Measures must be clinically relevant to engage clinicians.
- Composite measures provide a better assessment of system performance than multiple single-service measures.
- Composite measures with aligned incentives engage medical groups in improving systems and implementing team-based care.
- Data displays should not waste a viewer's time. It should take no longer than 30 seconds to understand the "call to action."

---

and calculating and validating performance rates, training of abstractors, maintenance of measurement specifications, and development and publication of results. Medical group costs relate to record retrieval, internal measurement and reporting, and quality improvement changes.

Performance improvement has been demonstrated for all composite measures. Optimal diabetes care (hemoglobin $A_1c \leq 8$, LDL cholesterol <130, blood pressure <130/85, not smoking, and daily aspirin) increased from 6.2 percent in 2000 to 18.4 percent in 2004. Optimal coronary artery disease care (LDL cholesterol <130, blood pressure <140/90 for age $\leq$60 and <160/90 for age >60, not smoking, and daily aspirin) increased from 21.3 to 51.0 percent in the same time period. The overall preventive care up-to-date rate (percentage of members within the sample who receive all preventive screenings appropriate to the member's age and gender) rose from 44 percent in 1997 to over 70 percent in 2004.

HealthPartners' performance measurement focuses on medical groups and comparative public reporting. Many, though not all, medical groups also report individual provider performance on the same measures internally but not publicly. The goal of medical group performance reporting is to achieve improvements in individual patient care and overall population health. In addition to the incentive created by public reporting, medical groups are eligible for bonus payments when performance targets are met. Key lessons learned from HealthPartners, Inc., are summarized in Box C-2.

Case Study 2: Internal Medicine Solo Practice

James P. Wilson is an internal medicine provider in Fort Walton Beach, Florida, who owns a small solo practice serving approximately 1,800 patients, 35 percent of whom are Medicare beneficiaries accounting for two-thirds of his 5,200 patient visits annually. A significant number of

Dr. Wilson's patients are retired military personnel who receive treatment ranging from preventive to chronic disease services.

In 1999, Dr. Wilson began participating in a quality improvement consortium, Acceleration Translation of Research into Practice (ATRIP), sponsored by the Agency for Healthcare Research and Quality and designed to maximize physicians' capacity to provide high-quality care through the use of information technology. ATRIP provides routine performance data and suggests ways to improve the use of templates and other features in the EHR. It also provides quarterly practice reports showing data trends in care for measures based on clinical practice guidelines. Dr. Wilson receives practice reports on more than 80 measures, including the following: diabetes, heart disease, stroke, asthma, infectious diseases, mental health, substance abuse, immunizations, and inappropriate prescribing for the elderly.

Dr. Wilson was using EHRs and developing his own quality measures when he joined the ATRIP consortium. One of the services provided by ATRIP is periodic site visits from staff members of the Medical University of South Carolina to help in implementing national practice guidelines. Assistance is provided in the development of templates, measurement structures, and patient information handouts. Computer hardware and software support is purchased locally on a contractual basis.

In 1994, Dr. Wilson purchased the electronic medical record, including hardware and software, for $24,000. He has received periodic upgrades to the software. In the last 6 months, he has spent $20,000 to upgrade the

---

**BOX C-3   Key Lessons Learned from
an Internal Medicine Solo Practice**

- A solo physician can successfully introduce electronic medical records and a quality-of-care program.
- Introducing electronic medical records is not simple and requires perseverance.
- Gaining buy-in from staff and giving them routine feedback and encouragement are vital.
- The physician and staff must remain very flexible in the face of unexpected technical problems.
- A learning network such as ATRIP permits expansion of the capabilities of electronic medical records and performance measurement, allowing serial analysis and comparison with national benchmarks.
- A consortium with similar practice guidelines and goals provides support to sustain enthusiasm.
- Risk management is an important benefit of electronic medical records.

server and three workstations and to purchase patient education software. Software support costs approximately $350 per month. Local computer specialists charge $60/hour, for an average total cost of $4,000 per year. A part-time employee loads data on blood chemistries and scans incoming mail, radiology reports, and paper forms.

Performance measurement has been demonstrated for Dr. Wilson's practice among patients with diabetes and cardiovascular disease. For example, the percentage of diabetic patients with hemoglobin A_1c below 7 increased from 20 percent in 2002 to 55 percent in 2003. Patients suffering from coronary heart disease who received lipid-lowering medications increased from 66 percent in 2002 to 83 percent in 2003. Patients with coronary heart disease whose LDL cholesterol was measured increased from 42 percent in 1999 to 70 percent in 2000. Patients in the general population (not with a specific disease) with cholesterol measured in the past 5 years increased from 50 percent in 1999 to 65 percent in 2000. Key lessons learned from Dr. Wilson's solo practice are summarized in Box C-3.

Case Study 3: Prime Care Family Practice

Prime Care Family Practice is a small internal medicine clinic located in Clinton, Oklahoma, that serves approximately 4,500 patients annually. The practice consists of one internist, a licensed practical nurse, and a medical technician. To improve their efficiency and track their patients' chronic conditions, they adopted EHRs for their office 5 years ago. Prime Care works voluntarily with its state Quality Improvement Organization (QIO), Oklahoma Foundation for Medical Quality, to improve patient care.

Six years ago, Prime Care began its involvement in quality improvement by initiating data collection using paper-based records to qualify for a recognition program in diabetes care. Currently, the practice routinely submits Medicare administrative claims data tracking such measures as diabetes, mammography, adult immunizations, and cardiovascular disease. These performance data are collected annually by the Centers for Medicare and Medicaid Services, and subsequently reported to Prime Care by the state QIO. The QIO also helps Prime Care choose quality areas for improvement.

In addition, the Oklahoma Foundation for Medical Quality offers technical support to Prime Care through educational programs designed to improve internal quality by increasing work efficiency and to help the practice treat its diabetic patients more effectively. For example, all staff members at Prime Care attended several diabetes education programs with the QIO. The QIO does not charge Prime Care for technical or educational assistance designed to help improve work efficiency or diabetes care.

Prime Care has invested $30,000 in software and hardware over the past 3.5 years and pays a $350 per month maintenance charge for its Web-based software. The adoption of EHRs, along with the use of a wireless tablet computer, saved Prime Care's internist 4 to 5 hours per day in documentation time. Additional costs include staff salaries and hiring of part-time staff, such as college students, to scan laboratory reports into the medical record so they can be entered and read electronically.

Performance improvement has been demonstrated by Prime Care in the management of diabetes. Examples of improvement in the practice's diabetes measures from September 2003 to August 2004 include hemoglobin A_1c (12 percent), complete lipid testing in-house (36 percent), eye consults in chart (44 percent), tobacco cessation counseling (44 percent), patient self-management (54 percent), and administration of pneumonia vaccines (61 percent). Additionally, it was found that only 8 percent of eligible patients had been referred for a mammogram. To address this problem, the practice scheduled times for its patients to receive mammograms at the local hospital every Friday, resulting in a 100 percent referral rate.

The practice is expanding its quality improvement efforts based on its experience with diabetes to address other chronic care areas, such as pain management and depression, in collaboration with other organizations. Prime Care's use of EHRs has led to an increase in revenue due to increased work efficiency. The practice received the Oklahoma Outpatient Quality Award for 2 consecutive years from Oklahoma's QIO, and earned dual recognition for diabetes and heart/stroke care from the National Committee for Quality Assurance. Key lessons learned from Prime Care Family Practice are summarized in Box C-4.

**BOX C-4   Key Lessons Learned from
Prime Care Family Practice**

- Incorporating technology into a practice, regardless of its size, can increase the practice's revenue, patient satisfaction, and employee satisfaction and performance.
- Frustration should be expected when initiating implementation of EHRs, but it is the only effective approach to chronic disease management in the long run.
- Staff should be educated in how to help manage patients with chronic disease through conferences or other educational programs to reduce provider burden.
- The investment is worth it because paper chart expenses run higher than what is expected using EHRs, and an increase in practice revenues may result.
- There is no perfect system, so practices should expect to learn from mistakes.

Case Study 4: Rochester Individual Practice Association

Founded in 1977, Rochester Individual Practice Association (RIPA) is a large nonprofit physician organization in Rochester, New York, that contracts with managed care companies to provide professional medical services. RIPA membership includes group practices and individual clinicians representing approximately 3,000 practitioners, consisting of 900 primary care providers and encompassing more than 20 specialties. Currently, RIPA contracts with Excellus Blue Cross Blue Shield and serves 300,000 Blue Choice enrollees for acute and chronic conditions.

In 2002, RIPA created an individual physician profiling program, the Value of Care Plan, which reports performance at the individual provider level three times a year. Data are collected in three areas of measurement and weighted as follows: patient satisfaction (20 percent); quality of care, comparing practice patterns with recommended care (40 percent); and efficiency (40 percent). Measures are collected using administrative data, and validation testing has shown them to be 92–95 percent accurate. Measures are based on communitywide guidelines established by the Rochester Health Commission, a nonprofit community-based organization representing all insurers, physician organizations, large employers, and hospital systems in Rochester.

As a part of RIPA's profiling system, registry data are available for family medicine, practitioners, obstetricians, and cardiologists with patients who have coronary artery disease, diabetes mellitus, and asthma, as well as those eligible for mammography. Each provider receives the following registry data: rate of patient adherence to expected care, costs of patient care, comparative data against the specialty average, and a target rate set by communitywide guidelines.

Technical support for RIPA, encompassing information technology and data analysis, is provided by Excellus Health Plans. RIPA and Excellus medical directors evaluate and propose measures, analyze variation patterns, and educate and meet with practitioners. Provider buy-in was obtained through the program's explicit goal of reducing underuse, misuse, and overuse, moving toward a more balanced, data-driven incentive system.

The estimated annual cost to RIPA and Excellus for supporting the profiling program is approximately $1.2 million which includes staff costs. Additional expenses are accrued for time spent correcting the patient-specific data and for developing and implementing improvement programs. The overall cost is $0.33 PMPM.

RIPA demonstrates improvement in a practitioner's performance that ultimately benefits the entire practice. For example, an opthalmologist requested data to improve his efficiency index. The efficiency index measure is the ratio of actual episode costs to the specialty average episode costs for

---

**BOX C-5   Key Lessons Learned from
Rochester Individual Practice Association**

- Employ a process to introduce measures that engages practitioners in creating and reporting measures that make clinical sense from the start.
- Deliver understandable reports.
- Anticipate practitioner concerns and solicit and address them.
- Set realistic targets for evidence-based measures.
- Make measure specifications available.
- Develop the performance measurement program with the advice and guidance of multispecialty physician committees.
- Make data issues actionable by developing tools to identify and address unnecessary variations, and do not assume that outliers are poor performers.
- Incorporate an appeal process in pay-for-performance programs.
- Make sure the plan and payer executives have a long-term commitment to the program.
- Do not rush a program—test measures for reliability and accuracy, educate practitioners about what is expected, and evaluate the reporting of results. Try to introduce measures over a year.

---

a given case mix. An episode is the cluster of medical services received by a given patient for a particular condition. The ophthalmologist switched his prescriptions to generics; the reduction in his efficiency index was 10 percent, resulting in a savings of $90,000. As a result, in 2003 RIPA provided similar data and counsel to more than 50 practitioners. By 2005, the method described above had saved the plan $1.4 million.

RIPA provides financial rewards to physicians for improved patient satisfaction, quality of care, and efficiency. These rewards, totaling $15 million, are distributed to RIPA providers each year and equal $4.00 PMPM. A busy internist may receive additional performance-based payments of $5,000–$15,000. The data are reported privately to each provider to improve care and are not publicly reported. Key lessons learned from RIPA are summarized in Box C-5.

Case Study 5: GreenField Health

Founded in 2001, GreenField Health in Portland, Oregon, is a small primary care practice with four internists serving 1,600 patients. It provides care to adults with all levels of health care needs, from preventive care to care for chronic conditions. GreenField's practice is divided into two main functions: (1) serving its patient base, and (2) participating in research and development on the design of medical practice systems, with a focus on new ways of interacting with and delivering services to patients. Currently, GreenField incorporates performance measurement as a part of its routine clinical practice to improve patient care.

Data for performance measures are generated by claims data linked to EHRs. GreenField has also designed a large registry in Microsoft Access, separate from the EHRs, that represents 10 distinct diseases or preventive screenings. Registry performance measures are generated and collected at the practice level, with quarterly reports reflecting evidence-based guidelines being provided to each physician. For example, a report provides information on a given diabetic patient for the following performance measures: hemoglobin A_1c, LDL cholesterol, blood pressure, eye exam, foot exam, and urine microalbumin.

One of GreenField's physicians provides technical support and also serves as information technology director for performance measurement. Approximately 3 weeks was required for him to develop the current performance measurement system. Additionally, this physician spends 2 to 3 hours per week maintaining the system and producing data reports. Provider support for quality and performance improvement was built into the recruitment process, which favored providers experienced in quality and performance measurement practices. Since 70 percent of GreenField's patients have access to e-mail accounts, a secure e-mail reminder is generated automatically from the registry; for example, a patient receives a reminder to schedule a hemoglobin A_1c test or an overdue eye exam.

The above technical functions have up-front costs, as does the reporting of results following data collection to support quality improvement efforts. The estimated cost for the entire system approaches $40,000 over the last 3 years. As a result of the use of the system, work efficiency has increased for the practice. It is now possible to contact 80 percent of patients by phone or e-mail; only 20 percent of patient contacts require a visit, which requires more time-intensive services.

Trend data produced by GreenField's patient registry document the results of internal quality improvement efforts that occurred from March 2004 to January 2005. For example, there was an estimated average decrease of 33 percent in the rate of diabetic patients with end-stage renal disease, a complication of uncontrolled diabetes mellitus. The average LDL cholesterol count for diabetics decreased approximately 10 percent from January 2004 to January 2005. Other diabetes quality measures showed similar positive trends. Key lessons learned from GreenField Health Care are summarized in Box C-6.

BOX C-6   Key Lessons Learned from GreenField Health

- Develop data systems even though they are time-consuming and expensive because the technology makes quality improvement feasible.
- Using internal data systems collect and manage data, with integrity to ensure that providers' performance information is valid.
- Do not expect that it will be easy to use data for quality improvement in practice. Having an infrastructure in place is necessary to improve identified deficiencies in care.
- Accept that performance will never be perfect.

Case Study 6: Community Medicine Associates

Community Medicine Associates (CMA) is a medium-sized primary care practice located in San Antonio, Texas, in which approximately 60–70 percent of the patient population is uninsured and lower-income. The practice consists of 33 primary care physicians and 11 midlevel nurse practitioners and physician assistants who provide care to more than 180,000 patients. Staff are hired and employed by the local Bexar County hospital district, which is connected to the larger university health system. CMA's mission is to care for county residents regardless of income level or insurance status.

CMA collects performance measurement data based on measures and criteria specified by the U.S. Preventive Services Task Force (USPSTF), a panel of experts in primary and preventive care that systematically reviews and develops recommendations for clinical preventive services.[1] CMA's preventive care and quality review committees convene annually to review and set performance measurement criteria guided by USPSTF practice goals. All measures are based on chart review, with the exception of adult immunizations, for which data are collected by a statewide registry. Each quarter, five quality measures—influenza vaccination, hemoglobin A_1c, systolic blood pressure, foot exam, and patient satisfaction—are reported to each physician group.

Technical assistance, such as that needed for changes and updates to CMA's registry database (created in Microsoft Access), is provided by a technician employed by the university health system. Chart abstraction is

---

[1]U.S. Preventive Services Task Force. 1996. *Guide to Clinical Preventive Services.* Baltimore, MD: Williams & Wilkins.

performed by a nurse who is the quality assurance coordinator for the practice. Physician support for performance measurement was greatly enhanced by CMA's quality incentive program. Bonuses involve a weighting scheme whereby a provider group receives a score for each quality indicator, ranging from 2 (highest level of care) to −2 (worst level of care).

CMA's estimated cost to implement performance measurement by chart review totals $14,330 per year. The quality assurance coordinator examines charts on a quarterly basis for more than 30 providers, reviewing a minimum of 15 charts per quality indicator. The overall cost for data collection is $2.76 PMPM, which encompasses staff salaries (including the cost of the medical director's time), database maintenance, and support costs.

Table C-4 shows CMA's improvement on performance measures for patients with heart disease and diabetes mellitus. For example, patients with congestive heart failure who were prescribed an ACE inhibitor during 2002–2004 increased by 10 percent. Similarly, the percentage of patients with coronary artery disease who were prescribed aspirin increased by 10 percent from 2002 to 2004. For diabetic patients, annual hemoglobin A_1c testing increased 6 percent from 2002 to 2004, while annual microalbuminuria testing increased by 13 percent over the same period. The greatest increase in performance for diabetes patients was a 32 percent increase in those having LDL cholesterol levels below 100 from 2002 to 2004.

Bonuses earned can amount to up to $5,000 per quarter, or $20,000 per year. The bonus structure is based primarily on productivity and billing

TABLE C-4 Community Medicine Associates' Illustrative Measures Improvement in Performance Measures for Patients with Heart Disease and Diabetes Mellitus

Measure	2002 (%)	2003 (%)	2004 (%)
Patients with congestive heart failure prescribed ACE inhibitor	87	97	97
Patients with coronary artery disease prescribed aspirin	74	74	84
Patients prescribed beta-blocker after myocardial infarction	81	79	100
Diabetes mellitus patients with annual hemoglobin A_1c test	91	91	97
Diabetes mellitus patients receiving annual microalbuminuria testing	71	78	84
Diabetes mellitus patients with LDL cholesterol below 100	58	65	90

BOX C-7 Key Lessons Learned from Community Medicine Associates

- Be sure to properly align economic incentives with performance measurement to motivate providers to aim for quality improvement.
- Set incentives at a high enough level to engage providers in the program. For example, the CMA bonus structure allows providers to increase their salary up to 15 percent per year.

---

compliance (70 percent), which rest entirely on billing correctly and not overbilling patients for services. The remaining 30 percent of the bonus covers patient satisfaction (10 percent), quality indicators (10 percent), and unit cost-efficiency (10 percent). Key lessons learned from CMA are summarized in Box C-7.

Case Study 7: North Texas Medical Group

North Texas Medical Group is a small primary care clinic located in Plano, Texas, serving approximately 14,000 patients annually. The practice consists of six providers who are board certified in internal medicine and family practice. Additional support staff include medical assistants, a physician assistant, and a nurse practitioner. North Texas Medical Group serves its patients' health needs, from preventive to chronic disease care.

Three years ago, the practice adopted EHRs for billing compliance as well as quality improvement purposes. The practice relies heavily on clinical guidelines for measuring its performance; when standard measures are not available, it relies on clinical judgment regarding best treatment practices to apply to its patient population. Data are collected using EHRs for the following measures: diabetes, hypertension, cholesterol, and use of the high-risk medication coumadin. Providers in the group receive feedback on their performance based on these measures on a monthly basis.

North Texas Medical Group designed its practice around EHRs and hired providers who were comfortable working in a technology-driven practice. Two full-time information technology staff were hired to manage the practice's databases, thus allowing providers to focus on patient care as opposed to technical issues. These technicians input laboratory data into database elements that can be read by EHRs.

The total investment made by the practice to date is approximately $250,000 for hardware and software. The estimated annual cost for the two technicians is $110,000. Additional costs include software support

---

**BOX C-8   Key Lessons Learned from
North Texas Medical Group**

- Incorporating technology into practice helps practitioners provide better care to patients.
- There is more control over patient data when the data are collected within the practice, instead of by outside sources. This control allows greater focus on quality improvement efforts specific to the care of patients within the practice.
- There may not be an economic balance between initial investments in technology and the consequences of not implementing EHRs; however, providers within the practice will be satisfied that they are providing the best possible care.

($40,000/year) and providers' time spent designing reports and undertaking quality improvement efforts.

An innovative use of performance measurement by the North Texas Medical Group is improved monitoring of blood testing for patients prescribed coumadin. The measure is the number of patients prescribed coumadin without blood test data in the preceding 30 days. Patients should be monitored for the amount of coumadin they receive because if the amount is not managed properly, the drug could prove fatal. By using its EHRs, the practice was able to demonstrate its ability to monitor the drug and achieve a modest improvement on the measure—from having 5 of 48 patients prescribed coumadin without blood tests in 2002 to 0 of 71 patients in 2004. Additionally, the practice achieved a 6 percent improvement from 2002 to 2004 in the number of patients diagnosed with diabetes, hypertension, dyslipidemia, or coronary disease who had their cholesterol measured in the preceding year.

North Texas Medical Group does not publicly report its data and uses its performance measurement activities exclusively for internal quality improvement purposes. Even though pay for performance is not currently a part of the practice, a small disincentive is used for the physician with the lowest percentage of treatment goals met each month—taking the other providers out to lunch. Key lessons learned from the North Texas Medical Group are summarized in Box C-8.

CASE STUDY QUESTIONS

The Institute of Medicine Performance Measures subcommittee is currently seeking examples of "real-life" case studies from entities who have successfully implemented performance measurement programs in physician practices. We are particularly interested in learning how more cumbersome measures (such as those requiring either chart review or registries) have been successfully implemented in ways that are acceptable to physicians while ensuring complete and valid data collection. We want to hear how you became successful and at what cost. Your organization has been identified as an innovator in this field. We would like to respectfully request from you, if willing, a succinct narrative of your initiative (no more than 2 pages single spaced) describing your implementation process, specifically addressing as many of the following questions as you are able to complete without major effort.

1. What kinds of data have you used for your performance measures in physician practices (i.e., claims data, chart review, paper-based registries, computer based registries, full EHR)?
2. Would you be able to give a brief "real-life" description of how one or more practices adopted chart review based measures? Paper-based registries for reporting measures?
3. How was the data collection system validated (i.e. field testing, provider engagement, feedback loop for refinement)?
4. What was the level of technical support that needed to be provided to physicians' offices?
5. How did you obtain provider buy-in (i.e., cultural and attitudinal change)?
6. What was the cost to individual practices (particularly for smaller practices less than 5 physicians) for implementing the performance measures that required either chart review or in-office registries?
7. What was the cost estimate to your organization as a whole for data collection? (Ideally this could be estimated "per-member per month" or per year.)
8. Can you provide illustrative examples of observed improvement?
9. Has improved performance been linked to any payment incentives? If yes, how?
10. Are data currently publicly reported?
11. Overall, what were your key "lessons learned"?

Appendix D

Ten Design Principles

Principle 1: Comprehensive Measurement

A performance measurement system should advance the core purpose of the health care system and foster improvements in all six quality aims identified in the *Quality Chasm* report (IOM, 2001): safety, effectiveness, patient-centeredness, timeliness, efficiency, and equity. The committee endorses the following statement of purpose, proposed by the President's Advisory Committee on Consumer Protection and Quality in the Health Care Industry:

> The purpose of the health care system must be to continuously reduce the impact and burden of illness, injury, and disability, and to improve the health and functioning of the people of the United States.

Principle 2: Evidence-Based Goals and Measures

A performance measurement system should be guided by a comprehensive set of evidence-based goals for improvement, where appropriate. The National Quality Coordination Board (NQCB) should identify explicit health care goals for the nation, assess progress toward achieving these goals; and continually update and modify the goals as circumstances, information, and needs change. As a starting point, the NQCB should adopt the priority areas for quality improvement identified by the Institute of Medicine (IOM, 2003), as endorsed and expanded by the National Quality Forum (2004), as national goals, and specify measures corresponding to these goals that encompass the care of patients across the lifespan (e.g., staying healthy, getting better, living with chronic illness, and coping with end of life) (FACCT, 1997).

Principle 3: Longitudinal Measurement

Standardized performance measures should characterize health and health care of a patient both within and across settings and over time. The NQCB should identify standardized measures that characterize the health and quality of care received by both individuals and populations. In general, the measures should not vary by type of health care provider or setting, but should characterize care across as well as within sites and settings. The set of standardized measures should provide the information needed to assess progress toward achieving the six quality aims and the national goals.

Principle 4: Supportive of Multiple Uses and Stakeholders

A national system for performance measurement and reporting should provide information for multiple uses, including provider-led improvement efforts, public reporting, payment and benefits design, and population health initiatives. This system should produce useful information for three purposes:

- *Accountability*—Information should be available to assist stakeholders in making choices about providers, including patients identifying a clinician, hospital, or other provider from which to seek services; purchasers and health plans selecting providers to include in their health insurance networks; and quality oversight organizations making accreditation and certification decisions.
- *Quality improvement*—The information provided should be of value to stakeholders responsible for improving the quality of care, including clinicians and administrators and governing board members of health care organizations.
- *Population health*—The information should be useful for stakeholders making decisions about access to services (e.g., public insurance benefits and coverage); those involved in communitywide programs and efforts to address racial and ethnic disparities and promote healthy behaviors; and public officials responsible for disease surveillance and health protection.

Principle 5: Measurement Intrinsic to Care

Performance measurement should be intrinsic to the care process. For most standardized measures (e.g., health care processes and some outcome measures), the data generated to calculate measures should be byproducts of the patient care process and should reside within an electronic health record system. For example, the data required to calculate standardized measures for assessing the quality of patient care provided to diabetics (e.g., cholesterol and hemoglobin A_1c levels) should be captured as a part of patient care encounters. This approach has several advantages: (1) it allows for the development of computerized decision-support systems (e.g., prompts to providers and patients that the patient is due for an annual retinal exam); (2) it enables more immediate calculation of measures and feedback to providers on performance; and (3) it minimizes the burden associated with special data collection processes. These data reflect the health care delivery system; in and of themselves they do not adequately address population and public health.

Principle 6: A Central Role for the Patient's Voice

The performance measurement system should also include direct reports and ratings from patients and family caregivers. Patients need a voice in the process of selecting measures and designing public reports. The input of patients and family caregivers should reflect their viewpoints on the quality and functionality of the care received. Caregivers' perceptions of the quality of care provided should also be incorporated into the measurement system.

Principle 7: Individual-, Population-, and Systems-Based Measurement

Measurement and measures should assess the health and health care of both individuals and populations and the many systems within which care is provided. A national system for performance measurement and reporting should include both measures of the quality of care provided by the personal health care system and measures of population health, health behaviors, and unmet health needs. The measure set should include measures of access and unmet service needs for the entire population of a community and for specific groups most likely to experience access limitations because of an inability to pay; high levels of uninsurance or underinsurance; racial, ethnic, class, cultural, and linguistic barriers; or geographic impediments. The measure set should also include measures of the efficiency of the local health system, such as resource use compared with that of other communities.

Principle 8: Shared Accountability

Measurement should not be constrained by the absence of a current, identifiable, single responsible agent. A national system should measure processes and outcomes of care important to patients and communities. Measurement should foster individual and shared accountability for health system performance. When no responsible agent can be identified, shared accountability by all agents within the health care system should be presumed, and responsible stewardship encouraged and induced. In many settings, this will require significant restructuring of how care is currently delivered.

Principle 9: A Learning System

A performance measurement system should be a learning system, continually evaluating its own performance and advancing knowledge regarding performance measurement. A national system for performance measurement and reporting should advance knowledge of (1) how environmental levers, such as purchasing, pay for performance, and quality oversight can best be used to motivate quality improvement; (2) the most effective strategies for redesigning care processes, including methods for transferring knowledge, implementing information technology, and forming effective care teams; and (3) the extent to which all quality efforts lead to improvements in the six quality aims.

Principle 10: Independent and Sustainable

A performance measurement and reporting system should be continually enhanced and financed in a way that ensures its independence and sustainability. This system should be dynamic and should evolve based on careful evaluation of its impact and advances in the science base. It should be adequately supported by both public- and private-sector stakeholders.

REFERENCES

FACCT (Foundation for Accountability). 1997. *The FACCT Consumer Information Framework: Comparative Information for Better Health Care Decisions.* [Online]. Available: *http://www.facct.org/information.html* [accessed June 4, 2002].
IOM (Institute of Medicine). 2001. *Crossing the Quality Chasm: A New Health System for the 21st Century.* Washington, DC: National Academy Press.
IOM. 2003. *Priority Areas for National Action: Transforming Health Care Quality.* Adams K, Corrigan JM, eds. Washington, DC: The National Academies Press.
National Quality Forum. 2004. *National Priorities for Healthcare Quality Measurement and Reporting.* [Online]. Available: *http://www.qualityforum.org/webprioritiespublic.pdf* [accessed January 19, 2005].

Appendix E

Methodology and Analytic Frameworks

The committee's selection of performance measures began with identifying leading performance measure sets[1] and classifying these measures within nationally endorsed frameworks for quality assessment and evaluation of health system performance. Table E-1 presents the frameworks that informed the committee's deliberations on the selection of performance measures. These analytic frameworks, briefly described below, are as follows: (1) Donabedian's model for assessing quality; (2) the Institute of Medicine's (IOM) six aims for quality improvement in health care; (3) the Foundation for Accountability's (FACCT) domains of consumer needs for health care; (4) the IOM's priority areas for national action, as adapted by the National Quality Forum (NQF); and (5) the Centers for Medicare and Medicaid Services' (CMS') priority chronic conditions for adults 65 and older.

The Donabedian Model

Donabedian's (1988) classic paradigm for assessing quality of care is based on a three-component approach—structure, process, and outcomes

---

[1]The committee defined leading performance measure sets as (1) those currently being used for public reporting, pay-for-performance, or quality improvement efforts at the national or regional level; (2) those recognized by leading national stakeholder groups; and (3) those whose owner had a rigorous process in place for assessing validity and reliability, as well as a mechanism for updating or retiring measures.

TABLE E-1 Analytic Frameworks Used by the Committee

Analytic Frameworks	Framework Components
Donabedian	Structure → Process → Outcomes
IOM six aims	Safe, effective, patient-centered, timely, efficient, and equitable
FACCT domains of consumer needs	Staying healthy, getting better, living with illness or disability, and coping with end of life
IOM priority areas as expanded by NQF[a]	*Infrastructure:* information technology (standardization and capacity); patient safety (including but not limited to health care–acquired infections and medication management and adherence)
	Processes of care: care coordination and communication, care at the end of life (focus on congestive heart failure and chronic obstructive pulmonary disease), immunizations (all ages), pain management, self-management/health literacy
	Health care conditions: asthma; cancer; pneumonia; depression; diabetes; children with special health care needs; frailty associated with old age (preventing falls and pressure ulcers, maximizing function, and developing advanced-care plans); hypertension; ischemic heart disease; kidney disease; mental illness; obesity; pregnancy, childbirth, and newborn care; stroke; and tobacco dependence (prevention and treatment)
CMS priority chronic conditions for adults 65 and over	Ischemic heart disease; cancer; chronic obstructive pulmonary disease/asthma; stroke, including hypertension; arthritis and nontraumatic joint disorders; diabetes mellitus; dementia, including Alzheimer's disease; pneumonia; peptic ulcer/dyspepsia; and depression and other mood disorders

[a]NQF endorsed the IOM's original 20 priority areas, and added the areas of kidney disease and information technology infrastructure.

(See Figure E-1). Donabedian's model proposes that each component has a direct influence on the next, as represented by the arrows in the following schematic (Donabedian, 1980):

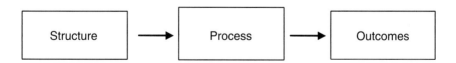

FIGURE E-1 Donabedian's model.

Structure refers to the attributes of the settings in which providers deliver health care, including material resources (e.g., electronic health records), human resources (e.g., staff expertise), and organizational structure (e.g., hospitals vs. clinics). For example, a cardiologist may use a disease registry to track whether a patient with cardiovascular disease is receiving drugs for lowering cholesterol.

Process of care denotes what is actually done to the patient in the giving and receiving of care. Building on the example above, the provider could review whether an eligible patient has been placed on an angiotensin-converting enzyme inhibitor to help prevent future heart attacks.

Health outcomes are the direct result of a patient's health status as a consequence of contact with the health care system. In the above example, the patient's receiving the preventive medications mentioned above could decrease the chance of dying from a heart attack.

IOM's Six Aims

The report *Crossing the Quality Chasm: A New Health System for the 21st Century* (IOM, 2001) calls for national action to address serious and well-documented quality shortcomings in the U.S. health care system. The report proposes a restructuring of the health care delivery system so that Americans will consistently receive the quality of care they deserve. To this end, the report recommends the adoption of six quality aims for improvement, defined as follows:

- *Safe*—avoiding injuries to patients from the care that is intended to help them
- *Effective*—providing services based on scientific knowledge to all who could benefit and refraining from providing services to those not likely to benefit (avoiding underuse and overuse, respectively)
- *Patient-centered*—providing care that is respectful of and responsive to individual patient preferences, needs, and values and ensuring that patient values guide all clinical decisions
- *Timely*—reducing waits and sometimes harmful delays for both those who receive and those who give care
- *Efficient*—avoiding waste, including waste of equipment, supplies, ideas, and energy
- *Equitable*—providing care that does not vary in quality because of personal characteristics such as gender, ethnicity, geographic location, and socioeconomic status.

FACCT's Consumer Information Framework

FACCT, closed in 2004, was a nonprofit organization committed to measuring health care quality and communicating the results to consumers in a meaningful way (FACCT, 1997). In 1997, FACCT developed a customer-centered framework for quality measurement that is based on what consumers conveyed as their health care needs across the lifespan, encompassing the following four domains:

- *Staying healthy*—helping people avoid illness and stay healthy through preventive care, reduction of health risks, early detection of illness, and education
- *Getting better*—helping people recover when they are sick or injured through appropriate treatment and follow-up
- *Living with illness or disability*—helping people with ongoing, chronic conditions (such as diabetes or asthma) take care of themselves, control symptoms, avoid complications, and maintain daily activities
- *Coping with the end of life*—caring for people and their families when needs change dramatically because of disability or terminal illness, with comprehensive services, caregiver support, and hospice care.

IOM's Priority Areas

The *Quality Chasm* report (IOM, 2001) recommended that no fewer than 15 priority areas be identified as the focus of quality improvement efforts, based on the premise that a limited number of chronic conditions account for the majority of the nation's health care burden and resource use. It was argued that by focusing on a discrete set of common chronic conditions, sizable improvements in the quality of care could be made over the next decade (IOM, 2003). An IOM committee was formed to respond to this recommendation. The committee selected 20 clinical priority areas on the basis of three overarching criteria (IOM, 2003):

- *Impact*—the extent of the burden—disability, mortality, and economic costs—imposed by a condition within the populations
- *Improvability*—the extent of the gap between current practice and evidence-based best practice and the likelihood that the gap could be closed and conditions improved through change in an area, and the opportunity to achieve improvements in the six quality aims
- *Inclusiveness*—the relevance of an area to a broad range of individuals with regard to age, gender, socioeconomic status, and ethnicity/race (equity); the generalizability of associated quality improvement strategies across

the spectrum of health care conditions; and the capability for change across a range of health care settings and providers.

NQF subsequently added two areas to the IOM's original list of 20—kidney disease and information technology infrastructure—and endorsed the resulting list of 22 areas.

CMS's Priority Chronic Conditions

A collaborative effort involving CMS, the Agency for Healthcare Research and Quality (AHRQ), the Food and Drug Administration, and other stakeholders recently identified 10 priority conditions (listed in Table E-1) that account for the majority of disease burden and service utilization for the Medicare population aged 65 and older (AHRQ, 2004). AHRQ has launched a $15 million initiative, with funding authorized under the Medicare Prescription Drug, Improvement, and Modernization Act of 2003, supporting research to investigate the effectiveness of interventions targeting these conditions, including prescription drugs. As a result of these efforts, CMS hopes ultimately to help providers and patients make more informed health care decisions.

COMMITTEE'S PROCESS FOR SELECTING PERFORMANCE MEASURES

The committee's analysis involved a series of steps that are listed below sequentially, although the actual process was far more iterative than linear:

1. Map measures from leading performance measure sets to a two-dimensional matrix.
2. Assess the current state of performance measurement and identify gaps.
3. Review measures in the matrix against the priority clinical areas.

Map Existing Measures to Matrix

To guide the selection of performance measures, the committee adopted a matrix building upon the IOM six aims and the FACCT domains representing patients' needs across the lifespan, as described above (FACCT, 1999). More than 800 measures of structure, process, and outcomes from more than 50 leading measurement sets were pooled and mapped against this two-dimensional matrix. When appropriate, the individual measures were maintained within the context of the original measure sets.

Assess Current State of Performance Measurement and Identify Gaps

The assignment of individual measures to matrix cells facilitated assessment of the current state of performance measurement and the identification of major gaps in existing measurement sets. The committee found that the majority of currently available measures evaluated effectiveness of care largely in acute or ambulatory settings. Conversely, there was a particular paucity of measures addressing the IOM aims of equity, efficiency, and patient-centeredness.

Review Measures Against Priority Clinical Areas

Following the initial mapping exercise, the committee took the additional step of checking against the 22 priority clinical areas to ensure the comprehensiveness of the performance measures now populating the matrix. Although some of these areas—such as pregnancy, childbirth, and newborn care—involve individuals outside the traditional boundaries of the Medicare population, the committee concluded that the recommended measurement system should represent the entire lifespan and spectrum of care to achieve the downstream goal of healthier older adults. The committee was also diligent in ensuring that the top chronic conditions affecting Medicare beneficiaries aged 65 and over were given due consideration.

Limitations to the Matrix

The matrix was a useful tool for cataloging leading performance measurement sets and identifying gaps in needed areas. However, the committee's analytic approach has some limitations. Assigning the measures to only one category or cell in the matrix often involved arbitrary judgment, since many of the measures, such as pain control, were applicable to multiple settings of care. Additionally, while most process and outcome measures fit neatly into the predefined categories of the matrix, some measures did not. An additional column was necessary to include structural measures characterizing the care system, such as a disease registry system. Thus enhanced, the matrix served as a functional starting point to help inform the committee's deliberations.

REFERENCES

AHRQ (Agency for Healthcare Research and Quality). 2004. *List of Priority Conditions for Research under Medicare Modernization Act Released.* [Online]. Available: *http://www.ahrq.gov/news/press/pr2004/mmapr.htm* [accessed February 1, 2005].

Donabedian A. 1980. Methods for deriving criteria for assessing the quality of medical care. *Medical Care Review* 37(7):653–698.

Donabedian A. 1988. The quality of care. How can it be assessed? *Journal of the American Medical Association* 260(12):1743–1748.

FACCT (Foundation for Accountability). 1997. *The FACCT Consumer Information Framework: Comparative Information for Better Health Care Decisions.* [Online]. Available: *http://www.facct.org/information.html* [accessed June 4, 2002].

FACCT. 1999. *FACCT: Quality Measures.* [Online]. Available: *http://www.facct.org/facct/site/facct/facct/Measures* [accessed September 17, 2004].

IOM (Institute of Medicine). 2001. *Crossing the Quality Chasm: A New Health System for the 21st Century.* Washington, DC: National Academy Press.

IOM. 2003. *Priority Areas for National Action: Transforming Health Care Quality.* Adams K, Corrigan JM, eds. Washington, DC: The National Academies Press.

Appendix F

Commissioned Paper

Improving the Quality of Quality Measurement

John D. Birkmeyer, Eve A. Kerr, and Justin B. Dimick

INTRODUCTION

With growing recognition that the quality of medical care varies widely across physicians, hospitals, and health systems, good measures of performance are in high demand. Patients and their families are looking to make informed decisions about where and by whom to get their care (Lee et al., 2004). Employers and payers need measures on which to base their contracting decisions and pay for performance initiatives (Galvin and Milstein, 2002). Finally, clinical leaders need measures that can help them identify "best practices" and guide their quality improvement efforts. An ever broadening array of performance measures is being developed to meet these different needs.

However, there remains considerable uncertainty about which measures are most useful. Current measures are remarkably heterogeneous, encompassing different elements of health care structure, process of care, and patient outcomes. Although each of these three types of performance measures has its unique strengths, each is also associated with conceptual, methodological, and/or practical problems. The clinical context (e.g., cancer screening vs. high risk surgery) is obviously an important consideration in weighing the strengths and weaknesses of different measures. So too is the underlying purpose of performance measurement. Measures that work well when the primary intent is to steer patients to the best hospitals or doctors (selective referral) may not be optimal for quality improvement purposes, and vice versa.

There is also disagreement about when a performance measure is "good enough." Most would agree that a measure is good enough when acting upon it results in a net improvement in quality. Thus, the direct benefits of implementing a particular measure cannot be outweighed by the indirect harms, e.g., resource and opportunity costs, antagonizing providers, incentivizing perverse behaviors, or negatively affecting other domains of quality. Although simple in concept, measuring these benefits and harm is often difficult and heavily influenced by which group—patients, payers, or providers—is doing the accounting.

Expanding on other recent reviews of performance measurement (Bird et al., 2005; Birkmeyer et al., 2004; Landon et al., 2003), this paper provides an overview of measures most commonly used to profile the quality of physicians, hospitals, or systems and their main limitations. We describe the trade-offs associated with structure, process, and outcome measures (see Table F-1). We address the question of "how good is good enough?" and make the case that the answer depends on the purpose of measurement—quality improvement or selective referral. Finally, we consider which measures are ready (or almost ready) for implementation right now and a research agenda aimed at improving performance measurement for the future.

OVERVIEW OF CURRENT MEASURES

A large number of performance measures has been developed for assessing health care quality. Tables F-2 and F-3 include a representative list of commonly used quality indicators and measurement sets. Almost all of these measures have been either endorsed by leading organizations in quality measurement and/or already applied in hospital accreditation, pay for performance, or public reporting efforts. A more exhaustive list of performance measures can be found on the Agency for Healthcare Research and Quality's (AHRQ's) National Quality Measures Clearinghouse Web site (www.qualitymeasures.ahrq.gov). Although the measures could be sorted on other dimensions, we consider them below according to whether they focus on ambulatory care (preventive care and chronic disease management) or hospital-based care (including surgery).

Ambulatory Care

Although not the only measurement set in ambulatory care, the Health Plan Employer Data and Information Set (HEDIS), developed by the National Committee on Quality Assurance is by far the most familiar (Table F-2). HEDIS measures focus largely on processes of care relating to preventive and other primary care services, but they also include measures of health plan stability, access to care, and use of services. The National Quality Forum (NQF) is endorsing a set of ambulatory care quality indicators devel-

TABLE F-1 Primary Strengths and Limitations of Structure, Process, and Outcome Measures

	Structure	Process	Outcomes
Examples	Procedure volume, intensivists managed ICUs	Majority of HEDIS performance measures for ambulatory care	Risk-adjusted mortality rates for CABG from state or national registries
Strengths	Expedient, inexpensive Efficient—one measure may relate to several outcomes More predictive of subsequent performance than other measures for some procedures	Reflect care that patients actually receive—buy-in from providers Directly actionable for quality improvement activities Don't need risk adjustment for many measures Positive "spillover" effect to other processes	Face validity Measurement alone may improve outcomes (i.e., Hawthorne effect)
Limitations	Limited number of measures, none for ambulatory care Generally not actionable Don't reflect performance of individual hospitals or providers	Sample size constraints for condition-specific measures May be confounded by patient compliance and other factors Variable extent to which process measures link to important patient outcomes Levels of metabolic control (e.g., intermediate outcomes) may not reflect quality of care	Sample size constraints Concerns about risk adjustment with administrative data Expense of clinical data collection

oped by other organizations based on the NQF Consensus Development Process (CDP). The set of measures under consideration includes many of the HEDIS measures, but also includes a longer list of more clinically relevant processes of care. These latter measures were developed with input from the American Medical Association's Physician Consortium for Performance Improvement in an effort to make them more clinically meaningful. Additionally, the U.S. Department of Veterans Affairs uses a set of measures that expand upon HEDIS to regularly and intensively monitor quality of ambulatory (and some inpatient) care (Kizer et al., 2000).

TABLE F-2 Quality Indicators for Ambulatory Care from the 2005 Version of the Health Plan Employer Data and Information Set (HEDIS)

	Measure
Immunization	
Childhood	Percentage of 2-year-olds with complete childhood immunizations
Adolescent	Percentage of 13-year-olds with complete adolescent immunizations
Acute Illness	
Upper respiratory tract infection	Percentage of children 3 months to 18 years with a diagnosis of upper respiratory infection who were not given antibiotics on or after 3 days from the diagnosis
Pharyngitis	Percentage of children 2 to 18 years old diagnosed with pharyngitis and given an antibiotic who received group A streptococcus testing
Screening	
Colorectal cancer	Percentage of adults 51 to 80 years old who had appropriate colorectal cancer screening
Breast cancer	Percentage of women aged 52 to 69 years old who had a mammogram within the last 2 years
Cervical cancer	Percentage of women aged 21 to 64 years old who had a Pap smear within the last 3 years
Chlamydia	Percentage of sexually active women aged 16 to 35 years old who had chlamydia testing within the last year
Glaucoma	Percentage of adults 65 years or older who received glaucoma screening in the past 2 years
Chronic Disease Management	
Hypertension	Percentage of patients with adequate blood pressure control (systolic <140 and diastolic <90)
Heart attack	1. Percentage of adults (35 years or older) discharged after heart attack with a beta-blocker 2. Percentage of adults (35 years or older) after heart attack still on a beta-blocker at 6 months
Hypercholesterolemia	Percentage of adult patients (18 to 75 years old) on cholesterol lowering medication after discharge for heart attack, coronary bypass surgery, or percutaneous coronary intervention
Diabetes	Percentage of patients age 18 through 75 with diabetes (type 1 or type 2) who met each of the recommended measures during the previous year (presented as 7 different measures): 1. HbA_1c checked 2. HbA_1c under control (<9.0%) 3. Lipid profile performed 4. Lipids controlled: LDL <130 5. Lipids controlled: LDL <100 6. Dilated retinal exam 7. Renal function checked
Asthma	Percentage of patients with persistent asthma 5 to 56 years old who are prescribed appropriate long-term medications (inhaled corticosteroids preferred but alternatives accepted)
Mental Illness	Percentage of patients 6 years and older who were hospitalized for mental illness and received appropriate follow up within 30 days

TABLE F-2 continued

	Measure
Depression	Appropriate antidepressant medication management for depression patients 18 or older: 1. Percentage of patients with 3 follow-up contacts during the 12-week Acute Treatment Phase 2. Percentage of patients on antidepressant medication for the entire 12-week Acute Treatment Phase 3. Percentage of patients who remained on treatment for a full 6-month trial
Low back pain	Percentage of patients aged 18 to 50 years old who received imaging studies for low back pain (Plain X-ray, CT scan, or MRI)
Smoking cessation	Percentage of smokers 18 or older who received smoking cessation advice
Influenza	Percentage of adults 50–64 years old who received the influenza vaccine
Physical activity level	Percentage of patients age 65 or older who were asked and advised about increasing physical activity in the prior year
Overall summary	Medicare Health Outcomes Survey
Access to Care	
Preventative/ambulatory services	Percentage of adults who received a preventative/ambulatory visit during the past 3 years
Primary care	1. Percentage of children aged 1 year to 6 years with a visit during the past year 2. Percentage of children aged 7 to 19 with a visit during the past 2 years.
Prenatal and postpartum care	1. Percentage of women who received a prenatal visit during the first trimester 2. Percentage of women who received a postpartum visit within 21 to 56 days
Dental care	Percentage of patients with a dental visit in the past year
Alcohol and drug dependence	1. Percentage of patients with a diagnosis of dependency with inpatient or outpatient treatment 2. Percentage who initiated treatment (intermediate step)
Claims timeliness	Percentage of all claims for the last year paid or denied within 30 days of receipt
Call answer timeliness	Percentage of calls during business hours answered with a live voice within 30 seconds
Call abandonment	Percentage of calls made during the prior year abandoned by a caller before meeting a live voice
Satisfaction with the Experience of Care	
Adult satisfaction	Consumer Assessment of Health Plans (CAHPS®) 3.0H Adult Survey
Child satisfaction	Consumer Assessment of Health Plans (CAHPS®) 3.0H Child Survey
Practitioner turnover	Percentage of physicians leaving the health plan each year
Years in business/ size of plan	Number of years in business and the total health plan membership

(continued on next page)

TABLE F-2   continued

	Measure
Use of Services	
Well-child visits	1. Percentage of children with a well-child visit during the first 15 months of life
	2. Percentage of 3-, 4-, 5-, and 6-year old children with a well-child visit within the past year
Adolescent well-care visit	Percentage of 12- to 21-year-olds with at least one primary care or OB/GYN visit during the past year
Frequency of procedures	Frequency of selected procedures that have wide regional variation
Inpatient utilization	Number of admissions for general hospital acute care
Ambulatory care	Number of ambulatory medical care visits
Inpatient utilization	Number of admissions for nonacute care (skilled nursing facilities, rehabilitation, transitional care, and respite)
Postpartum care	Number of discharges and average length of stay postpartum
Births and newborns	Number of births and average length of stay for newborns
Mental health utilization	1. Number of inpatient discharges and average length of stay
	2. Percentage of members receiving services
Outpatient drug utilization	Age-specific estimates of average numbers and cost of prescription drugs for each member per month
Chemical dependency utilization	1. Number of inpatient discharges and average length of stay
	2. Percentage of members receiving alcohol and other drug services

TABLE F-3   Performance Measures for Hospital-Based Care

	Endorser		Current Users		
	NQF	AHRQ	JCAHO	CMS	Leapfrog
Independent of Specific Diagnosis					
Critically ill patients					
Board-certified intensivist staffing					X
Medical or surgical inpatients					
Computerized physician order entry					X
Any surgical procedure					
Appropriate antibiotic prophylaxis (correct choice; given 1 hour pre-operatively; discontinued within 24 hours)	X		X	X	
Medical Diagnoses					
Acute myocardial infarction					
Smoking cessation counseling	X		X	X	

TABLE F-3 continued

	Endorser		Current Users		
	NQF	AHRQ	JCAHO	CMS	Leapfrog
Aspirin at arrival (within 24 hours)	X		X	X	
Aspirin at discharge	X		X	X	
Beta-blocker at arrival and discharge	X		X	X	
Thrombolytic agent (within 30 minutes)	X		X	X	
Percutaneous coronary intervention (within 30 minutes)	X		X	X	X
ACE inhibitor at discharge for patients with low left ventricular function	X		X	X	
Risk-adjusted mortality rates	X	X	X		
Congestive heart failure					
Smoking cessation counseling	X		X	X	
Standardized discharge instructions	X		X	X	
Assessment of left ventricular function	X		X	X	
ACE inhibitor at discharge for patients with low left ventricular function	X		X	X	
Risk-adjusted mortality rates		X			
Coronary artery disease					
Hospital volume—Percutaneous coronary interventions	X	X			X
Bilateral cardiac catheterization		X			
Gastrointestinal hemorrhage					
Risk-adjusted mortality rates		X			
Community acquired pneumonia					
Smoking cessation counseling	X		X	X	
Assessment of oxygenation at admission	X		X	X	
Blood cultures prior to antibiotics	X		X	X	
Antibiotics started within 4 hours	X		X	X	
Appropriate initial choice of antibiotics	X		X	X	
Pneumococcal screen or vaccination	X		X	X	
Influenza screen or vaccination	X		X	X	
Risk-adjusted mortality rates		X			
Hip fracture					
Risk-adjusted mortality rates		X			
Asthma					
Use of relievers (<18 years)	X				
Systemic steroids (<18 years)	X				
Acute stroke					
Risk-adjusted mortality rates		X			

(continued on next page)

TABLE F-3   continued

	Endorser		Current Users		
	NQF	AHRQ	JCAHO	CMS	Leapfrog
Obstetric Diagnoses					
Pregnancy and neonatal care					
Rates of 3rd and 4th degree perineal lacerations	X	X	X		
Risk-adjusted neonatal mortality	X		X		
Cesarean delivery in low risk women	X	X			
Vaginal births after cesarean delivery	X	X	X		
Birth trauma		X			
Hospital volume—Neonatal intensive care					X
Neonatal immunizations after 60 days	X				
Surgical Procedures					
Abdominal aneurysm repair					
Hospital volume		X			X
Risk-adjusted mortality rates		X			
Carotid endarterectomy					
Hospital volume		X			
Esophageal resection for cancer					
Hospital volume		X			X
Risk-adjusted mortality rates		X			
Coronary artery bypass grafting					
Hospital volume	X	X			X
Risk-adjusted mortality rates	X	X			X
Internal mammary artery use	X				X
Pancreatic resection					
Hospital volume		X			X
Risk-adjusted mortality rates		X			
Pediatric heart surgery					
Hospital volume		X			
Risk-adjusted mortality rates		X			
Hip replacement					
Risk-adjusted mortality rates		X			
Craniotomy					
Risk-adjusted mortality rates		X			
Cholecystectomy					
Laparoscopic approach		X			
Appendectomy					
Avoidance of incidental appendectomy		X			

JCAHO = Joint Commission on Accreditation of Healthcare Organizations; CMS = Center for Medicare and Medicaid Services; NQF = National Quality Forum; AHRQ = Agency for Healthcare Research and Quality; Leapfrog = The Business Roundtable's Leapfrog Group.

Hospital-Based Care and Surgery

NQF has endorsed a set of quality indicators for hospital-based care that cover several medical specialties (Table F-3). They focus primarily on process of care variables and thus most require access to clinical data. The Joint Commission on Accreditation of Healthcare Organizations and CMS have adopted many of these quality indicators for their accreditation and pay for performance efforts, respectively. For these two efforts, hospitals are responsible for collecting and submitting the data themselves.

The AHRQ has endorsed its own set of quality measures (Table F-3). In contrast to the NQF measures, which rely on collection of clinical data, AHRQ's Inpatient Quality Indicators were developed to take advantage of readily available administrative data. Because little information on process of care is available in these data sets, these measures focus mainly on structure and outcomes measures.

The Leapfrog group, a coalition of large employers and purchasers, has also created a set of quality indicators for its value-based purchasing initiative. Its original standards focused on three structural measures: hospital volume for high-risk surgery and neonatal intensive care; computerized physician order entry; and intensivist staffing for critical care units. Their recently updated standards have been expanded to include selected process and outcome measures. Hospitals voluntarily report their own procedure volumes and adherence to process measures. Risk-adjusted mortality rates for cardiovascular procedures are obtained from either state- or national-level clinical registries.

STRUCTURAL MEASURES OF QUALITY

Health care structure reflects the setting or system in which care is delivered. Many structural measures describe hospital-level attributes, such as the physical plant and resources or staff coordination and organization (e.g., RN–bed ratios, designation as Level I trauma center). Other structural measures reflect attributes associated with the relative expertise of individual physicians (e.g., board certification, subspecialty training or procedure volume).

Strengths

From a measurement perspective, structural measures of quality have several attractive features. First, many of these measures are strongly related to patient outcomes. For example, with esophagectomy and pancreatic resection, operative mortality rates at very-high-volume hospitals are as much as 10 percent lower, in absolute terms, than at lower volume centers (Dudley et al., 2000; Halm et al., 2002). In some instances, structural measures like procedure volume are considerably more predictive of subsequent hospital performance than any known processes of care or direct mortality measure (Figure F-1).

A second advantage is efficiency. A single structural measure may be associated with numerous outcomes. For example, with some types of cancer surgery, hospital or surgeon procedure volume is associated not only with lower operative mortality, but also with lower perioperative morbidity and higher late survival rates (Bach et al., 2001; Begg et al., 2002; Finlayson and Birkmeyer, 2003). Intensivist model ICUs are linked to shorter length of stay and reduced resource use, as well as lower mortality (Pronovost et al., 2002, 2004).

The third and perhaps most important advantage of structural variables is expediency. Many can be assessed easily with readily available administrative data. Although some structural measures require surveying hospitals or providers, such data are much less expensive to collect than measures requiring patient-level information.

Limitations

Among the downsides, there are relatively few structural measures that may be potentially useful as quality indicators. Their use in ambulatory care is particularly limited. Second, in contrast to process measures, most structural measures are not readily actionable. For example, a small hospital cannot readily make itself a high volume center, but it can increase how many of its surgical patients receive antibiotic prophylaxis. Thus, while selected structural measures may be useful for selective referral initiatives, they have limited value for quality improvement purposes.

Finally, structural measures generally describe groups of hospitals or providers with better performance, but they do not adequately discriminate performance among individuals. For example, in aggregate, high-volume hospitals have much lower mortality rates than lower volume centers for pancreatic resection. However, some individual high-volume hospitals may have high mortality rates, while some low-volume centers may have excellent performance (Shahian and Normand, 2003). In this way, structural measures are viewed as "unfair" by many providers.

PROCESS OF CARE MEASURES

Processes of care are the clinical interventions and services provided to patients. Although only occasionally applied as performance measures for surgery (e.g., appropriate use of perioperative antibiotics), process measures are the predominant quality indicators for both inpatient and outpatient medical care (Table F-2). In the latter setting, process measures

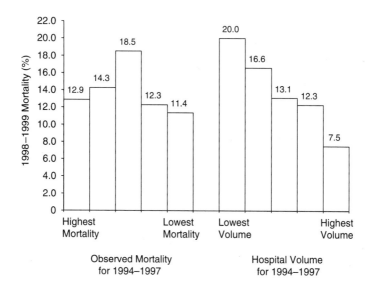

(a) Esophageal Cancer Resection

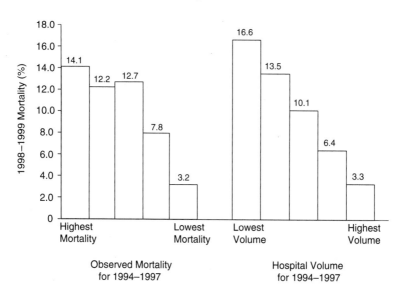

(b) Pancreatic Cancer Resection

FIGURE F-1 Relative usefulness of historical (1994–1997) measures of hospital volume and operative mortality in predicting subsequent (1998–1999) mortality. NOTE: Hospitals sorted by historical volume and mortality according to quintiles. Both historical and subsequent mortality rates are adjusted for Medicare patient characteristics.

are employed to reflect both preventive care (e.g., mammography in age-appropriate women) and chronic disease management (e.g., medication management for children with asthma; aspirin use for patients with coronary disease). Intermediate (or physiologic) outcomes (e.g., blood pressure control, glycemic control reflected by HbA_1C levels) could be considered with processes or with outcomes. However, because these measures that focus on improvement of intermediate outcome control share more properties with process measures, we consider them with other process of care measures here.

Strengths

Process of care measures are the only practical way to judge performance with most types of medical care. In contrast to surgery, few structural measures are strongly linked to patient outcomes in non-procedure-based care. Processes of care and intermediate outcomes are far more common and easier to measure than the end outcomes of ultimate interest (e.g., stroke, end-stage renal disease). Since processes of care reflect the care that physicians deliver, they have face validity and enjoy greater buy-in from providers. They are usually directly actionable and thus are a good substrate for quality improvement activities.

Although risk adjustment may be important for assessing intermediate outcomes (Greenfield et al., 2002; Hofer et al., 1999; Landon et al., 2003), it is not required for many process measures. For example, aspirin therapy for patients with coronary disease is a common performance measure. Since virtually all patients with coronary disease should be offered aspirin, there is little need to collect detailed clinical data about illness severity (assuming that the small number of patients with contraindications to aspirin is equally distributed across providers).

Finally, assessing performance with process measures may have a positive "spillover effect" to other practices within the targeted clinical condition. For example, Asch and colleagues found that the quality of medical care in the Department of Veterans Affairs health system was better than in a comparable national sample of private sector hospitals (Asch et al., 2004). Differences in quality were largest for processes of care actively profiled by the VA, but also extended to processes within the same clinical areas that were not explicitly profiled.

Limitations

The reliability of some process measures is limited by sample size constraints, particularly when used to profile performance for individual physicians. Imprecision may not be a major problem for preventive care measures that apply to a large proportion of a provider's panel. However, sample size limitations become more apparent for other process and intermediate outcome measures targeting specific conditions. For example, few individual providers see enough diabetic patients to measure laboratory test utilization or glycemic control with adequate reliability. Further, risk adjustment becomes particularly important when profiling intermediate outcomes, because it is likely that a provider's quality profile would be adversely affected by having just a few patients in their panel with poor glycemic control, for example, even after detailed case-mix adjustment (Hofer et al., 1999).

Additionally, process measures may sometimes reflect nonclinical factors that may confound performance assessment. For example, a physician may prescribe a cholesterol-lowering medication to a patient with hypercholesterolemia, but whether she fills the prescription and continues to take the medication will be influenced by her financial status, personal preferences, and cultural factors related to compliance. Relative to clinical variables, these factors are difficult to measure and account for with risk adjustment.

Perhaps the major limitation of process of care measures is the variable extent to which they link to patient outcomes. Some measures are "tightly linked" to outcomes, confirmed by high-level scientific evidence. For example, there is no doubt that patients discharged on beta-blockers after an acute myocardial infarction have lower mortality rates. Improvement efforts aimed at increasing beta-blocker use would no doubt translate to fewer deaths. In contrast, for community-acquired pneumonia, performance measures endorsed by NQF include early assessment of oxygenation and drawing blood cultures before administration of antibiotics. Both no doubt reflect sound clinical practice, but there is little evidence to suggest either would measurably reduce mortality or other important adverse events.

Weak relationships between processes and outcomes are sometimes attributable to the manner in which process measures are assessed. For example, lipid control in high-risk patients is clearly associated with lower cardiovascular morbidity and mortality. However, assessing the results of cholesterol tests requires expensive medical record review and profiling based on control alone is plagued by problems of risk adjustment and possible perverse incentives. Instead, administrative data are often used to simply count how many cholesterol tests were obtained. While it may be appropriate to encourage hypercholesterolemia screening, a better performance measure would record how often the physician prescribed and intensified appropriate therapy (or fully informed the patient about it). Indeed, in a study evaluating the use of such measures of medication intensification, Kerr and colleagues found that although 27 percent of patients had substandard quality based on a measure of cholesterol control, only 13 percent were classified as having substandard quality using a measure that took into account appropriate physician action in response to poor control (Kerr et al., 2003).

DIRECT OUTCOME MEASURES

Direct outcome measures reflect the "end result" of care, from a clinical perspective or as judged by the patient. Although mortality is by far the most commonly used measure, other outcomes which could be used as quality indicators include complications of care, hospital admission or readmission, and a variety of patient-centered measures of satisfaction, health status, or utility.

There are several ongoing, large-scale initiatives involving direct outcomes assessment. Although a few target one-time medical conditions (e.g., acute myocardial infarction), most relate to surgical care. A few proprietary health care rating firms and state agencies are assessing risk-adjusted mortality rates using Medicare or state-level administrative datasets. However, most of the momentum in outcomes measurement involves large clinical registries. Cardiac surgery registries in New York, Pennsylvania, and a growing number of other states are perhaps the visible examples. At the national level, the Society for Thoracic Surgeons and the American College of Cardiology have implemented systems for tracking morbidity and mortality with cardiac surgery and percutaneous coronary interventions, respectively. Although most outcomes measurement efforts have been procedure-specific (and largely limited to cardiac procedures), the National Surgical Quality Improvement Program (NSQIP) of the Department of Veterans Affairs (VA) assesses hospital-specific morbidity and mortality rates aggregated across a wide range of surgical specialties and procedures. Efforts to apply the same measurement approach outside the VA are currently under way.

Strengths

Direct outcome measures have at least two major advantages. First, direct outcome measures have obvious face validity, particularly for surgery, and thus are likely to get the greatest "buy-in" from hospitals and surgeons. Second, outcomes measurement alone may improve performance—the so-called Hawthorne effect. Surgical morbidity and mortality rates in VA hospitals have fallen dramatically since implementation of NSQIP in 1991 (Khuri et al., 2002). No doubt many surgical leaders at individual hospitals made specific organizational or process improvements after they began receiving feedback on their hospitals' performance. However, it is very unlikely that even a full inventory of these specific changes would explain such broad-based and substantial improvements in morbidity and mortality rates.

Limitations

Among the downsides, outcome measures are generally impractical for assessing the quality of most types of ambulatory medical care. Easily measured endpoints like mortality occur too infrequently or far downstream of the care being assessed. Patient-centered measures (e.g., health status) are much more difficult to collect and generally reflect illness severity in addition to provider quality.

Although outcome measurement is more practical and widely applied in surgery, hospital- or surgeon-specific outcome measures are severely constrained by small sample sizes. For the large majority of surgical procedures, very few hospitals (or surgeons) have sufficient adverse events (numerators) and cases (denominators) for meaningful, procedure-specific measures of morbidity or mortality. For example, Dimick and colleagues used data from the Nationwide Inpatient Sample to study 7 procedures for which mortality rates have been advocated as quality indicators by the AHRQ (Dimick et al., 2004). For 6 of the 7 procedures, a very small proportion of U.S. hospitals had adequate caseloads to rule out a mortality rate twice the national average. Although identifying poor-quality outliers is an important function of outcomes measurement, focusing on this goal alone significantly underestimates problems with small sample sizes. Discriminating among individual hospitals with intermediate levels of performance is more difficult.

Other limitations of direct outcomes assessment depend on whether outcomes are being assessed from administrative data or clinical information abstracted from medical records. For outcomes measurement based on clinical data, the major problem is expense. For example, it costs over $100,000 annually for a private-sector hospital to participate in NSQIP.

With administrative data, the adequacy of risk adjustment remains a major concern. High-quality risk adjustment may be essential for outcome measures to have face validity with providers. It may also be useful for discouraging gaming, e.g., hospitals or providers avoiding high-risk patients to optimize their performance measures. However, it is not clear how much the scientific validity of outcome measures is threatened by imperfect risk adjustment with administrative data. There is no disagreement that administrative data lack clinical detail and systematically underrepresent patient comorbidities and other clinical variables related to baseline risk (Finlayson et al., 2002; Fisher et al., 1992; Iezzoni, 1997; Iezzoni et al., 1992).

Instead, lack of clarity about the importance of risk adjustment reflects uncertainty about the extent to which case-mix varies systematically across hospitals and physicians. In some clinical contexts, case mix varies markedly. In medical care, for example, physician practices may be markedly different in terms of patients' diagnosis mix, illness severity, and socioeconomic status. Hospital case mix can vary similarly. Such factors can confound outcomes measures with even the best clinical data sources. For example, Rosenberg and colleagues found that even with identical efficiency and quality, a referral hospital with a 25 percent medical ICU transfer rate compared with another with a 0 percent transfer rate would appear to have 14 excess deaths per 1000 admissions—even after full adjustment for case mix and severity of illness (Rosenberg et al., 2003).

In contrast, for measures targeting narrower, more homogenous populations (e.g., patients undergoing the same surgical procedure), there is often surprisingly little variation in case mix. For example, we examined risk-adjusted mortality rates for hospitals performing CABG in New York State, as derived from their clinical registries. Unadjusted and adjusted hospital mortality rates were nearly identical in most years (correlations exceeding 0.90). Moreover, hospital rankings based on unadjusted and adjusted mortality were equally useful in predicting subsequent hospital performance (Figure F-2).

HOW GOOD IS GOOD ENOUGH?

Performance measures will never be perfect. Over time, analytic methods will be refined. Access to higher quality data may improve with the addition of clinical elements to administrative data sets or broader adoption of electronic medical records. However, some problems with performance measurement, including sample size limitations, are inherent and not fully correctable. Thus, clinical leaders, patient advocates, payers, and policy makers will not escape having to make decisions about when imperfect measures are good enough to act upon.

A measure should be implemented only with the expectation that acting will result in a net improvement in health quality. Thus, the direct benefits of implementing a particular measure cannot be outweighed by the indirect harms. Unfortunately, these benefits and harm are often difficult to measure and heavily influenced by the specific context and who—patients, payers, or providers—is doing the accounting. For this reason, there is no simple answer for where to "set the bar."

Matching the Measure to the Purpose

Instead, it may be more important to ensure a good match between the performance measure and the primary goal of measurement. The right

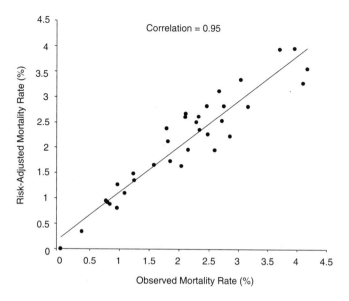

(a) New York State Hospitals (2001)

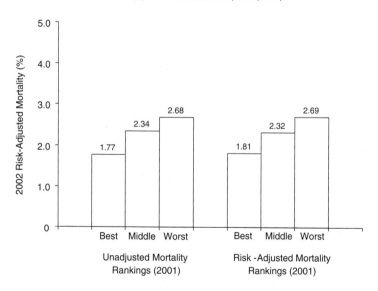

(b) New York State Hospitals

FIGURE F-2 Mortality associated with coronary artery bypass surgery in New York State hospitals, based on data from the state's clinical outcomes registry. (a) Correlation between adjusted and observed (unadjusted) 2001 mortality rates for all New York state hospitals. (b) Relative ability of adjusted and unadjusted mortality rates to predict performance in subsequent year.

measure depends on whether the underlying goal is (1) quality improvement or (2) selective referral—directing patients to higher quality hospitals and/or providers. Although many pay-for-performance initiatives have both goals, one often predominates. For example, the ultimate objective of the CMS pay-for-performance initiative with acute myocardial infarction, pneumonia, and congestive heart failure is improving quality at all hospitals. Conversely, the Leapfrog Group's efforts with selected surgical procedures and neonatal intensive care are primarily aimed at getting patients to hospitals likely to have better outcomes (selective referral).

For quality improvement purposes, a good performance measure—most often a process of care variable—must be actionable. Measurable improvements in the given process should translate to clinically meaningful improvements in patient outcomes. Although internally motivated quality improvement activities are rarely "harmful," their major downsides relate to their opportunity cost. Initiatives hinged on bad measures siphon away resources (e.g., time and focus of physicians and other staff) from more productive activities.

Advocates of pay for performance believe that financial incentives and/or public reporting can motivate greater improvements from hospitals or providers. However, adding "teeth" to quality improvement also increases the potential harms if hospitals or individual providers are unfairly rewarded or punished. They may also be harmful if physicians respond by gaming (e.g., avoiding the sickest patients) or optimizing performance measures at the cost of exposing some patients to undue risks or side effects (e.g., using four antihypertensive medications to achieve ideal blood pressure control in frail elderly patients). Given the current lack of empirical information about either marginal benefits or harms, it is not clear whether measures used in pay-for-performance initiatives should have a higher (or lower) bar than those used for quality improvement at the local level.

With selective referral, a good measure will steer patients to better hospitals or physicians (or away from worse ones). As one basic litmus test, a measure based on prior performance should reliably identify providers likely to have superior performance now and in the future. At the same time, an ideal measure would not incentivize perverse behaviors (e.g., surgeons doing unnecessary procedures to meet a specific volume standard) or negatively affect other domains of quality (e.g., patient autonomy, access, and satisfaction).

Measures that work well for quality improvement may not be particularly useful for selective referral, and vice versa. For example, appropriate use of perioperative antibiotics in surgical patients is a good measure for quality improvement. This process of care is clinically meaningful, linked to lower risks of surgical site infections, and directly actionable. Conversely, antibiotic use would not be particularly useful for selective referral purposes. It is unlikely patients would use this information to decide where to have surgery. More importantly, surgeons with high rates of appropriate antibiotic use may not necessarily do better with more important outcomes (e.g., mortality). Physician performance with one quality indicator is often poorly correlated with other indicators for the same or other clinical conditions (Palmer et al., 1996).

As a counterexample, the two main quality indicators for pancreatic cancer—hospital volume and operative mortality—are very informative in the context of selective referral. Patients would markedly improve their odds of surviving surgery by selecting hospitals highly ranked by either measure (Figure F-1). However, neither measure would be particularly useful for quality improvement purposes. Volume is not readily actionable; mortality rates are too unstable at the level of individual hospitals (due to small sample size problems) to identify top performers, identify best practices, or evaluate the effects of improvement activities.

Is Discrimination Important?

Many believe that a good performance measure must discriminate performance at the individual level. From the provider perspective in particular, a "fair" measure must reliably reflect the performance of individual hospitals or physicians. Unfortunately, as described earlier, small caseloads (and sometimes case-mix variation) conspire against this objective for most clinical conditions. Patients, however, should value information that improves their odds of good outcomes on average. Many measures meet this latter interest while failing on the former.

For example, Krumholz and colleagues used clinical data from the Cooperative Cardiovascular Project to assess the usefulness of Healthgrades' hospital ratings for acute myocardial infarction (based primarily on risk-adjusted mortality rates from Medicare data) (Krumholz et al., 2002). Relative to 1-star (worst) hospitals, 5-star (best) hospitals had significantly lower mortality (16 percent vs. 22 percent, $p<0.001$) after risk adjustment with clinical data. They also discharged significantly more (appropriate) patients on aspirin, beta-blockers, and ACE inhibitors, all recognized quality indicators. However, the Healthgrades' ratings poorly discriminated among any 2 individual hospitals. In only 3 percent of head-to-head comparisons did 5-star hospitals have statistically lower mortality rates than 1-star hospitals.

Thus, some performance measures which clearly identify groups of hospitals or providers with superior performance may be limited in their ability to discriminate individual hospitals from one another. There may be no simple solution to resolving the basic tension implied by performance measures that are unfair to providers yet informative for patients. However, it underscores the importance of being clear about both the primary purpose (quality improvement or selective referral) and whose interests are receiving top priority (provider or patient).

MEASURES READY OR NEAR-READY FOR IMPLEMENTATION

As described earlier, an ever broadening array of performance measures is being developed and promoted by various scientific and advocacy groups. However, there may be a price for this comprehensiveness in performance measurement. As the list grows longer, energy and resources devoted to performance measurement become more diluted and distinctions between important and unimportant measures are blurred. Thus, we believe that a first order of business should be prioritizing measures.

Condition- or Procedure-Specific Measures

Table F-4 lists several measures for ambulatory and hospital-based care that should receive high priority, based on consideration of issues outlined earlier in this paper and input from various experts in the field. While none of these quality indicators is perfect, all have a solid evidence base linking them to clinically important patient outcomes. Better performance with these measures would have important public health benefits—either because they apply to large populations at risk (e.g., use of statins for high-risk patients) or because they imply significant risk reductions for individual patients (e.g., high-risk surgical procedures). As described earlier, some of these measures are better applied in quality improvement efforts; others are more useful for selective referral.

Any short list of performance measures should be expected to evolve over time. New quality indicators should be added as clinical researchers identify new high leverage processes of care for specific conditions. Existing measures may also be dropped as a byproduct of success in quality improvement initiatives. For example, aspirin use in patients with acute myocardial infarction will become less useful as a performance measure as hospitals near 100 percent compliance. Even if few measures became "obsolete," rotating conditions and measures might be a useful approach to renewing interest in quality improvement initiatives while minimizing data collection burdens.

Broader Measures of Performance

In addition to condition- and procedure-specific performance measures, there is also interest in broader measures of quality for profiling health plans and organizations. At present, summary scores based on HEDIS measures may be the best tool for assessing quality with administrative data.

TABLE F-4 High Leverage Measures Ready or Near Ready for Implementation in Quality Improvement of Selective Referral Initiatives

	Quality Improvement	Selective Referral
Ambulatory Care		
Summary quality measures (e.g., HEDIS, Rand QA Tools)	X	X
Colorectal cancer screening	X	
Reducing cardiovascular events and death		
Blood pressure control or use of appropriate number of medications to control blood pressure	X	
Use of cholesterol-lowering medications (statins)	X	
Long-acting asthma medications (e.g., inhaled steroids) in adults and children with asthma	X	
Childhood immunizations (including influenza, pneumococcal, and varicella vaccination)		
Hospital-Based Care		
Intensivist-staffed ICUs		X
Acute myocardial infarction		
Time to thrombolysis or PCI	X	
Appropriate use of aspirin, beta-blockers, and ACE inhibitors	X	
Risk-adjusted mortality rates, CABG	X	X
Procedure volume, pancreatic resection and esophagectomy		X
Perioperative beta-blockage during noncardiac surgery (high-risk patients)	X	

These measures incorporate data from a wide range of clinical conditions and have the added advantage of familiarity. RAND's QA Tools measurement system is similarly broad in clinical scope, but scoring is based instead on clinical-level data (McGlynn et al., 2003a). The use of clinical data allows for more clinically meaningful process measures, with the primary downside of higher data collection costs.

The VA's NSQIP system provides broad measures of risk-adjusted morbidity and mortality at the hospital level and is marketed heavily to private-sector hospitals by the American College of Surgeons. To date, dissemination of NSQIP has been slowed by the relatively high cost of hospital participation. NSQIP does not currently collect process of care measures and its performance measures are not procedure-specific, limiting its usefulness as a platform for quality improvement. Both problems might be addressed in future versions. As with other national measurement efforts led by physician organizations (e.g., cardiac surgery and cardiology), NSQIP is based on confidential data reporting and performance feedback and thus not useful for public reporting and selective referral purposes.

A RESEARCH AGENDA FOR IMPROVING
PERFORMANCE MEASUREMENT

Although some of the limitations of specific performance measures are inherent, many measures could be substantially improved with better data sources and analytic methods. More broadly, performance measurement could be improved by the development of measures for often overlooked domains of quality. Although others have outlined a more comprehensive research agenda for improving performance measurement (Leatherman et al., 2003; McGlynn et al., 2003b), we describe below a few obvious areas in which progress is needed.

Getting to Better Data

The usefulness of many performance measures is limited by the quality or availability of appropriate data sources. Billing or other administrative data are ubiquitous, relatively inexpensive to use, and adequately robust for many performance measures. However, they often lack sufficient clinical specificity to define relevant patient subgroups (i.e., the denominator of patients appropriate for a given process measure), to conduct adequate risk adjustment, and to detect and discourage physicians from gaming measures. Although data obtained from medical records can often meet these needs, clinical data for performance measurement are very expensive and not widely available.

Future research should address how to meet the minimum data quality needs for various performance measures in the most cost-efficient manner possible. As a start, researchers might identify those measures for which current administrative data sets are sufficient. As described earlier, risk adjustment may not be as important as commonly assumed, particularly for outcome measures applied to relatively homogenous populations. To identify such instances, researchers could use existing clinical registries to highlight procedures or conditions for which adjusted and unadjusted mortality rates are sufficiently correlated.

Where better data are needed, future research could also explore the merits of two alternative approaches. The first would be to improve the accuracy and detail of administrative data by adding a small number of "clinical" variables to the billing record. These could include either specific process of care variables, laboratory values, or information most essential for risk adjustment purposes. With the latter, for example, Hannan and colleagues noted that risk adjustment models derived from administrative data for CABG would approximate the reliability of those from clinical data with the addition of only three variables (ejection fraction, reoperation, and left main stenosis). Similarly, information about laboratory values and medication prescriptions could facilitate construction of more clinically meaningful process measures (Hannan et al., 2003).

The second approach would be to reduce the costs of collecting clinical data. Although such costs may decline over time as medical records become electronic, this transition does not appear imminent at present at most U.S. hospitals. In the meantime, costs could be minimized by limiting data collection to only those elements necessary for process assessment and/or adequate risk adjustment. In some cases, these could be captured through extractable data fields in existing record systems. For example, blood pressure, which is routinely collected, could be recorded in an easily extractable manner. In many cases, sampling methods could be employed instead of full enumeration. Thus, rather than gathering process of care data on all patients, such information would be collected on the smallest subset of patients necessary to achieve adequate precision. For outcome measures, clinical data could be sampled for risk adjustment purposes or to monitor for gaming, while administrative data are used to assess the complete numerator and denominator.

Getting to Better Analytic Methods

No measure of process or outcomes is perfectly reliable—each contains some degree of measurement error. As described earlier, statistical "noise" is a large component of measurement error, which is compounded by small sample sizes when performance is assessed at the physician or even hospital level. However, process and outcome measures can also be unreliable because they are influenced by patient-related variables or other factors beyond the control of the hospital or physician whose performance is being assessed. To reduce problems with reliability, research aimed at advancing techniques in multilevel modeling and empirical Bayes' methods may help filter out noise (Gatsonis et al., 1993; Hayward and Hofer, 2001; Hofer et al., 1999; McClellan and Staiger, 2000; Miller et al., 1993). Better methods for determining how much of observed variation in a performance measure derives from provider-level factors versus patient factors may also be useful for understanding and accounting for measure reliability (Greenfield et al., 2002; Hofer et al., 1999).

Combining information across time and across dimensions of quality may be another means of developing more reliable estimates of provider performance. For example, McClellan and Staiger demonstrated the value of supplementing conventional 30-day mortality rates with information on 7-day and 1-year mortality and cardiac-related readmission rates in assessing hospital-specific mortality rates for acute myocardial infarction (McClellan and Staiger, 2000). As seen in Figure F-3, this approach yielded considerably more stable estimates of hospital performance. More importantly, the new estimates of hospital

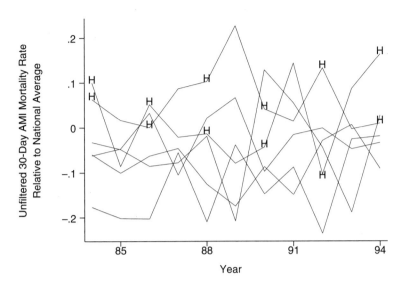

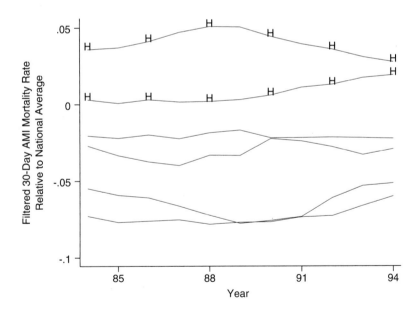

FIGURE F-3   30-day mortality rates for acute myocardial infarction at six hospitals in a large metropolitan region, relative to national average (1984–1994). Hospitals labeled "H" are high mortality outliers. Top: conventional 30-day mortality rates; Bottom: filtered 30-day mortality rates.

mortality were considerably more reliable in predicting subsequent hospital performance (Figure F-3). Future research could explore the effect of adding other structural variables (e.g., procedure volume for surgery) or process of care measures on the reliability of predicting future performance.

Broader Domains of Quality

For procedures, the large majority of performance measures currently reflects aspects of technical quality. Thus, they assess how well the procedure was performed, not whether it should have been performed in the first place. Prior research describing wide variation in the use of health services suggests that there may be greater variation in "decision quality" than in technical quality (Wennberg, 1996). Shared decision-making tools have been shown to reduce overuse of some procedures and may be an effective tool for improving decision quality in other areas (Sepucha et al., 2004; Wagner et al., 1995). Further research is needed to guide their broader implementation in clinical practice, to develop practical measures of decision quality, and to evaluate their usefulness as performances metrics.

In ambulatory care, performance measurement focuses primarily on individual components of care, not on how well these aspects of care are coordinated or their cumulative effects on patients' well-being (Coleman and Berenson, 2004). Patient-centered measures may help address some of these questions. However, further research is needed to assess how well they reflect true quality of care (and not patient factors) and thus their value as performance measures.

REFERENCES

Asch SM, McGlynn EA, Hogan MM, Hayward RA, Shekelle PM, Rubenstein LM, Keesey JB, Adams JP, Kerr EA. 2004. Comparison of quality of care for patients in the Veterans Health Administration and patients in a national sample. *Annals of Internal Medicine* 141(12):938–945.

Bach PB, Cramer LD, Schrag D, Downey RJ, Gelfand SE, Begg CB. 2001. The influence of hospital volume on survival after resection for lung cancer. *New England Journal of Medicine* 345(3):181–188.

Begg CB, Riedel ER, Bach PB, Kattan MW, Schrag D, Warren JL, Scardino PT. 2002. Variations in morbidity after radical prostatectomy. *New England Journal of Medicine* 346(15):1138–1144.

Bird SM, Sir David C, Farewell VT, Harvey G, Tim H, Peter C. S. 2005. Performance indicators: Good, bad, and ugly. *Journal of the Royal Statistical Society: Series A (Statistics in Society)* 168(1):1–27.

Birkmeyer JD, Dimick JB, Birkmeyer NJO. 2004. Measuring the quality of surgical care: Structure, process, or outcomes? *Journal of the American College of Surgeons* 198(4):626–632.

Coleman EA, Berenson RA. 2004. Lost in transition: Challenges and opportunities for improving the quality of transitional care. *Annals of Internal Medicine* 141(7):533–536.

Dimick JBM, Welch HGM, Birkmeyer JDM. 2004. Surgical mortality as an indicator of hospital quality: The problem with small sample size. *Journal of the American Medical Association* 292(7):847–851.

Dudley RA, Johansen KL, Brand R, Rennie DJ, Milstein A. 2000. Selective referral to high-volume hospitals: Estimating potentially avoidable deaths. *Journal of the American Medical Association* 283(9):1159–1166.

Finlayson EV, Birkmeyer JD. 2003. Effects of hospital volume on life expectancy after selected cancer operations in older adults: A decision analysis. *Journal of the American College of Surgeons* 196(3):410–417.

Finlayson EV, Birkmeyer JD, Stukel TA, Siewers AE, Lucas FL, Wennberg DE. 2002. Adjusting surgical mortality rates for patient comorbidities: More harm than good? *Surgery* 132(5):787–794.

Fisher ES, Whaley FS, Krushat WM, Malenka DJ, Fleming C, Baron JA, Hsia DC. 1992. The accuracy of Medicare's hospital claims data: Progress has been made, but problems remain. *American Journal of Public Health* 82(2):243–248.

Galvin R, Milstein A. 2002. Large employers' new strategies in health care. *New England Journal of Medicine* 347(12):939–942.

Gatsonis C, Normand SL, Liu C, Morris C. 1993. Geographic variation of procedure utilization. *Medical Care* 31(May Supplement):YS54–YS59.

Greenfield S, Kaplan SH, Kahn R, Ninomiya J, Griffith JL. 2002. Profiling care provided by different groups of physicians: effects of patient case-mix (bias) and physician-level clustering on quality assessment results. *Annals of Internal Medicine* 136(2):111–121.

Halm EA, Lee C, Chassin MR. 2002. Is volume related to outcome in health care? A systematic review and methodologic critique of the literature. *Annals of Internal Medicine* 137(6):511–520.

Hannan EL, Kilburn H, Lindsey ML, Lewis R. 2003. Clinical versus administrative data bases for CABG surgery. *Medical Care* 30(10):892–907.

Hayward RA, Hofer TP. 2001. Estimating hospital deaths due to medical errors: Preventability is in the eye of the reviewer. *Journal of the American Medical Association* 286(4):415–420.

Hofer TP, Hayward RA, Greenfield S, Wagner EH, Kaplan SH, Manning WG. 1999. The unreliability of individual physician "report cards" for assessing the costs and quality of care of a chronic disease. *Journal of the American Medical Association* 281(22):2098–2105.

Iezzoni LI. 1997. The risks of risk adjustment. *Journal of the American Medical Association* 278(19):1600–1607.

Iezzoni LI, Foley SM, Daley J, Hughes J, Fisher ES, Heeren T. 1992. Comorbidities, complications, and coding bias. Does the number of diagnosis codes matter in predicting in-hospital mortality? *Journal of the American Medical Association* 267(16):2197–2203.

Kerr EA, Smith DM, Hogan MM, Hofer TP, Krein SL, Bermann M, Hayward RA. 2003. Building a better quality measure: Are some patients with 'poor quality' actually getting good care? *Medical Care* 41(10):1173–1182.

Khuri SF, Daley J, Henderson WG. 2002. The comparative assessment and improvement of quality of surgical care in the Department of Veterans Affairs. *Archives of Surgery* 137(1):20–27.

Kizer KW, Demakis JG, Feussner JR. 2000. Reinventing VA health care: Systematizing quality improvement and quality innovation. *Medical Care* 38(6 Suppl 1):7–16.

Krumholz HM, Rathore SS, Chen J, Wang Y, Radford MJ. 2002. Evaluation of a consumer-oriented Internet health care report card: The risk of quality ratings based on mortality data. *Journal of the American Medical Association* 287(10):1277–1287.

Landon BE, Normand S-LT, Blumenthal D, Daley J. 2003. Physician clinical performance assessment: Prospects and barriers. *Journal of the American Medical Association* 290(9):1183–1189.

Leatherman ST, Hibbard JH, McGlynn EA. 2003. A research agenda to advance quality measurement and improvement. *Medical Care* 41(January Supplement):I-80–I-86.

Lee TH, Meyer GS, Brennan TA. 2004. A middle ground on public accountability. *New England Journal of Medicine* 350(23):2409–2412.

McClellan MB, Staiger DO. 2000. Comparing the quality of health care providers. *Frontiers in Health Policy Research* 3:113–136.

McGlynn EA, Asch SM, Adams J, Keesey J, Hicks J, DeCristofaro A, Kerr EA. 2003a. The quality of health care delivered to adults in the United States. *New England Journal of Medicine* 348(26):2635–2645.

McGlynn EA, Cassel CK, Leatherman ST, DeCristofaro A, Smits HL. 2003b. Establishing national goals for quality improvement. *Medical Care* 41(1 Supplement):I-16–I-29.

Miller ME, Hui SL, Tierney WM, McDonald CJ. 1993. Estimating physician costliness: An empirical Bayes approach. *Medical Care* 31(May Supplement):YS16–YS28.

Palmer RH, Wright EA, Orav EJ, Hargraves JL, Louis TA. 1996. Consistency in performance among primary care practitioners. *Medical Care* 34(September Supplement):SS52–SS66.

Pronovost PJ, Angus DC, Dorman T, Robinson KA, Dremsizov TT, Young TL. 2002. Physician staffing patterns and clinical outcomes in critically ill patients: A systematic review. *Journal of the American Medical Association* 288(17):2151–2162.

Pronovost PJ, Needham D, Waters HP, Birkmeyer C, Calinawan J, Birkmeyer J, Dorman TM. 2004. Intensive care unit physician staffing: Financial modeling of the Leapfrog standard. *Critical Care Medicine* 32(6):1247–1253.

Rosenberg AL, Hofer TP, Strachan C, Watts CM, Hayward RA. 2003. Accepting critically ill transfer patients: adverse effect on a referral center's outcome and benchmark measures. *Annals of Internal Medicine* 138(11):882–890.

Sepucha KR, Fowler FJ, Mulley AG. 2004. Policy support for patient-centered care: The need for measurable improvements in decision quality. *Health Affairs* Suppl Web Exclusive:VAR 54–62.

Shahian DM, Normand S-LT. 2003. The volume-outcome relationship: From Luft to Leapfrog. *Annals of Thoracic Surgery* 75(3):1048–1058v1.

Wagner EH, Barrett P, Barry MJ, Barlow W, Fowler FJ. 1995. The effect of a shared decisionmaking program on rates of surgery for benign prostatic hyperplasia. *Medical Care* 33(8):765–770.

Wennberg JE. 1996. *Dartmouth Atlas of Health Care*. Chicago, IL: American Hospital Publishing, Inc.

Appendix G

Starter Set of Measures

TABLE G-1 AQA Ambulatory Care Measures (26 measures)

Prevention Measures

1. Breast cancer screening — Percentage of women who had a mammogram during the measurement year prior to the measurement year

2. Colorectal cancer screening — Percentage of adults who had an appropriate screening for colorectal cancer. One or more of the following: FOBT during measurement year; flexible sigmoidoscopy during the measurement year or the four years prior to the measurement year; DCBE during the measurement year or the four years prior; colonoscopy during the measurement year or nine years prior

3. Cervical cancer screening — Percentage of women who had one or more Pap tests during the measurement year or the two years prior

4. Tobacco use — Percentage of patients who were queried about tobacco use one or more times during the two-year measurement period

5. Advising smokers to quit — Percentage of patients who received advice to quit smoking

6. Influenza vaccination — Percentage of patients (ages 50–64 years) who received an influenza vaccination (Note: NQF also preliminarily approved this measure for patients 65+)

7. Pneumonia vaccination — Percentage of patients who ever received a pneumococcal vaccine

Coronary Artery Disease (CAD)

8. Drug therapy for lowering LDL cholesterol — Percentage of patients with CAD who were prescribed a lipid-lowering therapy (based on current ACC/AHA guidelines)

9. Beta-blocker treatment after heart attack — Percentage of patients hospitalized with acute myocardial infarction (AMI) who received an ambulatory prescription for beta-blocker therapy (within 7 days

TABLE G-1   continued

	discharge) (Note: this measure was not reviewed by the NQF and therefore it is not approved)
10. Beta-blocker treatment—post–myocardial infarction	Percentage of patients hospitalized with AMI who received persistent beta-blocker treatment (6 months after discharge) (Note: this measure was not reviewed by the NQF and therefore it is not approved)
Heart Failure	
11. ACE inhibitor/ARB therapy	Percentage of patients with heart failure who also have LVSD who were prescribed ACE inhibitor or ARB therapy. Angiotensin receptor blocker (ARB) drugs are collected under this measure
12. LVF assessment	Percentage of patients with heart failure with quantitative or qualitative results of LVF assessment recorded
Diabetes	NOTE: These measures were not approved during the NQF expedited review, as NQF has taken previous action on diabetes measures
13. HbA$_1$c management	Percentage of patients with diabetes with one or more A$_1$c test(s) conducted during the measurement year
14. HbA$_1$c management control	Percentage of patients with diabetes with most recent A$_1$c level greater than 9.0% (poor control)
15. Blood pressure management	Percentage of patients with diabetes who had their blood pressure documented in the past year less than 140/90 mmHg
16. Lipid measurement	Percentage of patients with diabetes with at least one low density lipoprotein cholesterol (LDL-C) test (or ALL component tests)
17. LDL cholesterol level (<130 mg/dL)	Percentage of patients with diabetes with most recent LDL-C less than 100 mg/dL or less than 130 mg/dL
18. Eye exam	Percentage of patients who received a retinal or dilated eye exam by an eye-care professional (optometrist or ophthalmologist) during the reporting year or during the prior year if patient is at low risk for retinopathy. A patient is considered low risk if all three of the following criteria are met: (1) the patient is not taking insulin; (2) has an A$_1$c less than 8.0%; and (3) has no evidence of retinopathy in the prior year
Asthma	
19. Use of appropriate medications for people with asthma	Percentage of individuals who were identified as having persistent asthma during the year prior to the measurement year and who were appropriately prescribed asthma medications (e.g. inhaled corticosteroids) during the measurement year
20. Pharmacologic therapy	Percentage of all individuals with mild, moderate, or severe persistent asthma who were prescribed either the preferred long-term control medication (inhaled corticosteroid) or an acceptable alternative treatment

(continued on next page)

TABLE G-1 continued

Depression

21. Antidepressant medication management—Acute Phase — Percentage of adults who were diagnosed with a new episode of depression and treated with an antidepressant medication and remained on an antidepressant drug during the entire 84-day (12-week) Acute Treatment Phase

22. Antidepressant medication management—Continuation Phase — Percentage of adults who were diagnosed with a new episode of depression and treated with an antidepressant medication and remained on an antidepressant drug for at least 180 days (6 months)

Prenatal Care

23. Screening for Human Immunodeficiency Virus — Percentage of patients who were screened for HIV infection during the first or second prenatal visit

24. Anti-D immune globulin — Percentage of D (Rh) negative, unsensitized patients who received anti-D immune globulin at 26–30 weeks gestation

Quality Measures Addressing Overuse or Misuse

25. Appropriate treatment for children with upper respiratory infection (URI) — Percentage of patients who were given a diagnosis of URI and were not dispensed an antibiotic prescription on or 3 days after the episode date

26. Appropriate testing for children with pharyngitis — Percentage of patients who were diagnosed with pharyngitis, prescribed an antibiotic and who received a group A streptococcus test for the episode

TABLE G-2 HQA Acute Care Measures (20 measures)

NQF Endorsed Measures (39)	Hospital Quality Alliance Publicly Reported Measures on CMS' Hospital Compare
Acute Coronary Syndrome	
1. Aspirin at arrival for acute myocardial infarction (AMI)	√
2. Aspirin prescribed at discharge for AMI	√
3. Beta-blocker at arrival for AMI	√
4. Beta-blocker prescribed at discharge for AMI	√
5. AMI inpatient mortality	
6. Angiotensin converting enzyme inhibitor (ACEI) for left ventricular systolic dysfunction (LVSD)	√
7. Percutaneous coronary intervention (PCI) within 120 minutes of arrival for AMI	√
8. Thrombolytic agent within 30 minutes of arrival for AMI	√
9. PCI volume	
10. PCI mortality (risk-adjusted)	
11. Coronary artery bypass graft (CABG) using internal mammary artery	

TABLE G-2   continued

NQF Endorsed Measures (cont'd.)	Hospital Quality Alliance Publicly Reported Measures on CMS' Hospital Compare
12. CABG volume	
13. CABG mortality (risk adjusted)	
Heart Failure	
14. Left ventricular function (LVF) assessment	√
15. Detailed discharge instructions	√
16. ACEI for LVSD	√
Patient Safety	
17. Urinary catheter-associated urinary tract infection for intensive care unit patients	
18. Central line catheter-associated blood stream infection for intensive care unit patients	
19. Ventilator-associated pneumonia for intensive care unit patient	
20. Patient falls (per 1,000 patient days)	
Pediatric Conditions	
21. Use of relievers for inpatient asthma	
22. Use of systemic corticosteroids for inpatient asthma	
23. Neonate immunization administration	
Pneumonia	
24. Oxygenation assessment	√
25. Initial antibiotic consistent with current recommendations	√
26. Blood culture collected prior to first antibiotic administration	√
27. Influenza screen or vaccination	
28. Pneumonia screen or pneumococcal vaccination for adults over 65	√
29. Antibiotic timing	√
Pregnancy/Childbirth/Neonatal Conditions	
30. Vaginal birth after cesarean delivery rate	
31. Cesarean delivery rate	
32. Third- or fourth-degree laceration	
33. Neonatal mortality	
Smoking Cessation	
34. Smoking cessation advice/counseling for AMI patients	√
35. Smoking cessation advice/counseling for heart failure patients	√
36. Smoking cessation advice/counseling for pneumonia patients	√
Surgical Complications	
37. Timing of antibiotic administration (surgical patients)	√
38. Selection of antibiotic administration (surgical patients)	
39. Duration of prophylaxis (surgical patients)	√

√ Starter set measures.

TABLE G-3   HEDIS 2005 Measures

Effectiveness of Care

Childhood immunization status[H]	Estimates the percentage of children enrolled in managed care plans who turned 2 years old during measurement year and had the following vaccinations: 4 doses of DTP or DTAP (diphtheria-tetanus); 3 doses of OPV or IPV (polio); 1 dose MMR (measles-mumps-rubella); 2 doses of Hib (Haemophilus influenza type b), 3 doses of hepatitis B and one varicella vaccination
Adolescent immunization status[H]	Percentage of enrolled adolescents who turn 13 years old during the measurement year who had a second dose of MMR and three hepatitis B vaccinations, and one varicella vaccination by their 13th birthday
Appropriate treatment for children with upper respiratory infection (URI)[A]	Percentage of children 3 months–18 years of age who were given a diagnosis of URI and who did not receive an antibiotic prescription for that episode of care within 3 days of the visit
Appropriate testing for children with pharyngitis[A]	Percentage of children 2–18 years of age who were diagnosed with pharyngitis, prescribed an antibiotic and who received a Group A streptococcus test
Colorectal cancer screening[H]	Percentage of adults 50–80 years of age who have had appropriate screening for colorectal cancer. The screening criteria can be met with any one of four tests: a fecal occult blood test (FOBT) during the measurement year; a flexible sigmoidoscopy within the last 5 years (the measurement year or the 4 years prior to the measurement year); a double contrast barium enema within the last 5 years; or a colonoscopy within the last 10 years (the measurement year or the 9 years prior to the measurement year)
Breast cancer screening[H]	Percentage of women aged 52–69 years (as of Dec 31 of the measurement year) who had at least one mammogram in the past 2 years
Cervical cancer screening[H]	Percentage of women aged 21–64 years (as of Dec 31 of the measurement year) who were enrolled in a health plan and who had one Pap test in the past 3 years
Chlamydia screening in women[A]	Percentage of sexually active female plan members who had at least one test for chlamydia during the previous year. The measure is collected separately for women aged 16–20 and 21–25 years
Osteoporosis management in women who had a fracture[A]	Percentage of women 67 years of age and older who suffered a fracture and who had either a bone mineral density test or prescription for a drug to treat or prevent osteoporosis in the 6 months after the date of the fracture. Applies only to Medicare plans
Controlling high blood pressure[H]	In the percentage of enrolled adults aged 46–85 years who have diagnosed hypertension and whose blood

TABLE G-3 continued

	pressure was adequately controlled. Adequate control was defined as a blood pressure of 140/90 or lower. Both the systolic and diastolic pressure must have been at or under these thresholds for the person's blood pressure to be considered controlled
Beta-blocker treatment after a heart attack[H]	Percentage of members 35 years and older who were hospitalized and discharged alive during the measurement year with a diagnosis of a heart attack and who received a prescription for a beta-blocker upon discharge
Persistence of beta-blocker treatment after a heart attack[A]	The percentage of members 35 years and older who were discharged alive from July 1 of the year prior to the measurement year to June 30 of the measurement year with a diagnosis of a heart attack and who received persistent beta-blocker treatment. Persistent treatment is defined as receiving treatment for 6 mos after the discharge
Cholesterol management after acute cardiovascular event[H, C]	Percentage of health plan members 18–75 years of age who had evidence of an acute cardiovascular event and whose LDL-C was screened[H]; controlled to less than 130 mg/dL[C] in the year following the event; and controlled to less than 100 mg/dL[C]
Comprehensive diabetes care[H, C]	Percentage of members with type 1 and type 2 diabetes who were 18–75 years old and, during the measurement year, had a hemoglobin A_1c (HbA_1c) test [H]; an HbA_1c level greater than 9 [C]; a serum cholesterol level (LDL-C) screening [H]; a cholesterol level (LDL-C) controlled to less than 130mg/dL [C]; their cholesterol level controlled to less than 100 mg/dL [C]; an eye exam [H]; and a screening for kidney disease [H]
Use of appropriate medications for people with asthma[A]	Percentage of enrolled members 5–56 years of age who were identified as having persistent asthma and who were prescribed appropriate medication. Measure is also collected separately for children (aged 5–9), adolescents (aged 10–17), and adults (aged 18–56)
Follow-up after hospitalization for mental illness[A]	Percentage of members 6 years of age and older who had a follow-up visit after being discharged for an inpatient mental health stay. Includes hospitalizations for depression, schizophrenia, attention deficit disorder, and personality disorders. Measure looks at both 7-day and 30-day follow-up rates
Antidepressant medication management[A]	Three components of the measure estimate: **Optimal Practitioner Contacts:** Percentage of adult members who received antidepressant medication and had at least 3 follow-up visits during the 12-week

(continued on next page)

TABLE G-3   continued

	acute treatment phase after diagnosis of a new episode of depression **Continuation Phase:** Percentage of eligible members who remained on antidepressant medication continuously the 6 months after diagnosis of a new episode of depression **Acute Phase:** Percentage of adult members who remained on antidepressant medication during the entire 12-week acute treatment phase after diagnosis of a new episode of depression
Glaucoma screening in older adults[A]	The percentage of Medicare members 65 years and older without a prior diagnosis of glaucoma or glaucoma suspect who received a glaucoma eye exam in the last two years by an eye-care professional for early identification of persons with glaucomatous conditions. An eye-care professional is an ophthalmologist or optometrist
Use of imaging studies for low back pain[A]	This measure assesses whether imaging studies (plain X-ray, MRI, CT scan) are overused in evaluating patients with acute low back pain
Medical assistance with smoking cessation[S]	Three components: (1) Percentage of smokers or recent quitters who received advice to quit smoking from their practitioner; (2) Percentage whose practitioner discussed smoking cessation medications; and (3) Percentage whose practitioner discussed smoking cessation strategies
Flu shots for adults (ages 50–64)[S]	The percentage of commercial members 50–64 years of age as of September 1 of the measurement year who received an influenza vaccination between September 1 of the measurement year and the date on which the CAHPS 3.0H Adult Survey was completed
Flu shots for older adults[S]	The percentage of Medicare members 65 years of age and older as of January 1 of the measurement year who received an influenza vaccination from September 1–December 31 of the year prior to the measurement year
Pneumonia vaccination status for older adults[S]	The percentage of Medicare members 65 years of age and older as of January 1 of the measurement year who received a pneumococcal vaccine
Medicare Health Outcomes Survey[S]	This measure provides a general indication of how well a Medicare MCO manages the physical and mental health of its members. The survey measures each member's physical and mental health status at the beginning and the end of a 2-year period

TABLE G-3 continued

A 2-year change score is calculated and each member's physical and mental health status is categorized as better, the same, or worse than expected, taking into account risk adjustment factors. MCO-specific results are assigned as percentages of members whose health status was better, the same, or worse than expected

Management of urinary incontinence in older adults[S]

Discussing Urinary Incontinence. The percentage of Medicare members 65 years of age and older who reported having a problem with urine leakage in the last 6 months and who discussed their urine leakage problem with their current practitioner
Receiving Urinary Incontinence Treatment. The percentage of Medicare members 65 years of age and older who reported having a urine leakage problem in the last 6 months and who received treatment for their current urine leakage problem

Physical activity in older adults[S]

Discussing Physical Activity. The percentage of Medicare members 65 years of age and older who had a doctor's visit in the last 12 months and who spoke with a doctor or other health provider about their level of exercise or physical activity
Advising Physical Activity. The percentage of Medicare members 65 years of age and older who had a doctor's visit in the last 12 months and who received advice to start, increase, or maintain their level of exercise or physical activity

Access/Availability of Care

Adults' access to preventive/ ambulatory health services[A]

The percentage of enrollees 20–44, 45–64, and 65 years of age and older who had an ambulatory or preventive care visit. The MCO reports the percentage of:

- Medicaid and Medicare enrollees who had an ambulatory or preventive care visit during the measurement year
- Commercial enrollees who had an ambulatory or preventive care visit during the measurement year or the 2 years prior to the measurement year

Children and adolescents' access to primary care practitioners[A]

The percentage of enrollees 12–24 months, 25 months–6 years, 7–11 years, and 12–19 years of age who had a visit with an MCO primary care practitioner. The MCO reports:

- children 12–24 months and 25 months–6 years of age who had a visit with an MCO primary care practitioner during the measurement year

(continued on next page)

TABLE G-3 continued

	• children 7–11 and adolescents 12–19 years of age who had a visit with an MCO primary care practitioner during the measurement year or the year prior to the measurement year
Prenatal and postpartum care[H]	**Timeliness of Prenatal Care.** The percentage of deliveries that received a prenatal care visit as a member of the MCO in the first trimester *or* within 42 days of enrollment in the MCO
	Postpartum Care. The percentage of deliveries that had a postpartum visit on or between 21 and 56 days after delivery
Annual dental visit[A]	The percentage of enrolled members 2–21 years of age who had at least one dental visit during the measurement year. This measure applies only if dental care is a covered benefit in the MCO's Medicaid contract
Initiation and engagement of alcohol and other drug dependence treatment[A]	This measure calculates two rates using the same population of members with Alcohol and Other Drug (AOD) dependence:
	Initiation of AOD Dependence Treatment: The percentage of adults diagnosed with AOD dependence who initiate treatment through either:
	• an inpatient AOD admission, **or** • an outpatient service for AOD dependence *and* additional AOD services within 14 days
	Engagement of AOD Treatment is an intermediate step between initially accessing care (initiation treatment) and completing a full course of treatment. This measure is designed to assess the degree to which members engage in treatment with two additional AOD services within 30 days after initiation
Claims timeliness[A]	The percentage of all claims received by the MCO or its claims processing centers January 1 through December 1 of the measurement year that were paid or denied within 30 calendar days of receipt. This includes all MCO claims delegates (e.g., keying centers, clearinghouses)
Call answer timeliness[A]	The percentage of calls received by the MCO's member services call centers (during member services operating hours) during the measurement year that were answered by a live voice within 30 seconds
Call abandonment[A]	The percentage of calls received by the MCO's member services call centers (during member services operating hours) during the measurement year that were abandoned by the caller before being answered by a live voice

TABLE G-3 continued

Satisfaction with the Experience of Care

CAHPS 3.0H Adult Survey[S]	This measure assesses commercial and Medicaid members' satisfaction with the MCO. Results summarize member experiences through ratings, composites, and individual question summary rates Four global rating questions reflect overall satisfaction with the following:

- Rating of All Health Care
- Rating of Health Plan
- Rating of Personal Doctor
- Rating of Specialist Seen Most Often

Six composite scores summarize responses in key areas:

- Claims Processing
- Courteous and Helpful Office Staff
- Customer Service
- Getting Care Quickly
- Getting Needed Care
- How Well Doctors Communicate

CAHPS 3.0H Child Survey[S]	This measure assesses parents' satisfaction with their child's MCO. Results summarize member experiences through ratings, composites, and individual question summary rates Four global rating questions reflect overall satisfaction with the following:

- Rating of All Health Care
- Rating of Health Plan
- Rating of Personal Doctor
- Rating of Specialist Seen Most Often

Six composite scores summarize responses in key areas:

- Claims Processing
- Courteous and Helpful Office Staff
- Customer Service
- Getting Care Quickly
- Getting Needed Care
- How Well Doctors Communicate

Children with Chronic Conditions[S]	This measure assesses parents' satisfaction with their child's MCO for the population of children with chronic conditions. Six composites summarize satisfaction with basic components of care essential for successful treatment, management, and support of children with chronic conditions:

- Access to Prescription Medicines
- Access to Specialized Services
- Family Centered Care: Personal Doctor or Nurse Who Knows Child

(continued on next page)

TABLE G-3 continued

	• Family Centered Care: Shared Decision Making • Family Centered Care: Getting Needed Information • Coordination of Care
ECHO 3.0H Survey for MBHOs[S]	A standardized survey that assesses MBHO enrollee experiences with behavioral health care, including mental health and chemical dependency services Results are summarized through ratings, composites, and question summary rates: **Global Question Rating.** • Rating of Counseling and Treatment **Composite Scores.** • Getting Treatment Quickly • How Well Clinicians Communicate • Access to Treatment and Information from the MBHO • Informed About Treatment Options **Question Summary Rates.** • Office Wait Times • Informed About Medication Side Effects • Received Information About Managing Condition • Informed About Patient Rights • Ability to Refuse Medicine or Treatment
Health Plan Stability[A]	
Practitioner turnover[A]	From the MCO provider database: • the percentage of primary care physicians affiliated with the MCO as of December 31 of the year prior to the measurement year who were *not* affiliated with the MCO as of December 31 of the measurement year • the percentage of nonphysician primary care practitioners affiliated with the MCO as of December 31 of the year prior to the measurement year who were *not* affiliated with the MCO as of December 31 of the measurement year For the Medicaid product line only, the MCO also reports the same percentages for the following practitioners: • OB/GYN and other prenatal care practitioners • chemical dependency practitioners • mental health practitioners • dentists
Years in business/total membership[A]	The number of years since **licensure** (the number of years that each product line has existed) and the number of members enrolled as of December 31 of the measurement year. The number of years of operation

TABLE G-3 continued

should be considered when evaluating the MCO's financial profile. For example, a new MCO may have a greater level of debt than a more mature MCO, and financial profiles may vary according to MCO type (e.g., staff model HMO, POS, IPA)

Use of Service[A]

Frequency of ongoing prenatal care[H]	The percentage of Medicaid deliveries between November 6 of the year prior to the measurement year and November 5 of the measurement year and received <21 percent, 21–40 percent, 41–60 percent, 61–80 percent or ≥81 percent of the expected number of prenatal care visits, adjusted for gestational age and the month that the member enrolled in the MCO. This measure uses the same denominator and deliveries as the Prenatal and Postpartum Care measure. For these deliveries, the MCO: • identifies the actual number of prenatal care visits rendered while they were enrolled in the MCO • identifies the number of expected visits • calculates the ratio of received-to-expected visits • reports an unduplicated count of deliveries had <21 percent; 21–40 percent, 41–60 percent, 61–80 percent or ≥81 percent of the number of expected visits, adjusted for the month the member enrolled and the MCO and gestational age. The MCO reports five rates
Well-child visits in the first 15 months of life[H]	The percentage of enrolled members who turned 15 months old during the measurement year and who had the following number of well-child visits with a primary care practitioner during their first 15 months of life: zero; one; two; three; four; five; six or more
Well-child visits in the third, fourth, fifth, and sixth years of life[H]	The percentage of members who were three, four, five, or six years of age during the measurement year who received one or more well-child visits with a primary care practitioner during the measurement year
Adolescent well-care visits[H]	The percentage of enrolled members who were 12–21 years of age who had at least one comprehensive well-care visit with a primary care practitioner or an OB/GYN practitioner during the measurement year
Frequency of selected procedures[A]	This measure provides a summary of the number and rate of several frequently performed procedures—myringotomy, tonsillectomy, nonobstetric dialation and curettage, hysterectomy, cholecystectomy, laminectomy/diskectomy, angioplasty, cardiac catheterization, coronary artery bypass graft, pros-

(continued on next page)

TABLE G-3 continued

	tatectomy, reduction of fracture of femur, total hip replacement, total knee replacement, partial excision of large intestine, carotid endarterectomy These procedures often show wide regional variation and have generated concern regarding potentially inappropriate utilization *For Medicaid members,* the MCO reports the absolute number of procedures and the number of procedures per 1,000 member months *For commercial and Medicare members,* the MCO reports the absolute number of procedures and the number of procedures per 1,000 members per year
Inpatient utilization—general hospital/acute care[A]	This measure summarizes utilization of acute inpatient services in the following categories: • total services • medicine • surgery • maternity Nonacute care, mental health and chemical dependency services, as well as newborn care, are excluded. Medical and surgical services are reported separately because the factors influencing utilization in these two categories vary. This method also facilitates comparisons between ambulatory surgery utilization (refer to the Ambulatory Care measure) and inpatient surgery utilization
Ambulatory care[A]	This measure summarizes utilization of ambulatory services in the following categories: • outpatient visits • emergency department visits • ambulatory surgery/procedures performed in hospital, outpatient facilities or freestanding surgical centers • observation room stays that result in discharge (observation room stays resulting in an inpatient admission are counted in the Inpatient Utilization—General Hospital/Acute Care measure)
Inpatient utilization—nonacute care[A]	This measure summarizes utilization of nonacute inpatient care in hospice, nursing home, rehabilitation, SNF, transitional care and respite. These data exclude services with a principal diagnosis of mental health and chemical dependency
Discharge and average length of stay—maternity care [A]	Utilization of maternity-related care for enrolled females who had live births during the measurement year, reported for total deliveries, vaginal deliveries and Cesarean section (C-section) deliveries

TABLE G-3 continued

Births and average length of stay, newborns[A]	This measure summarizes utilization information about newborns discharged during the measurement year and reports information for total newborns, well newborns and complex newborns
	Newborns are identified and reported separately from maternity members. **Newborn care** is care provided from birth to discharge to home. If a newborn is transferred from one hospital to another and has never gone home, the care is still newborn care. Newborn care that is rendered after the baby has been discharged should be reported in Table IPU-A (Inpatient Utilization—General Hospital/Acute Care)
	Include newborns delivered in an inpatient setting and at birthing centers. For newborns delivered in birthing centers, count one day of stay
	Some MCOs do not keep separate records on well newborns that leave the hospital at the same time as their mothers. The MCO must develop a methodology to estimate the number of well newborns for whom the MCO does not produce separate discharge records. For example, the mother's length of stay can be used as a proxy for the well newborn's length of stay. The MCO must provide documentation for the approach used
Mental health utilization—inpatient discharges and average length of stay[A]	This measure summarizes utilization of inpatient mental health services, stratified by age and sex
Mental health utilization—percentage of members receiving services[A]	The number and percentage of members receiving the following during the measurement year:
	• any mental health services (includes inpatient, intermediate or ambulatory)
	• inpatient mental health services
	• intermediate mental health services
	• ambulatory mental health services
	Report in each category the number of members who received the respective service and, of all enrollees with a mental health benefit, the percentage who received the respective service; report this information by age and sex. This measure gives an overview of the extent to which different levels of mental health services are utilized
Chemical dependency utilization—inpatient discharges and average length of stay[A]	This measure summarizes utilization of inpatient chemical dependency services, stratified by age and sex

(continued on next page)

TABLE G-3 continued

Identification of alcohol and other drug services[A]	The number and percentage of members with an alcohol and other drug (AOD) claim. AOD claims contain a diagnosis of AOD abuse or dependence and a specific AOD-related service during the measurement year, in the following categories:

• any chemical dependency services (includes inpatient, intermediate, ambulatory)

Reported by age and sex:

• the number of members in each category who received the service
• from all enrollees with a chemical dependency benefit, the percentage of members who received the service

Outpatient drug utilization[A]	A summary of the data on outpatient utilization of drug prescriptions (total cost of prescriptions; average cost of prescriptions per member per month [PMPM]; total number of prescriptions; average number of prescriptions per member per year [PMPY]) during the measurement year, stratified by age

Cost of Care
Informed Health Care Choices
Health Plan Descriptive Information[A]

Board certification[A]	The percentage of the following physicians who are board certified:

• primary care physicians
• OB/GYN physicians
• pediatric physician specialists
• geriatricians
• all other physician specialists

Board certification refers to the various specialty certification programs of the American Board of Medical Specialties and the American Osteopathic Association. The MCO should report separately for each product as of December 31 of the measurement year

Total enrollment by percentage[A]	This measure provides an overview of the mix of MCO membership. The MCO reports the percentage of total member months contributed by each product by age and sex during the measurement year

• Medicaid: Members enrolled through a contract between the state Medicaid agency and the MCO. Members eligible for Medicaid and Medicare should be counted under both products
• Commercial: Members enrolled through an employer group policy or individual policy
• Medicare: Members enrolled through a contract between CMS and the MCO. Members eligible

TABLE G-3   continued

	for both Medicare and Medicaid should also be counted under Medicare if the MCO has a Medicare contract • Other: Members not classified as Medicaid, commercial, or Medicare
Enrollment by product line[A]	This measure reports the total number of members enrolled for each product line stratified by age and sex • Medicaid is reported in the member months contributed by enrollees during the measurement year, it is stratified by Medicaid eligibility category, age and sex. The MCO may report this information only if it is provided by the state Medicaid agency • Medicare and commercial are reported in the number of member years contributed by enrollees during the measurement year, stratified by product line, age, and sex
Unduplicated count of Medicaid members[A]	Provides state Medicaid agencies with information that enables them to calculate by age, sex, and Medicaid eligibility category the average number of months Medicaid beneficiaries spent in the MCO. The MCO reports an unduplicated count of the number of all Medicaid members enrolled during any part of the measurement year, stratified by age, sex, and eligibility category
Diversity of Medicaid membership[A]	The number and percentage of Medicaid members enrolled at any time during the measurement year by race/ethnicity, Hispanic origin, and spoken language. The MCO may report this information only if is furnished to them by their state Medicaid agencies
Weeks of pregnancy at time of enrollment in the MCO[H]	The percentage of all enrolled women who delivered a live birth during the measurement year by the weeks of pregnancy at the time of their enrollment in the MCO, according to the following categories: • prior to pregnancy (280 days or more prior to delivery) • the first 12 weeks of pregnancy, including the end of the 12th week (279–196 days prior to delivery) • the beginning of the 13th week through the end of the 27th week of pregnancy (195–91 days prior to delivery) • the beginning of the 28th week of pregnancy or after (90 days or fewer prior to delivery)

Medicare Advantage PPOs—data collection requirements.
[A]Administrative data.
[H]Hybrid (administrative specifications, optionally augmented by chart record abstraction).
[C]Chart abstraction—2008 target.
[S]Survey data.

TABLE G-4 MDS Publicly Reported Measures on CMS' Nursing Home Compare (15 measures)

Long-Term Measures

1.	Activities of daily living	Percentage of residents whose need for help with daily activities has increased
2.	Pain	Percentage of residents who have moderate to severe pain
3 & 4.	Pressure sores	Percentage of high-risk residents who have pressure sores
		Percentage of low-risk residents who have pressure sores
5.	Restraint use	Percentage of residents who were physically restrained
6.	Depressed or anxious	Percentage of residents who are more depressed or anxious
7.	Incontinence	Percentage of low-risk residents who lose control of their bowels or bladder
8.	Indwelling catheters	Percentage of residents who have/had a catheter inserted and left in their bladder
9.	Bedfast	Percentage of residents who spent most of their time in bed or in a chair
10.	Ambulation/locomotion	Percentage of residents whose ability to move about in and around their room got worse
11.	Urinary tract infections	Percentage of residents with a urinary tract infection
12.	Weight loss	Percentage of residents who lose too much weight

Short-Stay Measures

13.	Delirium symptoms	Percentage of short-stay residents with delirium
14.	Pain	Percentage of short-stay residents who had moderate to severe pain
15.	Pressure sores	Percentage of short-stay residents with pressure sores

TABLE G-5 OASIS Publicly Reported Measures on CMS' Home Health Compare (11 measures)

1.	Improvement in ambulation/ locomotion	Patients who get better at walking or moving around in a wheelchair safely
2.	Improvement in transferring	Patients who get better at getting in and out of bed
3.	Improvement in toileting	Patients who get better getting to and from the toilet
4.	Improvement in pain interfering with activity	Patients who have less pain when moving around
5.	Improvement in bathing	Patients who get better at bathing
6.	Improvement in management of oral medications	Patients who get better at taking their medications correctly (by mouth)
7.	Improvement in upper body dressing	Patients who get better at getting dressed
8.	Stabilization in bathing	Patients who stay the same (don't get worse) at bathing
9.	Acute care hospitalization	Percentage of patients who had to be admitted to the hospital
10.	Emergent care	Percentage of patients who need urgent, unplanned medical care
11.	Improvement in confusion frequency	Patients who are confused less often

TABLE G-6 NHQR's ESRD Measures (5 measures)

Process	Percentage of dialysis patients registered on a waiting list for transplantation
	Percentage of patients with treated chronic kidney failure who receive a transplant within 3 years of renal failure
Outcome	Percentage of hemodialysis patients with urea reduction ratio of 65 or greater
	Percentage of patients with hematocrit of 33 or greater
	Patient survival rate

Appendix H

Commissioned Paper

Efficiency/Value-Based Measures for Services, Defined Populations, Acute Episodes, and Chronic Conditions

Kyle L. Grazier

INTRODUCTION

This paper was commissioned by the Institute of Medicine (IOM) to provide an overview of "value-based" or efficiency measurement in health care. It will define selected terms; provide a brief history of the development of these measurement sets; assemble information on the efficiency measurement sets in current use; identify challenges to applying these in practice and research; and identify gaps in efficiency measurement.

DEFINITION OF EFFICIENCY

Central to this work is the manner in which "efficiency" and "value based" are defined. Among others, the economics, statistics, management science, and health services research literatures have contributed variations on these definitions that differ in their specificity to health care and their generalizability beyond the economic costs of health care services. Specifically, definitions differ as to whether the mix of inputs includes quality, and the mix of outputs includes health, health status, or mortality.

Economic efficiency is commonly expressed as the relationships between a given quantity and quality of output using a bundle of inputs that minimizes the cost of production. Several different combinations of capital, labor, and raw materials (where each of these can have multiple dimensions, e.g., physician labor, nurse labor, etc.), could feasibly be used as inputs to produce a particular quantity and quality of output. Generally, only one of these combinations will have the lowest cost associated with that input bundle.

Palmer and Torgerson's (1999) definition of efficiency includes both health care inputs and health outcomes. The goals for measurement determine which aspect of efficiency is emphasized. They suggest that "allocative efficiency" should dictate policy decisions focused on resource distribution (Palmer and Torgerson, 1999). This aspect of efficiency requires that a specific outcome be defined in advance, after which a choice is made among alterative interventions or resources based on their relative costs. The resulting costs may not reflect the most efficient combination of inputs and outputs but it does allow for an allocation strategy. An example: If one is interested in promoting one of two surgical interventions, and the identified criteria for selection is a fixed minimum postsurgical mortality rate, then one can compare the relative costs of each to achieve a fixed mortality threshold.

To assess "productive efficiency," one maximizes "health outcome for a given cost," or minimizes "cost for a given outcome." For example, one chooses different combinations of inputs to achieve the best health outcome for a given cost. "Technical efficiency" is achieved if the physical mix of labor and capital inputs achieves the maximum output. For instance, if surgical procedure A and surgical procedure B produce the identical defined outcomes of hospital discharge in 3 days, but procedure A uses less labor but identical amounts of capital, then procedure B is considered technically inefficient.

The measurement of the individual inputs and outputs in the efficiency function also vary by setting, goals, and the availability of data. The definition of costs or economic resources has been relatively consistent in services research: direct and indirect monetary resources that contribute to the institution's costs of providing a service. However, as the goals of measurement change to incorporate an understanding of *system* resources, then the physician's resource use is included, as are out-of-pocket direct costs, and even indirect costs of lost workplace productivity and reductions in general economic production. Such expansive cost constructs can inhibit practical solutions due to conceptual and data complexities. For the most part, this paper focuses on the service-related resource costs consumed in the delivery of medical care within the health care system.

Over a decade ago, the IOM defined quality as "the degree to which health services for individuals and populations increase the likelihood of desired health outcomes and are consistent with current professional knowledge" (IOM, 1990). But as many authors have noted recently, the definition of quality, as in quality care or quality improvement, has not reached national consensus (Berwick, 2002; McGlynn, 1995; McGlynn et al., 2003; McKee, 2001; Palmer and Torgerson, 1999; Wennberg et al., 2002). Complicating these efforts are the paucity of "gold standards" for health outcomes, definitive levels of health that are measurable, valid, and reliable.

Patient, population, and clinical characteristics introduce variations in outcomes. In addition, the choice of services and the process for delivering them have limited clinical evidence of their efficacy and effectiveness. Finally, deficits in management costing have limited the ability to measure accurately the resources consumed in the care delivery process and the quantitative outcomes.

In the discourse on performance measurement in health care, "efficiency" is used in many contexts and for many purposes. Policymakers at national, local, plan, and purchaser levels are deliberating how to maximize health-related outcomes of their enrollees, beneficiaries, or employees receiving services, while minimizing costs for a standard outcome. Maximizing efficiency or reducing expenditures may compete for attention with a target morbidity rate.

These challenges influence which measures of value and efficiency to evaluate or support; which methods to endorse for practitioners, services, and resources; and how to implement and integrate efforts to improve intermediate and longer-term population-, firm-, or patient-specific outcomes. Despite these many challenges, considerable effort has advanced thinking and action in the research and practice arenas.

While there is not yet consensus on the definition of "efficiency" or "value based," this paper will incorporate both the Institute of Medicine (IOM) landmark report's definition of efficiency (eliminating waste) and the theoretical economics definition of efficiency (IOM, 2001; Palmer and Torgerson, 1999). For these purposes, efficiency will be broadly defined as the mix of health care resource inputs that produce optimal quantity and quality of health and health care outputs. In short, the bias is toward measuring the production efficiency of relative health care resources among individual, institutional, and groups of providers.

It is important to note here that there are several current initiatives and programs to assess, improve, promote, and reward improvements in and delivery of quality health care (AHRQ, 2004; Bridges to Excellence, 2004; Kerr et al., 2004; Leapfrog Group, 2005). Other consortia of employers, purchasers, and health plans are planning programs to measure and reward institutional performance in effectiveness and efficiency (Leapfrog Group, 2005; PBGH, 2005; Worthington, 2004). Although this paper addresses the broader definition of efficiency to include "value," and therefore, quality inputs and outcomes, no attempt will be made to discuss all measures of quality, performance, or effectiveness currently in use.

MOTIVATIONS FOR VALUE-BASED MEASURES AND MEASUREMENT

Policy makers, researchers, providers, and others are motivated to seek value-based or efficiency measures for various reasons. In the past two decades, the quality of the available data and the rigor of the analysis have advanced our ability to measure the economic outputs that are derived from resource inputs. As a result, numerous health care institutions and researchers are willing to invest in value-based measurements, with a clear focus on quality-adjusted outcomes. Many purchasing groups, health plans, insurers, and consumer groups are at least as concerned, if not more so, with the cost-*efficiency* of services. Algorithms for assessing relative efficiency of providers vary in their transparency to the user, but are widespread among health plans and physician group practices. Outputs from these types of analyses trigger decisions on appointing and reappointing physicians within a practice or network; form the basis for monetary incentive packages for providers and groups; and generally are aimed at the containment and management of contract and practice costs of physicians delivering inpatient and outpatient, general and specialty care in solo, single-, or multispecialty practices.

The following purposes for efficiency measurement have been documented in the literature (Berwick, 2002, 2003; Fiscella et al., 2000; Franks et al., 1993; Galvin and McGlynn, 2003; Iezzoni et al., 1992b, 1994a; IOM, 1990; Kerr et al., 2004; Leatherman et al., 2003; McGlynn, 2003a,b; McGlynn and Brook, 2001; McGlynn and Halfon, 1998; McGlynn et al., 2003; Nauert, 1996; NCQA, 2004; Shahian and Normand, 2003; Schield et al., 2000; Siu et al., 1992).

While extensive, the list is not exhaustive:

- Improve quality of care
- Encourage payer involvement
- Integrate responsibility for employment, payment, health status
- Reduce waste
- Re/appoint/certify medical staff for network participation
- Increase financial risk associated with practice decisions
- Alter practice patterns
- Assist in cost containment
- Encourage/steer selection of efficient health plans
- Allocate service resources differently
- Deploy alternative labor and capital
- Track/evaluate relationships to health management, health status, survival

MEASUREMENT CONSIDERATIONS

Validity

There are generic guidelines for selecting measurement criteria, not all of which can be met in the current efforts to measure efficiency. Regardless of the goals for measuring efficiency, the measure used for efficiency or value must be valid. Unfortunately, gold standards for health care efficiency don't exist, complicating efforts to establish the validity and reliability of a measure.

Surrogates for validity in measuring practice efficiency include the notion of "accuracy" of the programs and "consistency" or "stability" across practices and providers (Thomas et al., 2004b). Technical accuracy is highlighted by holding constant an outcome, and comparing inputs, namely costs, across physicians of the same specialty. By varying the methods used in measuring the inputs, and comparing the consistency of the outputs, production efficiency is captured. By establishing the "stability" of the output measure over time, over different types of physician specialties and patient panel sizes, one can learn more about potential variation in the inputs and outputs, and the financial and health consequences.

Unit of Analysis

Currently, the majority of practice efficiency measurement tools rely on the physician as the unit of analysis, rather than the physician group, individual patient, or community member. The purpose of this physician-focused measurement is to establish the economic resources consumed by the physician in the delivery of care, relative to physician peers. The visit, service, or case descriptors attempt to bundle patient and clinical care characteristics into discrete, homogeneous categories. These categories are then used to help define the services a patient might expect to receive when presenting with the characteristics defined by a particular resource category (Franks and Fiscella, 2002; Franks et al., 2003). However, there is still considerable variation in which variables contribute to "case" categories and resource use, and the algorithms for assigning the costs of those resources to providers.

Attribution of Resource Use

Attributing patient-specific resource use to an individual physician is particularly complicated when services are delivered as part of a team of providers, over an extended period of time, for complex or persistent conditions.

Under a gatekeeper model, primary care physicians are held responsible for all services delivered, whether provided by the physician, referred to another approved physician, or provided by other clinical staff within the practice. Although the underlying risk-sharing arrangement within a primary care practice may not be known, many efficiency tools assume that all consumed resources can be attributed to the primary care physician. When evaluating the resources used by nonprimary care physicians, or "specialists," attributing responsibility for services across the providers is usually based on a formula. These formulas differ in their attribution decision rules, and vary the amounts of resources assigned to a responsible provider proportionally or nonproportionally to the primary care, nonprimary care, or total resources consumed across the episode.

Data

The data sources for these efforts have traditionally included encounter and claims data supplied through an employer, insurer, or plan's administrative data systems. In some cases, the administrative data have been validated against medical records, but these efforts have been inconclusive in determining which source is better than another for these purposes (Hannan et al., 2003). Claims or encounter data at this time are generally more accessible and less expensive to analyze than medical charts or patient surveys, although efforts to identify quality and value metrics continue to explore these sources as well as electronic medical records and online order entry systems (Birkmeyer et al., 1999, 2002, 2003; Fisher et al., 1990a,b, 1992; Malenka et al., 1994; Thomas et al., 2004a).

Different types and amounts of data can be extracted from the same claims data set (Baron et al., 1994; Fisher et al., 1992). Many profiling tools capture and use in their algorithms different numbers of diagnoses, procedures, and different time periods for services. Current episoding algorithms vary in the numbers of episode categories to which diagnoses and procedures are assigned. They also differ in the length of the "clean periods," those time periods during which no services for the condition are received, thus triggering the end of one episode and the beginning of another.

It is common in profiling methods to aggregate all costs of care that appear with an episode and attribute this total to a provider. But there is also variation in the complexity or severity of the case or in patient characteristics that are not captured in episode categories defined by time of service (Iezzoni et al., 1992a,b, 1994b). Several risk adjustment methods that have been perfected for other purposes as well as for physician efficiency profiling are applied to episodes to explain better the resources identified as inputs in the model.

Risk Adjustment

Risk adjustment is used to adjust claims profiles to account for differences in the health status (and thus expected resource use) of patients served. Without proper adjustment, practice patterns of physicians whose patient panels include greater than average proportions of elderly patients or patients with severe or chronic disease could appear, incorrectly, to reflect inappropriately high levels of resource use (such as office visits, ancillary services, prescription medications, specialist referrals, and hospital days). Different risk-adjustment methodologies—all purporting to "do" the same thing—can produce quite different results. Research on hospital profiling demonstrates that comparative judgments about provider performance can be influenced significantly by the specific risk measurement methodology utilized (Iezzoni, 1997).

There are several models of risk adjustment that have been tested over time and on various data sets. The vast literature reflects the range of purposes, data sources, algorithms, analytic models, and outputs associated with risk adjustment methods (Thomas et al., 2004a). Researchers and policy makers see a growing role for risk adjustment payment models, financing policies, and performance measurement. Patient interviews, surveys, claims records, medical records, or some combination of these have been suggested as sources for data on health or medical risk (Ash et al., 2001; Grazier and Thomas, 2002; Hornbrook and Goodman, 1996; Newhouse et al., 1997; Pope et al., 2004; Street, 2003; Worthington, 2004; Zhao et al., 2001). The costs associated with collection are weighed against the quality and volume of the information from each source.

There are many physician profiling and efficiency tools based solely on administrative data, although even in these cases there are significant differences in the data fields used in the algorithms that define risk categories; models may include age, sex, one or more primary, principal, or secondary procedures and diagnoses, and pharmacy National Drug Codes (NDC) (Ash et al., 2001; de Brantes, 2002; de Brantes et al., 2003; Goldman et al., 2004; Grazier and Thomas, 2002; Pope et al., 2004; Thomas et al., 2002; Worthington, 2004; Zhao et al., 2001). Many efficiency-profiling packages also require specific record layouts and field definitions.

Resource Costs

Service or resource costs used in efficiency measurement are seldom collected from institutional management accounting processes; instead they rely on the monetary data appearing in the claim record; these include paid charges, allowable charges, or relative value adjusted charges. In some cases, to remove the effects of price variations in the reported charges, charges are standardized to a regional or local mean value for similar procedures or practices. In cases in which detecting price variations and their impact on practice is central to the profiling effort, actual recorded paid charges are used without standardizing for market differences.

Thresholds

Physician profiling tools assess the extent to which "costs" of the resources used for an individual type of patient or panel of patients exceeds a predetermined percentile, a group-specific median or mean, a national specialty group consensus level, other national benchmarks, or a relative value based on annual budgets or financial targets. Patient or episode cost outliers can influence many of the algorithms for assessing efficiency. Case outliers are often examined separately from the pool to determine what factors affect their occurrence. The width of the threshold bands determines in part how stable efficiency rankings are over time and across specialties.

Outputs

The output from efficiency measurement for individual physicians is most commonly the ratio of the observed costs to the expected costs (Thomas et al., 2004a,b). The closer a physician comes to using (spending) resources at levels expected for the clinical risk of the patient or panel of patients, the more efficient he or she is assumed to be. While use of the observed/expected cost ratio is prevalent, users should be cautious when applying the ratio to physicians with small patient panels, since misclassification is in many cases related to panel group size. Use of a measure of the difference between the standardized expected costs and the standardized observed costs for a patient or panel could dampen this small sample bias.

MEASURES OF "VALUE-BASED" METRICS (EFFICIENCY MEASURES)

In 2003, the National Quality Forum (NQF) endorsed national voluntary consensus standards for hospital care performance measures. The initial 39 measures were "intended to promote both public accountability and quality improvement." The Institute for Healthcare Improvement, through several programs and as described in several white papers as part of their innovation series, has initiated efforts among hospitals to improve the outcomes and experiences of patients and providers on medical/surgical units. Although not specifically designed to measure efficiency, they promote the potential increased value to patients and providers through use of the measures (Institute for Healthcare Improvement, 2005). The IOM, NQF, the Agency for Healthcare Research and Quality (ARHQ), and the National Committee for Quality Assurance (NCQA) singularly and as part of consortia have produced topics, criteria, and measures for clinical conditions and priority areas for health care quality improvement activities (AHRQ,

2004; IOM, 2005; NCQA, 2004; NQF, 2005). These works continue to contribute measures of quality into the value-based efficiency measurement equation. The report on measuring provider efficiency, a collaborative effort of the Leapfrog Group and the Bridges to Excellence, notes "reporting performance on efficiency should be linked to reporting performance on quality to better understand, measure and communicate the value that is delivered by physicians and hospitals" (Bridges to Excellence, 2004; NCQA, 2004).

Other organizations and sponsors have begun or are considering using data collected for earlier purposes, such as quality measures for accreditation or internal monitoring, for value measurement. The NCQA monitors health plan performance by collecting and analyzing the Health Plan Employer Data and Information Set. As noted earlier, it has convened technical panels to design efficiency measures for implementation among member health plans. The AHRQ is providing guidance based on its own research as to how best to use the quality indicators that they make publicly available for performance and potentially efficiency measurement (Remus and Irene, 2004). The Joint Commission on Accreditation of Healthcare Organizations (JCAHO) is considering reporting some of its measures collected during accreditation processes. AHRQ reports "JCAHO will be replacing hospital performance reports with quality reports in 2004."

Table H-1 presents some of the measures of value and efficiency that have been proposed or are in use either by or under the sponsorship of several of the above-named organizations. Few of the existing measures endorsed by national organizations are specifically for measuring efficiency; however, some programs are included if they noted in their documentation their preparations for expansion of quality measurement to "efficiency" or "value."

GAPS IN THE LITERATURE AND EMPIRICAL WORK

Health care value can be viewed as a set of individual and conflated components (e.g., quality, cost, population health, clinical measurement, payment methods, practice patterns, and delivery system). The dynamic nature of the research in each of these areas leads to frequent, important contributions. Recent advances stimulate efforts to identify and fill the gaps remaining in our knowledge of value-based metrics, and in related policies and practices. Several remaining challenges are being addressed in demonstrations, experiments, and practice; some have not yet been rigorously examined; and many remain ripe for rigorous study.

Standardization in the Measures Used to Assess Efficiency

Standardization has been a necessary step in the advancement of numerous technologies and in improvements in production. The need for standardized measures of quality, effectiveness, and efficiency has been documented extensively.

Most commercial products on the market and many of those in development by NCQA and others measure efficiency by comparing actual observed expenses with expected expenses incurred in the delivery of services. In some cases, the effect of prices is removed. The price-adjusted (or standardized) measure assumes that "paid amount" noted on claims reflects volume, type of services, and price. Unless the intent was to assess the impact of price variation on provider efficiency, the ratio of observed to expected costs would be standardized to remove this variation. To accomplish this, standard or average regional prices for similar services are applied to the services data. Recent studies have recommended that both price-adjusted and unadjusted observed versus expected costs be measured and compared with one another (Bridges to Excellence, 2004; Leapfrog Group, 2005; Thomas et al., 2004a). NCQA efforts to create an efficiency indicator for health plans include examining both standardized and unadjusted efficiency measures, to understand better the extent of variation in outcomes due to regional or price differences.

Physicians are obvious stakeholders in the standardization of these measures, and many complain that efficiency performance is being measured and interpreted differently within and across health plans, insurers, health systems, and consumer groups. Policymakers must consider the cost to the plans or practices of imposing one particular episoding and/or risk adjustment commercial product, rather than specifying standardized input and output measures. Transparency in methods and algorithms aids evaluation of the logic and components that could and should contribute to a standard. To advance understanding and promote progress in standard setting, product details need to be revealed; examples of information needed for this purpose include: the underlying logic and processes of the algorithms used for preparing data for the application, and for episoding and risk adjustment; standard errors and statistical significance of output measures; outlier threshold levels; frequency and types of omitted cases; total member panel size and number of valid episodes per physician per time period; and the attribution method used within specialty and across specialties.

Inclusion of Quality Dimensions in the Measures

Significant progress has been made in identifying process and outcomes components of quality care, particularly for certain conditions treated in certain settings. Experts in clinical care and measurement recommend that recently piloted processes be expanded and that current larger-scale empirical work be tested on other samples and in other venues.

For instance, clinical quality measures for diabetes care and heart/stroke care included in Bridges to Excellence/NCQA Provider Recognition Programs are available for use in assessing efficiency performance (Tom Lee, personal communication, 2004). The End of Life metrics developed by the Dartmouth Atlas team (Wennberg et al., 2002) have been proposed as a proxy for hospital system efficiency (Eugene Nelson, personal communication, 2004). Active research programs and demonstrations by the NQF, the NCQA, Bridges to Excellence, the Leapfrog Group, research groups, and others are rapidly advancing the measurement of quality using medical records and administration data. These efforts need to be shared and combined on an ongoing basis into the measurement of health care value.

Validated Clinical (Medical Service, Pharmacy) and Financial Data

A number of studies have examined the validity of self-reported data, medical records, and administrative data and found that, with some caveats, claims data are adequate for many purposes related to value measurement. Although recent, these studies may not be generalizable to future information systems in which the electronic medical record, integrated services/ encounter data, and advanced cost accounting systems are the norm. Concurrent with efforts to measure efficiency and performance are demonstrations and experiments in facility-based standardized records and information systems that can form the basis for reliable measurement of services, quality, and providers across sites and health systems (Physician Practice Connections for the Bridges to Excellence rewards program, Physician Office Link, the product of a collaboration between NCQA and Bridges to Excellence).

Although these efforts will undoubtedly lead to important answers and recommendations, ongoing empirical work should include sampling and analysis of:

(1) medical records for office visits and inpatient stays to validate data that appear on and are extracted from claims-based files and similar administrative records;

(2) cost data collected from multiple sources, including facility-specific, payer-specific records of billed charges, allowed charges, paid charges, and retroactive adjustments to assess the validity of resource measures;

(3) physician or group panel member characteristics including age, sex, race/ethnicity, and zipcode (to measure average socioeconomic status) relative to the service area or plan population. This can serve several purposes.

It would allow for relative assessments of a provider's practice case mix, which differs from the case or severity mix of treated patients, and plays an important role in determining the efficiency of a provider with a "sicker" panel of patients versus a sicker panel of "potential" patients. Researchers have made a strong case recently for the relevance of these characteristics to patterns of use, treatment, costs, and outcomes.

To ensure that data provide information on the persons who use services and those who do not, several population-based characteristics and patient- and service-specific data elements are needed, sometimes from several sources.

There are facility- and service-specific standardized forms and conventions for data collection. These include the UB-92 and HCFA 1500 forms for inpatient and professional services, and procedure, diagnosis, and pharmacy coding schemes (CPT, HCPCC, NDC, ICD) for clinical services delivered. What appears on claims records and what is extracted from them as part of measurement algorithms can differ across claims administrators, payers and product designers. Provider characteristics, including specialty and details on physicians' panels, referrals patterns, and physician payment algorithms are normally not readily available from administrative data sources. Cost data are also collected and presented variably in claims records and billing forms, requiring scrutiny of the definitions of data elements and the cost adjustment processes used by systems administrators. Validation studies are required prior to using these different data sources.

Multiyear, Multisystem, Linked, Population-Based Data that Captures:

- Acute and chronic care episodes
- Pharmacy data
- Population characteristics (age, sex, race/ethnicity)
- Provider characteristics
- Service delivery and payment model (FFS, HMO, PPO, POS, etc.)

Due to temporal variation in services delivery, claims reporting, episode construction, and services utilization, measuring value requires longitudinal data for several units of analysis. It also requires the capacity to link the units through a unique personal (e.g., member, patient, or provider) identifier. Although there is no published research on the optimal time frame for collecting physician experience data to ensure validity of the performance measures, actuarial models of medical care utilization indicate the importance of at least two years of claims experience to estimate with moderate confidence future utilization behavior.

While one year of claims data may allow for detection of acute care episodes, it may omit lengthy or complex episodes, particularly if the profiling algorithm truncates those cases that show no end date within the contract year or capture only episodes with clean periods at both ends.

One year of data is also likely to omit those patients who consistently incur high costs from year to year, whether because of severe and persistent illnesses, or due to high-frequency moderately resource-intensive service needs. Analysis of three years of claims and exposure data from the Society of Actuaries medical claims study (Grazier and G'Sell, 2004) indicates that for claimants with annual claims expense of more than $25,000, over 13 percent have annual claim costs in the subsequent two years of over $25,000; for those with annual claims in one year exceeding $50,000, almost 25 percent have total annual claims exceeding $25,000 in the subsequent year; and for those with annual claims cost exceeding $100,000, over 30 percent have claims exceeding $25,000 in subsequent years. While these data are for patients and not per physician, the effect of such cases on a panel from one year to the next could be misinterpreted if multiple years of data were not captured in the algorithms.

More than one year of data would be needed to establish a fuller picture of use, and to accommodate "clean periods" for episodes that span the limits of inforce coverage contracts or reflect care for chronic conditions. In the White Paper released by Bridges to Excellence (2004), authors recommended "at least two years of data, based on incurred claims" to "develop a statistically reliable determination of provider efficiency."

Recent research on measuring efficiency and quality has used administrative claims and member data either from commercial carriers or employers, or beneficiary claims data from fee-for-service Medicare. Because of the different payment models reflected in these data sets, care should be taken to ensure internal and external consistency. Within commercial population data, health mainenance organziation (HMO), exclusive provider organization, preferred provider organization (PPO), and traditional indemnity covered care may be captured differently. For instance, HMO encounter data may not incorporate professional fees with the inpatient/hospital records, while traditional-coverage-generated data may have both. Commercial claims data cannot be directly combined with Medicare data, without adjusting for beneficiary, coverage, and charge differences across the payers.

Most claims systems used by commercial carriers or those developed in-house separate pharmacy data systems. If quality is to be incorporated into efficiency measurement, then pharmacy data should be incorporated into the measurement and assessment of the appropriateness of resources (Goldman et al., 2004). If it were combined, then pharmacy data can be edited and aggregated and then linked by unique member identifiers across commercial data sets. If comparable pharmacy data are not available, such as in

Medicare claims, then pharmacy data should be removed from both sets prior to combination for analysis. Most large employers are requiring their third-party administrators or their health coverage carriers to collect and link pharmacy with medical claims information for analysis.

Identifying Validity of Measures Across Different Physician Specialties

- Primary care
- Inpatient specialty
- Ambulatory care, doctor office/group specialty

Very few studies are available to inform the use of efficiency metrics for different physician specialties. Primary care providers have been the subjects of physician cost profiling algorithms for almost a decade. Several vendor products are available for specialist profiling, using similar methods as those used for primary care. One study examined the reliability of different profiling algorithms for different types of specialists, and cautioned policymakers in using the outputs from such algorithms. More recent recommendations include evaluating only those physicians who are responsible for a fixed proportion of cases, and for whom peer specialists are available within the system or region for comparison. While national benchmarks are often used to compare specific results, transparency in those benchmarks is necessary to determine their appropriateness for these purposes.

Results of research to date have been confounded by complexities in capturing the underlying referral and payment allocation mechanics of plans or practices. It has also been limited in many cases to cost efficiency measurement, and not necessarily value.

Attribution of Resource Use to Provider, Site, Patient, Geographic Unit

- Fractional vs. fixed attribution methods
- Inpatient vs. outpatient
- Individual provider vs. team vs. health system

There are few studies that systematically examine the impacts of using different thresholds of responsibility for resources consumed. In one study, total resources were assigned proportionately to participating specialists if the specialist was responsible for 30, 50, or 80 percent of the total resources used. The selected threshold for inclusion obviously limits the numbers of physicians that can be measured. It also influences the apparent efficiency of the provider.

In the 2004 White Paper (Andrianos and Stam, 2004; Bridges to Excellence, 2004; Leapfrog Group, 2005), "Episodes were attributed to providers who had the highest professional claims within an episode, exceeding a minimum threshold for 25 percent of eligible clinician fees (eligible clinician fees included all professional fees, excluding hospital based physicians)." This was based on analysis performed by the authors to alter the attribution rules in increments of 10 percent, from 0 percent to 100 percent for the "minimum portion of total professional dollars in the episode required to be delivered by the attributed clinician." They concluded, "very little data is lost as the threshold changes from 0 percent to 30 percent, whether we consider episode volume, number of attributed clinicians, or total dollars. In this large sample of commercial claims, more than 88 percent of all episodes featured only one clinician eligible to be the attributed clinician."

More research is required on attribution threshold and distribution methods.

Consensus on the Basis for Selection of Service or Provider for Measurement

- Most prevalent conditions treated
- Highest cost episodes
- Highest volume of episodes
- Highest total costs

Research on quality and efficiency has progressed at different rates for different dimensions of value, and for different types of facilities, practitioners, and diseases. Users of value-based metrics may have different goals for their use.

Measurement of processes and outcomes associated with quality care for patients with certain conditions, such as cardiovascular disease, diabetes, and Chronic Obstructive Pulmonary Disease (COPD), is highly advanced. Adding cost and efficiency dimensions to that research may expedite our understanding of the potential for these types of approaches. Current purchaser-based initiatives on pay for performance may lend themselves to additional study of the incremental value and cost of using alternative algorithms to assess provider relative efficiency.

In addition to the many goals driving selection of the unit of measurement, there are also likely to be changes in the quality of the data available for analysis. How we measure and to whom we attribute resources may change as cost data improve in quality and availability within and across integrated systems.

Given that no consensus across stakeholders exists and that no one dominant basis for selecting physicians has been established, value-based measurement research should continue to study the marginal value of applying these metrics to current alternatives: primary care or other specialty physicians; inpatient and ambulatory care or office-based services; on the basis of disease or condition prevalence, panel health risk, total costs, or attributable costs.

Risk-Adjustment Methods

- Episode-based measures
- Encounter-based measures
- Provider-based measures

Episode grouping algorithms are integral to several existing commercial vendor and public sector products, as well as products and processes under development. The empirical support and logic behind this approach to understanding the package of resources used to treat a patient with certain conditions has positioned episode systems as superior to other alternatives. However, further analysis is necessary to compare episoding algorithms, including the use and length of "clean periods" for different conditions; the parsing of clinician conditions into episodes; and the effect of delivery system and payment method on resources assigned per episode.

By risk-adjusting episodes, total resource use can be considered in light of clinical condition and severity. Risk adjustment has received considerable attention in the literature; however, no dominant clinical risk-adjustment system has surfaced for episodes or non-Medicare cases. Research is still needed on the optimal method for determining clinical risk as it relates to the quality and efficiency of services and for adjusting for it using valid and reliable methods. Trade-offs among methods that utilize different or increasing numbers of variables from multiple data sources need to be made explicit.

Consensus in the Principles Behind and the Goals of Value-Based Measurement

The large number of stakeholders with interests in value-based metrics forces policymakers to recognize and prioritize the goals of such measurement. A consensus can streamline decisions on choice of methods and measures. For instance, agreement that high-quality, efficient allocation of resources to the public demands that value-based methods include measure of population health status. As another example, consensus as to the importance of the principle of fairness in the application of these metrics across plans, providers, and over time implicitly imposes a commitment to evaluate the consistency of the processes and the validity of the measures.

More broadly, the process of sharing values and selecting priorities through multiple stakeholder discussions can more rapidly integrate lessons learned and promote progress toward multiple goals.

CONCLUSION

The goals of value-based health care measurement are to improve practice, ensure high-quality care, and reduce underuse, overuse, and misuse of health care resources. Methods are available that permit identification of many primary care and other specialists who treat the most prevalent illnesses, the highest cost caseload, and the highest volume of services delivered. Administrative data are sufficiently ubiquitous to provide a ready palette for careful analysis when internal service records are not adequate or available. Multiple years of linked data improve identification of full episodes of care, evaluation of chronic care delivery models, and reliability of patient or member risk levels. Risk adjustment methods continue to be refined and evaluated. Efficiency metrics are still under development and testing, requiring some redundancy in use. Both standardized and nonstandardized observed costs should be further modeled.

It is critical when using any method that identifies or ranks the most or least efficient physicians or hospitals that those using these systems understand the underlying practice philosophy and service system within which the provider operates. If services were delivered by primary care teams, through care managers, or under indemnity or other insurance models in which patients have more choice in supply sensitive services, then profiling algorithms either must reflect these variations or highlight inputs and metrics for additional attention.

Further research and demonstrations on these and other features of a value-based metric system are under way.

REFERENCES

AHRQ (Agency for Healthcare Research and Quality). 2004. *What Consumers Say About the Quality of Their Health Plans and Medical Care, National CAHPS® Benchmarking Database 2003, Chartbook Volume 1: Composites and Ratings.* Rockville, MD: AHRQ.

Andrianos J, Stam D. 2004. *Study of Professional Episode Attribution Thresholds Summary: Vast majority of episodes involve only one managing clinician.* [Online]. Available: *http://www.regence.com/research/docs/professionalEpisodeAttributionStudy.pdf* [accessed November 9, 2004].

Ash A, Yang Z, Randall PE, Kramer MS. 2001. Finding future high-cost cases: Comparing prior cost versus diagnosis-based methods. *Health Services Research* 26(6):194–206.

Baron JA, Lu-Yao G, Barrett J, McLerran D, Fisher ES. 1994. Internal validation of Medicare claims data. *Epidemiology* 5(5):541–544.

Berwick DM. 2002. A user's manual for the IOM's "Quality Chasm" report. *Health Affairs* 21(3):80–90.

Berwick DM. 2003. Improvement, trust, and the healthcare workforce. *Quality and Safety in Health Care* 12(Suppl.1):i2–i6.

Birkmeyer JD, Lucas FL, Wennberg DE. 1999. Potential benefits of regionalizing major surgery in Medicare patients. *Effective Clinical Practice* 2(6):277–283.

Birkmeyer JD, Siewers AE, Finlayson EV, Stukel TA, Lucas FL, Batista I, et al. 2002. Hospital volume and surgical mortality in the United States. *New England Journal of Medicine* 346(15):1128–1137.

Birkmeyer JD, Stukel TA, Siewers AE, Goodney PP, Wennberg DE, Lucas FL. 2003. Surgeon volume and operative mortality in the United States. *New England Journal of Medicine* 349(22):2117–2127.

Bridges to Excellence (BTE). 2004. *Measuring Provider Efficiency*. A Collaborative multi-stakeholder effort. Version 1.0.

de Brantes FS. 2002. Bridges To Excellence: A program to start closing the quality chasm in healthcare. *Journal of Healthcare Quality* 24(2):2–11.

de Brantes FS, Galvin RS, Lee T. 2003. Bridges to Excellence: A business case for quality. *Journal of Clinical Outcomes Management* 10(8):431–438.

Fiscella K, Franks P, Gold MR, Clancy CM. 2000. Inequality in quality: Addressing socioeconomic, racial, and ethnic disparities in health care. *Journal of the American Medical Association* 283(19):2579–2584.

Fisher ES, Baron JA, Malenka DJ, Barrett J, Bubolz TA. 1990a. Overcoming potential pitfalls in the use of Medicare data for epidemiologic research. *American Journal of Public Health* 80(12):1487–1490.

Fisher, ES, Malenka DJ, Wennberg JE, Roos NP. 1990b. Technology assessment using insurance claims: Example of prostatectomy. *International Journal of Technology Assessment in Health Care* 6(2):194–202.

Fisher ES, Whaley FS, Krushat WM, Malenka DJ, Fleming C, Baron JA, et al. 1992. The accuracy of Medicare's hospital claims data: Progress has been made, but problems remain. *American Journal of Public Health* 82(2):243–248.

Franks P, Fiscella K. 2002. Effect of patient socioeconomic status on physician profiles for prevention, disease management, and diagnostic testing costs. *Medical Care* 40(8):717–724.

Franks P, Nutting PA, Clancy CM. 1993. Health care reform, primary care, and the need for research. *Journal of the American Medical Association* 270(12):1449–1453.

Franks P, Fiscella K, Beckett L, Zwanziger J, Mooney C, Gorthy S. 2003. Effects of patient and physician practice socioeconomic status on the health care of privately insured managed care patients. *Medical Care* 41(7):842–852.

Galvin RS, McGlynn EA. 2003. Using performance measurement to drive improvement: A road map for change. *Medical Care* 41(Suppl. 1):I48–I60.

Goldman D, Joyce GF, Escarce JJ, Pace JE, Solomon MD, Laouri M, Landsman PB, Teutsch SM. 2004. Pharmacy benefits and the use of drugs by the chronically ill. *Journal of the American Medical Association* 291(19):2344–2350.

Grazier KL, G'Sell WA. 2004. *Group Medical Insurance Claims Database Collections and Analysis*. Schaumburg, IL: Society of Actuaries.

Grazier KL, Thomas JW. 2002. *A Comparative Evaluation of Risk-Adjustment Methodologies for Profiling Physician Practice Efficiency*. A report to the Robert Wood Johnson Foundation.

Hannan EL, Doran DR, Rosenthal GE, Vaughn MS. 2003. Provider profiling and quality improvement efforts in coronary artery bypass graft surgery: The effect on short-term mortality among Medicare beneficiaries. *Medical Care* 4(10):1164–1172.

Hornbrook M, Goodman M. 1996. Chronic disease, functional health status and demographics: A multi-dimensional approach to risk adjustment. *Health Services Research* 31(3):283–307.

Iezzoni LI. 1997. The risks of risk-adjustment. *Journal of the American Medical Association* 278:1600–1607.

Iezzoni LI, Foley SM, Daley J, Hughes J, Fisher ES, Heeren T. 1992a. Comorbidities, complications, and coding bias. Does the number of diagnosis codes matter in predicting in-hospital mortality. *Journal of the American Medical Association* 267(16):2197–2203.

Iezzoni LI, Foley SM, Heeren T, Daley J, Duncan CC, Fisher ES, et al. 1992b. A method for screening the quality of hospital care using administrative data: Preliminary validation results. *QRB Quality Review Bulletin* 18(11):361–371.

Iezzoni LI, Daley J, Heeren T, Foley SM, Fisher ES, Duncan C, et al. 1994a. Identifying complications of care using administrative data. *Medical Care* 32(7):700–715.

Iezzoni LI, Daley J, Heeren T, Foley SM, Hughes JS, Fisher ES et al. 1994b. Using administrative data to screen hospitals for high complication rates. *Inquiry* 31(1):40–55.

Institute for Healthcare Improvement. 2005. [Online]. Available: *http://www.ihi.org/IHI/* [accessed November 15, 2004].

Institute of Medicine (IOM). 1990. *Medicare: A Strategy for Quality Assurance*, Vol. II. Washington, DC: National Academy Press.

IOM. 2001. *Crossing the Quality Chasm: A New Health System for the 21st Century*. Washington, DC: National Academy Press.

IOM. 2005. *Pathways to Better Health Services: Measuring Quality*. Washington, DC: The National Academies Press.

Kerr EA, McGlynn EA, Adams J, Keesey J, Asch SM. 2004. Profiling the quality of care in twelve communities: results from the CQI study. *Health Affairs* 23(3):247–256.

Leapfrog Group. 2005. *The Leapfrog Group*. [Online]. Available: *http://www.leapfroggroup.org/home* [accessed November 2, 2005].

Leatherman ST, Hibbard JH, McGlynn EA. 2003. A research agenda to advance quality measurement and improvement. *Medical Care* 41(Suppl. 1):I80–186.

Malenka DJ, McLerran D, Roos N, Fisher ES, Wennberg JE. 1994. Using administrative data to describe casemix: A comparison with the medical record. *Journal of Clinical Epidemiology* 47(9):1027–1032.

McGlynn EA. 1995. Quality assessment of reproductive health services. *Western Journal of Medicine* 163(Suppl. 3):19–27.

McGlynn EA. 2003a. Introduction and overview of the conceptual framework for a national quality measurement and reporting system. *Medical Care* 41(Suppl. 1):I-1–I-7.

McGlynn EA. 2003b. Selecting common measures of quality and system performance. *Medical Care* 41(Suppl. 1):I-39–I-47.

McGlynn EA, Brook RH. 2001. Keeping quality on the policy agenda. *Health Affairs* 20(3): 82–90.

McGlynn EA, Halfon N. 1998. Overview of issues in improving quality of care for children. *Health Services Research* 33(4 Pt. 2):977–1000.

McGlynn EA, Cassel CK, Leatherman ST, DeCristofaro A, Smits HL. 2003. Establishing national goals for quality improvement. *Medical Care* 41(Suppl. 1): I-16–I-29.

McKee M. 2001. Measuring the efficiency of health systems. The world health report sets the agenda, but there's still a long way to go. *British Medical Journal* 323(7308):295–296.

Nauert R. 1996. The quest for value in health care. *Journal of Health Care Finance* 22(3):52–61.

NCQA (National Committee for Quality Assurance). 2004. *State of Health Care Quality*. Washington, DC: National Committee for Quality Assurance.

Newhouse JP, Beeuwkes Buntin M, Chapman JD. 1997. Risk adjustment and Medicare: Taking a closer look. *Health Affairs* 16(5):26–43.

NQF (National Quality Forum). 2005. *National Priorities for Healthcare Quality Measurement and Reporting*. [Online]. Available: *http://www.qualityforum.org/webprioritiespublic.pdf* [accessed January 19, 2005].

Palmer S, Torgerson DJ. 1999. Economic notes: Definitions of efficiency. *British Medical Journal* 318(7191):1136.

PBGH (Pacific Business Group on Health). 2005. *Value Based Purchasing.* [Online]. Available: *http://www.pbgh.org/programs/value_based_purchasing.asp* [accessed October 24, 2005].

Pope GC, Kautter J, Randall PE, Ash AS, Ayanian JZ, Iezzoni LI, Ingber MJ, Levy JM, Robst J. 2004. Risk adjustment of Medicare capitation payments using the CMS-HCC model. *Health Care Financing Review* 25(4):119–141.

Remus D, Irene F. 2004. *Guidance for Using the AHRQ Quality Indicators for Hospital-level Public Reporting or Payment.* [Online]. Available: *http://www.qualityindicators.ahrq.gov* [accessed October 26, 2005].

Schield JM, Bolnick HJ, Murphy JJ. October 2000. *Evaluating Managed Care Effectiveness: A Societal Perspective.* Paper presented to the Society of Actuaries, Schaumburg, IL. [Online]. Available: *http://www.soa.org/ccm/content/?categoryID=1079102* [accessed January 10, 2005].

Shahian DM, Normand SL. 2003. The volume-outcome relationship: From Luft to Leapfrog. *Annals of Thoracic Surgery* 75(3):1048–1058.

Siu AL, McGlynn EA, Morgenstern H, Beers MH, Carlisle DM, Keeler EB, et al. 1992. Choosing quality of care measures based on the expected impact of improved care on health. *Health Services Research* 27(5):619–650.

Street A. 2003. How much confidence should we place in efficiency estimates? *Health Economics* 12(11):895–907.

Thomas CP, Wallack SS, Lee S, Ritter GA. 2002. Impact of health plan design and management on retirees' prescription drug use and spending, 2001. *Health Affairs* Suppl Web Exclusives:W408–W419.

Thomas JW, Grazier KL, Ward K. 2004a. Comparing accuracy of risk-adjustment methodologies used in economic profiling of physicians. *Inquiry* 41(2):218–231.

Thomas JW, Grazier KL, Ward K. 2004b. Economic profiling of primary care physicians: Consistency among risk-adjusted measures. *Health Services Research* 39(4 Pt. 1):985–1003.

Wennberg JE, Fisher ES, Skinner JS. 2002. Geography and the debate over Medicare reform. *Health Affairs* Supp Web Exclusives:W96–W114.

Worthington AC. 2004. Frontier efficiency measurement in health care: A review of empirical techniques and selected applications. *Medical Care* 61(2):135–170.

Zhao Y, Randall PE, Ash AS, Calabrese D, Ayanian J, Slaughter JP, Weyuker L, Bowen B. 2001. Measuring population health risks using inpatient diagnoses and outpatient pharmacy data. *Health Services Research* 26(6 Pt. 2):180–193.

TABLE H-1   "Value-Based" and Efficiency Metrics

Measures	Definition: Input:Output	Stated Purpose/Function	Health Care Setting
Disease-specific (e.g., CVD) cost-episodes per person	Person or patient annual episode specific costs for CVD services: health-related process or outcome measures	Measure guideline concordance; aggregate resources consumed; attribute resource use to provider; compare across physician groups; pay for performance	Acute care hospital
Agreement between pairs of efficiency rankings using the weighted kappa statistic	Relative practice efficiency rankings	Physician efficiency profiling; nine clinical specialties selected, based on numbers of episodes managed, numbers of physicians in the specialty, and whether the specialty was medical or surgical	Mixed group model/IPA HMO
NCQA plan efficiency measurement	Relative resource consumption across plans	Measure and report relative resource consumption, risk adjusted for underlying population risk	Health plans
Process and outcome measures related to transitional care (across settings) (Mary Naylor)			Multiple settings: home care, hospital, ED, nursing home

Required Enhancements/ Methods	Data Sources	Output Measure
Risk adjustment using ETGs	Hospital-reported data; payer claims paid charges for procedure codes (CPT-9-CMxxxx, . . .) for episode length of time	Patient health status; provider payment; patient disposition; patient, provider satisfaction
Two different episode definition systems—ETGs and MEGs; three cost outlier tests: Winzorized at 10% and 90%; Winzorized at 90%; and Winzorized at 80%	Four years of claims and membership data	Two measures of costs were used in the analyses: Actual costs, as recorded by the HMO, and standard costs, determined by assigning the same costs to all procedures of the same type
	Plan costs (total costs vs. disease specific costs)	
		30-day rehospitalization; Emergent care for wound infections (Source: OASIS, OBQM)
		Emergent care for improper medication administration, medication side effects (Source: OASIS, OBQM)
		Emergent care for hypo/ hyperglycemia (Source: OASIS, OBQM)
		Discharge to the community needing wound care or medication assistance (Source: OASIS, OBQM)
		Acute care hospitalization (Source: OASIS/OBQI)

(continued on next page)

TABLE H-1 continued

Measures	Definition: Input:Output	Stated Purpose/Function	Health Care Setting
"Risk-adjustment accuracy" across primary care physicians	Group R^2 analyses	Compare six different risk-adjustment methods in terms of capacity to explain variations in annual claims cost among HMO members	Physicians in HMO/IPA
Identification of high-outlier PCPs (family practitioners, general internists, and general practitioners, pediatricians)			
Bridges to Excellence/NCQA Provider Recognition Programs: clinical quality measures for diabetes care (Diabetes Care Link); clinical quality measures for heart/stroke care Provider Recognition Programs Cardiac Care Link; adoption of electronic medical records and other office systems:		Measure quality processes and outcomes; reporting; recognition and possible financial rewards	Hospitals

Required Enhancements/ Methods	Data Sources	Output Measure
		Unexpected nursing home admission (Source: OBQM)
		Discharge to the community (Source: OASIS/OBQI)
		Emergent care (Source: OASIS/OBQI)
Outlier removal	HMO, one state; member and adjudicated claims files (inpatient, outpatient/ professional, and pharmacy) for calendar years 1997 and 1998 for the 156,280 continuously enrolled members	Reasonably consistent estimates of member level expected costs, across a broad range of panel sizes
		Identification of high-outlier PCPs ranged from 54% to 58% for adult care physicians (family practitioners, general internists, and general practitioners), and from 67% to 77% for pediatricians, when rankings were based on the standardized cost difference measure which accounts for physician panel size
	Hospital sampling, self-report	Rates of adherence

(continued on next page)

TABLE H-1 continued

Measures	Definition: Input:Output	Stated Purpose/Function	Health Care Setting
Physician Office Link: Clinical Information Systems/Evidence-Based Medicine (See Bridges to Excellence)			
Leapfrog Group: Computer physician order entry (CPOE) systems	Presence of systems; use	Electronic prescribing systems that intercept errors	Hospitals
Evidence-based hospital (EHR) Safety Standard	Combination of outcome, process and volume	Adoption of clinical processes for high-risk procedures; volume of procedures per year; direct outcome measures (i.e, risk-adjusted mortality) for coronary artery bypass graft and percutaneous coronary interventions, using robust and approved measurement systems for the EHR Safety Standards	
ICU physician staffing	Operate adult and/or pediatric ICUs that are managed or comanaged by intensivists who: 1. Are present during daytime hours and provide clinical care exclusively in the ICU and, 2. At other times can— at least 95% of the time, (i) return ICU pages within five minutes and (ii) arrange for a FCCS-certified nonphysician effector to reach ICU patients within five minutes	Patients are cared for exclusively by critical-care specialists or teams that are closer on hand for both fine-tuning routine care and dealing with emergencies	

Required Enhancements/ Methods	Data Sources	Output Measure
Upfront capital	Voluntary hospital self-report; data survey	Explicit: extent to which standards are met, relative to other hospitals; implicit: costs of adverse drug events: mortality, morbidity; other costs
An EHR standard does not apply to hospitals that do not perform the procedure or treat the condition. Patients under 18 are excluded	Hospitals to report their volume and process or performance information for these procedures and conditions by responding to the Leapfrog Hospital Patient Safety Survey on the Leapfrog Website	
	Hospitals with adult or pediatric ICUs to respond to the Leapfrog Group	Presence/absence of intensivists in ICU; organization of closed/open ICU
	Voluntary online survey	

(continued on next page)

TABLE H-1   continued

Measures	Definition: Input:Output	Stated Purpose/Function	Health Care Setting
Leapfrog Group: Expert Panel-Endorsed Process Measures	Cases meeting endorsed process measure: eligible cases (meeting criteria for inclusion)	Establish, monitor, and report measures of process-oriented quality	Hospitals
IHI Whole System Measures: efficiency	Costs per capita; hospital specific standardized reimbursement		
The Agency for Healthcare Research and Quality Quality Indicators (QIs) are measures of health care quality	Prevention QIs identify hospital admissions that evidence suggests could have been avoided, at least in part, through high-quality outpatient care	National tracking or quality improvement	
	Inpatient QIs reflect quality of care inside hospitals including inpatient mortality for medical conditions and surgical procedures		
	Patient Safety Indicators also reflect quality of care inside hospitals, but focus on potentially avoidable complications and iatrogenic events		

Required Enhancements/ Methods	Data Sources	Output Measure
Exclude transferred patients; expired patients	Hospital: random sample of at least 60 cases with the condition; principal or secondary discharge diagnosis	Rate of adherence to endorsed process measures of quality
Measure health care quality using administrative data; update for ICD codes		Currently being considered for uses other than tracking quality improvement; namely provider payment and public reporting

Appendix I

Commissioned Paper

Transitional Care Performance Measurement

Eric A. Coleman

INTRODUCTION

Whether our goals are to improve quality, enhance patient-centered care, ensure patient safety, or implement cost containment practices, the time has come to focus our attention on performance measurement for transitional care. The absence of measurement in this area remains a significant barrier to achieving these goals. Lack of attention to transitional care is the result of multiple factors: accountability is poorly defined, financial incentives are not aligned, information systems are not well connected across settings, each setting requires the use of unique databases and documentation, and most practitioners have received minimal training for cross-site collaboration (Coleman, 2003; Coleman and Berenson, 2004; Coleman and Fox, 2004). Yet despite these potential barriers, transitional care is an essential and cross-cutting area of health care for persons with complex health care needs, including older adults, children with special health care needs, and disabled populations. As such, performance in this area needs to be measured. Currently, there exists an array of promising measures that, if implemented nationally, could bring the requisite attention needed to stimulate quality improvement in transitional care, define accountability, realign financial incentives, and foster interoperable electronic health information systems.

Definitions

A recent position statement defines transitional care as a set of actions designed to ensure the coordination and continuity of health care as patients transfer between different locations or different levels of care within the same location. Representative locations include (but are not limited to) hospitals, subacute and postacute nursing facilities, the patient's home, primary and specialty care offices, assisted living, and long-term care facilities. Ideally, transitional care is based on a comprehensive plan of care and the availability of health care practitioners who are well trained in chronic care and have current information about the patient's goals, preferences, and clinical status. It should include logistical arrangements, education of the patient and family, and coordination among the health professionals involved in the transition (Coleman and Boult, 2003).

Transitional care is distinguished from discharge planning in that the former encompasses both the sending and the receiving aspects of the transfer. Transitional care is primarily concerned with the relatively brief time interval that begins with preparing a patient to leave one setting and be received in the next. Many transitions are unplanned, result from unanticipated medical problems, occur in "real time" during nights and on weekends, and happen so quickly that formal and informal support mechanisms cannot respond in a timely manner.

While the focus of this background paper is on the "hand-offs" of care that occur as patients with complex care needs move across settings, it is important to acknowledge that transitional care shares key attributes with both coordination of care and continuity of care (Institute of Medicine, 2001, 2004). A comprehensive discussion of the latter two care domains is beyond the scope of this report. However, the intersection between transitional care, coordination of care, and continuity of care will be highlighted in this report.

Transitional Care in Context

Transitional care highlights a fundamental disconnect within the U.S. health care delivery system. The focus of transitional care is inherently patient-centered, attempting to ensure that the health care needs of patients with complex care are met irrespective of where care is delivered. But our health care delivery system, whether examined by payment, quality improvement initiatives, accreditation, performance measurement, or how clinicians define their practice, is increasingly setting-centered. In many respects, the term "health care system" is a misnomer. There are few mechanisms in place for coordinating care across settings, and often no single practitioner or team assumes responsibility during patients' transitions. As was discussed during the December 1st 2004 Workshop, Dr. Mark Miller, Executive Director of MedPAC, acknowledged that organizing payment and quality setting by setting is not satisfactory. He expressed, however, that there exists a high level of interest in better coordination of these activities across settings.

It has become increasingly rare for a single physician or nurse care manager to take responsibility for coordinating care across settings during a care transition. Nationwide, practitioners are limiting the scope of their practice to a single setting such as the hospital, nursing home, or ambulatory clinic (Katz et al., 2000; Wachter and Goldman, 2002). Further, health care professionals frequently transfer patients to settings in which they have never practiced. They are often unfamiliar with the capacity of these settings for delivering care and may transfer patients to these settings inappropriately. As hospitals struggle with problems of overcapacity, they are frequently diverting patients to care settings where their personal physician does not practice and where the patient's prior medical records are unavailable (Bazzoli et al., 2003; Brewster et al., 2001). Few health delivery systems currently have access to an electronic health record system, and even fewer have a system with connectivity to rehabilitation or skilled nursing facilities or home health care (ASTM International et al., 2003; Institute of Medicine, 2003; Kramer et al., 2004).

Further, institutions and physicians assume minimal financial risk for ensuring safe and effective care transitions. Aside from capitation, most payment approaches do not penalize providers for inappropriate discharges or transfers. An Office of Inspector General report determined that in 1996 and 1997, 34,500 hospital patients were discharged and readmitted on the same day, with accompanying payments of nearly $226 million (U.S. DHHS, 2000). However, within Medicare's statutory framework, Conditions of Participation explicitly include requirements concerning continuity of care and discharge planning for hospitals, home health agencies, rehabilitation and skilled nursing facilities. For hospitals, the Joint Committee on Accreditation of Healthcare Organizations (JCAHO) has deemed status from the Centers for Medicare and Medicaid Services (CMS) to provide oversight for these Conditions of Participation. In 2002, more than 90 percent of all hospitals nationwide received the highest score of 5/5 (i.e., "substantial compliance") for these accreditations items. As will be discussed further in the next section, these findings are in sharp contrast to the growing evidence base that demonstrates there are serious quality problems in transitional care. Equally important, from a measurement standpoint, such high ratings for these items may indicate the need for revision.

Our understanding of the health care utilization patterns and accompanying influence on health care expenditures for the population of persons with complex care needs is increasing. The Robert Wood Johnson Foundation-funded Partnership for Solutions poll provides important insights. For the 125 million persons with chronic conditions in this country, there is a strong relationship between the number of chronic conditions, the number of prescriptions filled, the rates of unnecessary hospitalization, and average per capital health care spending (Partnership for Solutions, 2002). Although persons with 5 or more chronic conditions average 15 office visits and fill 50 prescriptions per year, they frequently do not receive adequate information regarding medication administration, illness management, and follow-up testing and procedures (Partnership for Solutions, 2002). Focusing on the Medicare beneficiary population, this poll revealed that beneficiaries with 2 or more chronic conditions see 7 different physicians per year, fill 20 prescriptions, and account for 95 percent of Medicare expenditures (Wolff et al., 2002). Within this subgroup, beneficiaries with 5 or more conditions account for two-thirds of Medicare spending.

Transfers among care settings are common. Twenty-three percent of hospitalized patients over the age of 65 are discharged to another institution, and 11.6 percent are discharged with home health care (Agency for Healthcare Research Quality, 1999). An estimated 19 percent of patients discharged from a hospital to an SNF are readmitted to the hospital within 30 days (Kramer et al., 2000). One study tracked posthospital transitions for 30 days in a large, nationally representative sample of Medicare beneficiaries. Transitions in this study were defined as transfers to or from an acute hospital, skilled nursing or rehabilitation facility, or home with or without home health care. Overall, 46 unique care patterns were identified during this relatively brief 30-day time period. Sixty-one percent of care episodes resulted in one transition, 18 percent in two transitions, 9 percent in three transitions, 4 percent in four or more transitions, and 8 percent resulted in death (Coleman et al., 2004a).

Finally, a discussion of the context within which transitional care occurs would not be complete without describing the factors that contribute to patients' vulnerability. Not surprisingly, transitions in patients' care settings parallel transitions in their physical health status. As such, these patients are not only adjusting to new settings but also to new or worsening health symptoms or changes in their ability to carry out daily functional tasks (Mor et al., 1989). Those patients in institutional settings often adapt to the environment by becoming dependent and complacent while their needs are being addressed; however, upon discharge to home, patients and family members are abruptly expected to assume a considerable self-management role in the recovery of their condition, with little support or preparation. The prevalence of transient or permanent cognitive impairment and limited health literacy among patients experiencing care transitions only exacerbates this challenge to preparing for self-care (Gazmararian et al., 1999; Kiely et al., 2003). Finally, family caregivers are both the first and last line of defense for ensuring safe and effective care transfers for these vulnerable patients. Their contributions in this area are vastly underestimated as they compensate for the many deficiencies of our current health care system. It is difficult to discuss family caregiving without discussing the challenges of coordinating care across settings. Conversely, it is nearly impossible to discuss the challenges of coordinating care across settings without recognizing the essential role of family caregivers.[1]

EVIDENCE FOR SERIOUS QUALITY PROBLEMS DURING CARE TRANSITIONS

An expanding evidence base demonstrates that serious quality problems exist for patients undergoing transitions across sites of care. Qualitative studies performed in the United States as well as Canada, Europe, and Australia, have produced remarkably consistent results. These studies have shown that patients are often unprepared for their self-management role in the next care setting, receive conflicting advice regarding chronic illness management, are often unable to reach an appropriate health care practitioner who has access to their care plan when questions arise, have minimal input into their care plan, and are annoyed by having to repeatedly provide the same information to each new set of practitioners. Family caregivers voice feelings of frustration that they are often excluded from care planning meetings, despite their central role in the execution of this care plan. They are also dissatisfied with having to perform tasks that their health care practitioners have left undone (Coleman et al., 2002; Grimmer et al., 2000; Harrison and Verhoef, 2002; Levine, 1998; vom Eigen et al., 1999; Weaver et al., 1998).

A recent report by the California Health Care Foundation (CHCF) reinforces these qualitative findings. CHCF surveyed over 36,000 patients to learn of their experiences during their recent stays in 200 California hospitals (approximately one-half of all hospitals in the state). Patients' experience with transition to home was the lowest of all patient-rated hospital measures (CHCF, 2004).

Quantitative studies have documented that patient safety is jeopardized due to high rates of medication errors and lack of appropriate follow-up care (Beers et al., 1992; Dudas et al., 2001; Forster et al., 2003; Moore et al., 2003). During care transitions, patients receive medications from different prescribers who rarely have access to patients' comprehensive medication list (Partnership for Solutions, 2002). As such, no one clinician is ideally positioned to monitor the entire regimen and intervene to reduce discrepancies, duplications, or errors. Thus although much of the recent national attention on medication errors has been setting-specific, the lack of coordination between prescribers across settings may pose an even greater

---

[1]At the time of the writing of this report, the National Family Caregiving Association has partnered with the University of Colorado Health Sciences Center to seek Congressional appropriations to commission an Institute of Medicine (IOM) report that would address the need to more formally support the role of family caregivers in general and in the context of coordination of care across settings in particular.

challenge. Forster and colleagues found that 19 percent of patients discharged from the hospital experienced an associated adverse event within 3 weeks (Forster et al., 2003); 66 percent of these were adverse drug events. Moore and colleagues examined three types of discontinuity among older patients transferred from the hospital: medication, test result follow-up, and initiation of a recommended work-up. They found that nearly 50 percent of hospitalized patients experienced at least one discontinuity and that patients who did not have a recommended work-up initiated were six times more likely to be re-hospitalized (Moore et al., 2003). In contrast to the studies led by Foster and Moore, which were conducted in tertiary academic health centers, researchers at the University of Colorado Health Sciences Center studied older patients receiving care from multiple community settings and found that 15 percent had at least one medication problem (Coleman et al., 2004b).

Significant lapses in information transfer also threaten patient safety. Each time a patient's medical record is recreated, it increases the chance for a medical error to occur. Further, inadequate information transfer potentially increases health care expenditures. Re-creation of essential information is inefficient and can lead to redundant ordering of laboratory tests, diagnostic imaging, and procedures. Studies by van Walraven and colleagues have documented not only failures in information transfer, but they have also documented that the information that is transferred is frequently incomplete and even inaccurate (van Walraven et al., 2002a,b). Leaders from the American Medical Directors Association have shown that despite requirements articulated by Medicare Conditions of Participation, skilled nursing facilities to not receive a discharge summary from the hospital approximately 28 percent of the time (Coleman et al., 2003).

Each of the types of qualitative and quantitative problems described above conspire to increase rates of recidivism to high-intensity care settings when patients' care needs are not met, increase the frequency of medical errors, and increase costs of health care (Beers et al., 1992; Boockvar et al., 2004; Coleman et al., 2004c; Moore et al., 2003; van Walraven et al., 2002a). In a national study examining 30-day post–hospital care patterns in a representative sample of Medicare beneficiaries, between 12 and 25 percent of all care patterns were categorized as complicated, requiring return to higher intensity care settings (Coleman et al., 2004a).

PERFORMANCE MEASUREMENT AS A POTENTIAL DRIVER FOR QUALITY IMPROVEMENT IN TRANSITIONAL CARE

The underlying premise behind this report is that the absence of performance measurement for transitional care is one of the most significant barriers to quality improvement. Lack of financial incentives and accountability make these "hand-offs" of care extremely vulnerable to medical errors, service duplication, and unnecessary utilization. And yet without processes in place to measure performance, the serious quality problems discussed in the prior section will remain undetected, and consequently, ignored. From this perspective, integrating transitional care into national performance measurement activities could have a profound impact as a primary driver of quality improvement.

Fortunately, there are a number of points of leverage addressed by transitional care from which to build such an initiative. These include national attention to the problem of patient safety in general and medication safety in particular, national efforts towards making the health care system more patient-centered (CMS, 2004; Hibbard et al., 2004; IOM, 2000, 2001), cost containment, and expansion of health information technology. Greater attention to transitional care could foster each of the efforts but before this can happen, performance measurement will be needed. In other words, performance measurement could drive improved quality, patient safety, cost containment, and development and dissemination of health information technology.

Recent developments demonstrate that this position is achievable. JCAHO has identified medication reconciliation across settings as one of its top patient safety goals (CMS, 2004). In response, hospitalist physicians have begun to develop quality improvement initiatives and protocols for information transfer (discussed further in a subsequent section entitled "Current Transitional Care Efforts Among Leading Quality Improvement Organizations"). JCAHO has also recently implemented a new tracer methodology employed during on-site surveys designed to assess standards compliance by following a few, select active patients through the organization's health care process in the same sequence experienced by patients. In so doing, surveyors may assess the relationships between disciplines and important functions during these care activities (JCAHO, 2004b). Criteria for selecting tracer conditions include: patients who have received complex services (often those close to discharge), patients who cross different programs (such as behavioral health and hospital), and patients whose care or condition relate to organizational systems (such as medication management or infection control). Although currently in the planning stages, there is some interest in expanding the tracer methodology across settings, such as from a JCAHO accredited hospital to a JCAHO accredited nursing home.

In the realm of health information technology, national leaders in geriatric care coordination and electronic health information systems met with Dr. David Brailer who leads the Office of the National Coordinator for Health Information Technology with the Department of Health and Human Services. The discussion centered primarily around how to incorporate information into electronic health information systems that was not only meaningful to patients with complex care needs, but also of use for capturing performance measurement as an essential step towards quality improvement. Another critical step that was discussed was to encourage interoperability of electronic health information systems across settings, including nursing homes and home health care agencies.

An advisory meeting on transitional care performance measurement was held at CMS in August, 2004.[2] The meeting included representation from CMS, National Quality Forum (NQF), National Committee for Quality Assurance (NCQA), AARP, Associates in Process Improvement, National Family Caregivers Association, PeaceHealth, University of Colorado Health Sciences Center, and Commonwealth Fund. Overall, there was a high level of interest in advancing quality improvement in the area of transitional care in general and the utility of the University of Colorado Health Sciences Center's Care Transitions Measure (CTM) in particular (the CTM is discussed in detail below in the section on Leading Performance Measures). Although the Advisory Committee acknowledged that the 8th Scope of Work for the nation's Quality Improvement Organizations (QIOs) does not address this topic directly, there was discussion on how to best partner with QIOs to weave transitional care performance measurement into existing activities, such as advancement of health information technology and hospital and nursing home performance. At the recommendation of the Advisory Committee, researchers at the University of Colorado Health Sciences Center have initiated a process of collaboration with QIOs, including a "kick-off" WebEx presentation for which 46 QIO staff members attended, and direct participation in four QIO projects that directly pertain to transitional care. In general the QIOs seems motivated to move out of their setting-centric focus.

Finally, performance measurement could be an important driver to increase demand for the growing number of evidence-based interventions that have been found to improve the quality of transitional care (Coleman et al., 2004c; Naylor et al., 1999; Rich et al., 1995; Stewart et al., 2000). In other words, once health care providers and delivery systems are asked to measure their performance, undoubtedly some will prove to have deficiencies. The fact that interventions have already been developed, tested, and implemented in clinical practice could facilitate advancement through the quality improvement cycle.

---

[2]Dr. Eric Coleman from the University of Colorado convened and chaired this meeting that served to advise a performance measurement/quality improvement project supported by the Commonwealth Fund of New York.

Key Measurement Considerations

The following section addresses key measurement considerations for pursuing a performance measurement agenda focused on transitional care (Box I-1). Some of these considerations are unique to the topic of transitional care while other considerations are applicable to most measurement efforts.

A first consideration is to resist the temptation to oversimplify measurement in this area. To embrace transitional care is to embrace complexity. A "hemoglobin A_1c equivalent" does not currently exist for transitional care, nor is it likely that a single summative measure available from administrative or laboratory data will be able to adequately capture the transitional care experience for patients with complex care needs.

A second consideration is the perspective from which performance should be assessed. For example, should performance be measured from the standpoint of the patient, the sending care team, the receiving care team, or the broader health care system? The challenges faced when measuring performance in this area were raised earlier in this report. They include identifying who is accountable for care across settings, poorly aligned financial incentives, and the fact that few if any practitioners move across settings with the patient. Given these realities, no single approach to defining the perspective represents a "gold standard." Some health care systems have chosen to define and measure care processes that are to take place at the time of transfer for both the sending and receiving care teams (Coleman and Fox, 2004). Others have reasoned that because patients and their family caregivers are often the only common thread weaving across disparate health care settings, they are uniquely positioned to re-

---

BOX I-1   Key Measurement Considerations

1. Resist the temptation to oversimplify measurement in this area.
2. Choose the perspective from which performance should be assessed.
3. Determine whether measurement should be a separate activity or integrated into a larger effort.
4. Examine what type of data sources needed for measurement.
5. Select the health care settings for which transitional care measures will apply.
6. Decide whether all patients undergoing care transitions should be assessed or only those identified as high-risk.
7. Agree on the focus for quality improvement (i.e., structure, process, or outcome).
8. Explore whether there is a role for case-mix adjustment.

port on the care they have received (Coleman et al., 2004d; Grimmer and Moss, 2001; Hendriks et al., 2001). Finally, broader measures of health utilization that attempt to examine the problems that arise during care hand-offs from a more systems-oriented focus have also been explored (Coleman et al., 2004a).

A third consideration concerns whether performance measurement in transitional care should be a separate dedicated activity or whether it should be integrated into a larger effort. As stated in the Introduction, transitional care is a cross-cutting area within health care and, as such, measurement in this area perhaps should not occur in isolation. Rather, to promote adoption, transitional care measurement may be best served by incorporating relevant items into existing measurement activities. Illustrative examples of this approach are highlighted in an upcoming section entitled "Current Transitional Care Efforts Among Leading Quality Improvement Organizations."

A fourth consideration examines the types of data sources needed for measurement. To date, data have been gathered through patient report, administrative data, chart review, and on-site survey. Both researchers and leading quality improvement organizations have raised concerns with each approach. For instance, do patients have the ability to evaluate their transition-related experiences at a time when their judgment may be compromised by acute illness? Can examination of administrative data or claims capture the patient's experience? If processes of care are not documented in a patient's record, is this because they were not done, they were not documented, or there was a failure in communication between the sending and receiving site that was necessary to prompt the care process? In other words, how can the receiving clinician be expected to document that a revision in a patient's medication regimen occurred in a prior setting if that information was not transferred? Enhanced interoperability of electronic health information systems could potentially overcome some of these limitations. However, for the present time, if a reasonable immediate goal is to incorporate assessment of transitional care performance into existing efforts, then the types of data required will need to simply mirror these activities.

A fifth consideration focuses on what health care settings should transitional care measures apply. To date, most measurement activity has focused on transfer out of the hospital. As was pointed out by Dr. Elliott Fisher during the December 1st 2004 Workshop, one problem with this approach is that it does not reward high-quality care that averts the hospitalization in the first place. Yet in order to promote broader quality improvement efforts, priority needs to be given to measures that can be employed across multiple settings. Initially, researchers from the University of Colorado Health Sciences Center embarked on the task of creating a series of "modular" measures for transitional care. As part of this effort, a measure would be constructed to assess transitional care from hospital to nursing home, nursing home to home health care, home health care to primary care, and so forth. The research team abandoned this approach as their experiences strongly suggested that there exists a core set of items that "transcend the transition" or are important irrespective of the transition in question. These items reflect the same domains that the qualitative studies cited earlier identified: patient preparation (both for what to expect and readiness for self-care), information transfer, medication management and/or reconciliation, and follow-up appointments and testing.

A sixth consideration is whether to assess all patients undergoing care transitions or only those identified as high-risk for poor-quality or complicated care transitions. There are some conditions that traditionally lead to multiple transfers among care settings, such as acute stroke, congestive heart failure, and hip fracture (Coleman et al., 1999). Tools have been developed to identify patients at risk for complicated care transitions (Coleman et al., 2004a). JCAHO's tracer methodology (described earlier) has included patients who undergo orthopedic procedures for joint replacement. As experience with measurement in this area has been limited, assessing all patients undergoing transitions may allow health care leaders the opportunity to gain a comprehensive view of the quality of transitional care that could better inform targeting for successive efforts.

A seventh consideration examines the type of quality that is being measured, including structure, process, and outcome. To date, process measures represent the vast majority of efforts and relationships between care processes and outcomes are becoming increasingly salient (Coleman and Berenson, 2004; Coleman et al., 2004d). In discussions with adult and pediatric health care leaders, a number of structural items have also been put forth. For example, the Colorado Foundation for Medical Care (QIO serving Colorado and other mountain states) has initiated a quality improvement project that aims to enhance communication around skin integrity and pressure ulcers between hospitals and nursing homes in Denver. A number of different strategies have been employed but one approach in particular appears to stand out as being most effective—the opportunity for the hospital nurse and nursing home nurse to exchange information via a 5-minute telephone call. Thus despite efforts to create new paper forms or implement a common language for communication of a patient's skin integrity, a structural modification in a nurse's daily workflow that facilitates this person-to-person dialog may be worthy of assessment. Similarly, pediatric health care leaders conveyed another structural modification that could be assessed—creating time during business hours for the "back-office" staff to help children with special health care needs and their families obtain referrals, schedule appointments, communicate with teachers and nurses at school and arrange for durable medical equipment.

A final consideration is case-mix adjustment, an important area with particular relevance to potential pay-for-performance initiatives. As this topic has been central to larger discussion of the Subcommittee, this section will concentrate on its relevance to assessing transitional care. As was discussed at the December 1st 2004 Workshop, process of care measures may not require formal case-mix adjustment techniques. As noted, the majority of transitional care measures assess processes of care. As such, case-mix adjustment has not served as a primary focus in this area. Hospital Consumer Assessment of Health Providers and Systems (HCAHPS) testing has demonstrated that the following three items are most critical for risk adjustment for the entire 25-item measure (i.e., not specific to the two discharge to home items that are detailed in the next section): age, education, and self-rated health status. Key case-mix adjustment variables have been identified for examining at recidivism, such as return to the hospital or emergency department after a transfer to a lower-intensity care setting (Coleman et al., 2004a).

LEADING PERFORMANCE MEASURES SETS ASSESSING QUALITY OF CARE DURING TRANSITIONS

Performance measures were identified through a comprehensive review of the medical literature, discussions with leaders within quality improvement organizations, discussions with academic experts, and searches of the Internet (primarily focused on the Web sites of quality improvement entities and supplemented with leading search engines). Identified measures are summarized in the table. If written materials or articles did not provide the complete requisite information to complete the table, attempts were made to contact the primary author. In some cases, the author chose not to respond.

Overall, there has been a recent proliferation of measures in this area. Initially, most attempts at quality measurement focused on post-hospitalization recidivism (either return to the hospital or to the emergency department). Now there is an expanding array of patient-centered measures and process of care measures that show promise for implementation in performance measurement initiatives. However, a number of caveats remain. There is growing interest in examining completeness and accuracy of information transfer across disparate care settings. Although the physical transfer of information across settings represents an important step towards quality improvement, even more important is how the available information is incorporated into a continuous care plan and used to improve health outcomes. Further, measurement efforts that focus on the quality of the "hand-off" across settings may lose sight of the fact that in some cases, high-quality care might obviate the need for a transition altogether. For example, having a patient remain in the hospital for an additional 1–2 days to receive rehabilitation before going home may make a transfer to a skilled nursing facility (and its accompanying risks for medical errors and iatrogenesis) unnecessary. Finally, to date the National Quality Forum has not approved any of these measures. However, a steering committee is being convened with a focus on care coordination for hospital and ambulatory care.

Performance measures focused on transitional care can be categorized into four general types or "buckets" including process of care measures, patient-reported measures of their experiences during transitions, outcomes of care, and accreditation measures. These measures reflect many of the key domains identified in the qualitative studies reviewed earlier, namely patient/caregiver preparation for self-care, information transfer, medication reconciliation, follow-up testing, or appointments with primary care or specialty clinicians.

The first bucket includes process of care or task-oriented measures. Representative measures include the Assessing Care of Vulnerable Elders (ACOVE) developed by RAND and UCLA and funded by Pfizer and the Anderson/Helms Referral Data Inventory (RDI). The ACOVE items examine whether certain tasks around communication across settings were achieved (Wenger and Young, 2003). The RDI was initially designed to assess the completeness of home health care referrals but has since been expanded to include other care settings (Anderson and Helms, 1995). A summative score is generated to reflect the completeness (but not the accuracy) of information transfer. Medication reconciliation is increasingly recognized as an important activity for patient safety by organizations such as the Institute for Healthcare Improvement (2004) and JCAHO (discussed further below). Within this process, pre- and posttransition care regimens are reconciled to reduce redundancy and prescribing errors.

The second bucket includes patient-reported measures of care experiences during care transitions. Representative measures include the HCAHPS developed by CMS and the Agency for Healthcare Research and Quality (AHRQ), the Patients' Evaluation of Performance in California (PEP-C-II) and the CTM. HCAHPS was designed to serve as a voluntary measure of hospital performances, ideally adopted across the country (Agency for Healthcare Research and Quality, 2003). As such it primarily focuses on the care delivered during the hospital stay but also includes two items that reflect the discharge experience. The PEP-C-II incorporates items from the NRC—Picker group and has been used for public reporting in a collaborative effort between the CHCF and the California Institute for Health System Performance (CHCF, 2004). Similar to HCAHPS, this measure primarily focuses on the overall hospital experience but includes select items on the transition to home. Researchers from the University of Colorado Health Sciences Center developed the CTM with an explicit and unique focus on the care transition experience (Coleman et al., 2004d). The CTM can be administered either as a 15-item and a 3-item (subset) measure, both of which have been shown to discriminate among hospitals and predict rehospitalization or return to the emergency department.

The focus of the third bucket is on outcomes, usually in the form of utilization of or recidivism to high-intensity health care services such as the hospital or emergency department. To date, this strategy has been the least developed. One approach, developed in the Medicare Current Beneficiary Survey, defines complicated care transitions as an interruption in the movement from higher intensity care settings (where there is presumably greater functional dependency and medical instability) to lower intensity care settings (Coleman et al., 2004a).

The fourth bucket includes accreditation measures, such as those used by JCAHO. The relevant JCAHO activities that pertain to transitional care are discussed in greater detail in the following section.

There are other potential approaches to assessing quality in this area that either do not fit into one of the buckets above or have not yet been attempted, for example, the completion or updating of an adult patient's Personal Health Record (ASTM International et al., 2003) or information to support a child's Medical Home within pediatric care (American Academy of Pediatrics, 2003). Inclusion of a completed Physician Orders for Life-Sustaining Treatment (Oregon Health and Science University, 1996) in the transfer information that accompanies a patient across settings could be converted into a measurement activity. Areas addressed may include: resuscitation, medical interventions, antibiotic usage, artificially administered fluids, and nutrition. Finally, a number of measures have been developed to assess the transition from pediatric to adult medical providers among teenagers (Reiss and Gibson, 2002).

CMS currently reimburses clinicians for a number of care coordination and care oversight activities that, if modified, could serve as a template for more formal performance measurement for transitional care. For example, Care Plan Oversight (CPT code 99374 for home health care) involves physician development and/or revision of care plans, review of subsequent reports of patient status, review of related laboratory and other studies, communication (including phone calls) for purposes of assessment or care decisions with health care professionals, family members, surrogate decision makers, and/or key caregivers involved in patient's care, integration of new information into the medical treatment plan, and/or adjustment of medical therapy within a calendar month. In addition, Discharge Day Management (CPT code 99238 if <30 minutes or 99239 if >30 minutes) includes final examination, discussion of hospital stay, instructions for continuing care, and preparation of discharge records. Further strengthening of these codes to ensure greater accountability, foster more effective communication, and encourage more overt collaboration with family caregivers, combined with routine auditing, could represent important step towards financially rewarding high-quality transitional care.

In summary, the table illustrates the wide array of potential approaches that could be used for the purpose of transitional care performance measurement. Although great strides have been made in the area of transitional care performance measurement, collectively these measures stand to improve in a number of key areas. Each of the measures presented have relatively limited experience in testing in diverse populations. Most self-reported measures have not been formally tested in patient populations with transient or permanent cognitive impairment and as a consequence, do not have established protocol for when a proxy respondent is needed. Very few of these measures have been used in quality improvement initiatives and as a result, the accountable party remains undefined. There are few examples whereby these measures have been tested "head-to-head" to understand their strengths and limitations. While measures may have been evaluated based on psychometric characteristics, the majority of measures have not been tested in "real-world" settings to determine whether scores are associated with positive or negative outcomes nor have the developers shown whether scores discriminate among different health care institutions. Finally, despite their integral role in facilitating safe and effective care transitions, the "voice" of family caregivers is not well represented among existing measures.

CURRENT TRANSITIONAL CARE EFFORTS AMONG LEADING QUALITY IMPROVEMENT ORGANIZATIONS

The NQF has initiated (January 2005) a new steering committee on coordination of care within and out of the hospital. As mentioned earlier, NQF has not approved any measures in this area; however, a call for measures has been issued with a due date of mid-January 2005. Also previously mentioned was NQF's participation in the transitional care performance measurement meeting held at CMS in August 2004, during which there was considerable interest expressed for the University of Colorado Health Sciences Center's CTM. CMS has held a series of listening sessions on the 39 NQF consensus standards for hospital care and care coordination was identified as a priority area among stakeholders. NQF has endorsed set of safe practices that recommends health care institutions should "ensure that care information, especially changes in orders and new diagnostic information, is transmitted in a timely and clearly understandable form to all of the patient's current health care providers who need that information to provide care." NQF is in the process of exploring nursing care sensitive measures that may include items pertinent to transitional care.

The Leapfrog Group Hospital Patient Safety Survey incorporates the NQF-endorsed safe practices described above and provides a series of steps, based on awareness, accountability, ability, and actions to address the problem. This guide sets the stage for performance measurement to be developed and implemented by each participating individual hospital but does not offer specific measurement tools or items.

The experiences of the CHCF have been described earlier. CHCF surveyed over 200 hospitals using PEP-C-II and HCAHPS items for the purpose of public reporting. Hospital-level performance can be identified on their Web site.

Due to constraints in how performance data are obtained, NCQA has not developed specific measures in the area of transitional care in general. However, they have implemented a measure that examines follow-up after hospitalization for mental illness. This item estimates the percentage of health plan members who had a follow-up visit after being discharged from an inpatient mental health stay for depression, schizophrenia, attention deficit disorder, and personality disorders (National Committee for Quality Assurance, 2004). The measure looks at both 7-day and 30-day follow-up rates. CMS has asked NCQA to assemble an advisory group[3] related to the "Doctor Office Quality-Information Technology" (DOQ-IT) project (Centers for Medicare and Medicaid Services, 2004). This pilot project, mandated by the Medicare Modernization Act, is aimed at paying for performance specifically related to physician office practices that implement changes in their use of information technology. It is conceivable that this new technology could be designed in such a way to facilitate information transfer and coordination across settings.

Bridges to Excellence has three programs under way: Physician Office Link, Diabetes Care Link, and Cardiac Care Link. Perhaps most relevant to transitional care, the Physician Office Link enables physician office sites to qualify for bonuses based on their implementation of specific processes to reduce errors and increase quality. They can earn up to $50 per year for each patient covered by a participating employer or plan. In addition, a report card for each physician office describes its performance on the program measures and is made available to the public. However, to date, transitional care has not been an explicit focus of this program.

---

[3]Dr. Eric Coleman is a member of this advisory group.

Nationwide, QIOs are involved with transitional care to an extent. The 8th Scope of Work focuses on providing health information technology assistance to physicians' offices that could have application in improving communication and coordination across settings (CMS, 2004). QIOs are also in a position to examine "sentinel events" including consumer appeals for inappropriate or early hospital discharges and hospital readmissions for the same diagnosis. As described earlier, the Colorado Foundation for Medical Care has an initiative aimed at improving communication across hospitals and nursing homes regarding skin integrity and pressure ulcers. Lumetra, the QIO serving California, has initiated a Continuity of Care Collaborative that focuses on improving cross-setting communication for older patients following surgical repair (either elective or nonelective) of the hip. Members of the Collaborative are exploring measurement strategies around pain control (outcome) and completeness of information transfer (process) from both the perspective of the sending and receiving care providers. Delmarva, the QIO serving Delaware, Maryland, and Virginia, has been interested in transitional care as it relates to home health care. The Illinois Foundation for Quality Health Care is the quality improvement organization that has decided to work on a collaborative with the home health agencies focusing on acute hospitalizations. As of December 2004, 14 requests for the University of Colorado Health Sciences Center's CTM have been received from 11 different QIOs (including those mentioned above).

HealthGrades has adopted AHRQ Patient Safety Indicators and released a report in July 2004 entitled *HealthGrades Quality Study: Patient Safety in American Hospitals.* However, among the 16 indicators, none were directly related to transitional care.

The Society for Hospital Medicine (SHM), with funding from the John A. Hartford Foundation, has initiated a project aimed at improving hospital discharge. In April 2005, SHM will hold a series of workshops that will review the evidence base, best practices, and conduct a modified Delphi consensus building process. The objective is for SHM members to take these idealized evidence-based practices back to their respective hospitals to implement quality improvement projects. The timing of this interest reflects the implementation of the JCAHO patient safety measures and Tracer Methodology described in detail below. Initiatives such as these will likely generate considerable demand for performance measures.

Funded by The Robert Wood Johnson Foundation and housed at America's Health Insurance Plans, the Care Management Workgroup (comprised of medical directors and operations leaders of leading health care delivery systems) recently completed a report aimed at educating health care delivery systems on evidence-based transitional care and best practices

(Coleman and Fox, 2004). In addition to performance measurement, the report focuses on aligning financial incentives, ensuring accountability, implementing approaches to information transfer, and supporting patients, caregivers, and clinicians. To date, over 2200 reports have been requested.

The American Academy of Pediatrics (AAP) advocates for a Medical Home for children with special health needs (American Academy of Pediatrics, 2003). Communication of a core set of information and a common shared care plan across settings is a central component of the Medical Home. AAP also realizes that high-quality care for this population must include reimbursed time to review home health care orders for completeness and accuracy and to communicate changes in medications. At present, a comprehensive medication review and communication to involved practitioners can consume approximately 15 minutes which exceeds the time dedicated to a face-to-face visit. Analogous to the care oversight codes allowed under Medicare, pediatricians believe there should be codes for generating the care plan, sharing the information with family and involved clinicians and also communicating with the schools. Documentation of these activities could be a performance measure.

Finally, the JCAHO has deemed status for hospital discharge planning and continuity of care. Under statute, this requires JCAHO to assess the following representative care practices (Box I-2).

Encouraged by its Public Advisory Group, JCAHO has expressed interest in revising and strengthening its accreditation items in this area. To this end, JCAHO measurement leaders have held a series of telephone meetings with researchers from the University of Colorado Health Sciences Center to explore a possible collaboration.

In January 2004, JCAHO implemented a new approach to the survey process, Tracer Methodology (JCAHO, 2004b). This new approach includes the following elements: (a) following the course of care and services provided to a particular patient; (b) assessing relationships among disciplines and important functions; (c) evaluating the performance of relevant processes related to patient care; and (d) identifying potential vulnerabilities in care processes. It is now part of the typical 3-day on-site hospital survey process, and in most instances, a typical team of three surveyors is expected to complete approximately 11 tracers. The Tracer Methodology has not yet been extended beyond the hospital setting but it has potentially important implications for discharge planning and transitions. In particular, this approach can follow a particular patient, assessing how the patient fares along a continuum of care. It can assess how well the hospital staff has ascertained posthospital needs of a particular patient, the planning for discharge that has occurred, and, through patient interviews, assess the patient's understanding about the postacute care aspects of his or her care.

**BOX I-2   Hospital Discharge Planning
and Continuity of Care Practices**

- The hospital must identify at an early stage of hospitalization all patients who are likely to suffer adverse health consequences upon discharge if there is no adequate discharge planning.
- The hospital must arrange for the initial implementation of the patient's discharge plan.
- As needed, the patient and family members or interested persons must be counseled to prepare them for posthospital care.
- The hospital must transfer or refer patients, along with necessary medical information, to appropriate facilities, agencies, or outpatient services, as needed, for follow-up or ancillary care.

JCAHO has expressed an interest in using the University of Colorado Health Sciences Center's three-item CTM to assess how well the hospital prepared patients to return to self-care at home.

JCAHO has adopted the accurate and complete reconcile medications across the continuum of care for one of its 2005 National Patient Safety Goals (JCAHO, 2004a). Full implementation will occur by January 2006. For 2005, hospitals will be encouraged to develop a process for obtaining and documenting a complete list of the patient's current medications upon the patient's admission to the organization and with the involvement of the patient. This process includes a comparison of the medications the organization provides to those on the list. A complete list of the patient's medication is communicated to the next provider of service when it refers or transfers a patient to another setting, service, practitioner or level of care within or outside the organization. The Institute for Healthcare Improvement, with researchers from Luther Midlefort-Mayo Health System in Wisconsin, has sponsored learning collaboratives for participating health care systems in this area (Institute for Healthcare Improvement, 2004).

CHALLENGES TO APPLYING THESE MEASURES FOR THE PURPOSES OF QUALITY IMPROVEMENT, PAY FOR PERFORMANCE, AND PUBLIC REPORTING

Challenges to implementing performance measurement for transitional care center around the misalignment of financial incentives, the unexplored accountability, the difficulty sorting out failed "hand-offs" from worsening illness, the limited utility of administrative data, and the lack of training and support for clinicians in this area. These challenges are not insurmountable and in several cases, implementing performance measurement would be the exact stimulus needed to overcome these challenges.

Currently providers are not at financial risk for poor-quality transitional care. Few penalties exist for poor performance. For example, the hospital attending physician receives additional payment on the day of discharge irrespective of how well prepared the patient is to resume self-care. Alternatively it could be argued that providers are financially rewarded for poor quality to the extent that this care leads to recidivism and additional billing opportunities. While performance measurement in general and pay-for-performance in particular could positively influence the alignment of financial incentives, there will likely be significant resistance from the health care industry in defense of the status quo.

There has been limited experience exploring what aspects of transitional care health plans, institutions, and clinicians can be held accountable. Existing Medicare Conditions of Participation articulate these responsibilities but these have not been strongly enforced. Accountability also raises unprecedented questions as to whether two institutions that have no formal or fiscal relationships can be held jointly accountable for a failed transition. It also raises questions pertaining to the definition of an episode of care. However, as was alluded to above, this is a case in which answers to key questions such as these would follow once progress is made towards promoting greater accountability by enacting performance measurement.

Pay-for-performance discussions ultimately lead to discussions regarding case-mix adjustment. Currently performance measures oriented towards outcomes may not be sophisticated enough to discern whether a poor-quality care transition experience was due to a failed "hand-off" or simply a matter of disease progression. Experience with case-mix adjustment has been limited. This situation may argue for preferentially relying on process-oriented and patient experience-oriented measures versus more outcome-oriented measures. It may also argue for a two-staged approach in which, initially, health systems or institutions are paid for doing certain tasks rather than being paid for how they performed. For example, payment for timely transfer of a discharge summary, followed by timely transfer of a discharge summary that meets certain criteria for content and accuracy.

To date, pay-for-performance activities have focused on a set of measurement items that could be easily audited using administrative data sources. Yet as detailed earlier, the leading performance measurement instruments do not fit this profile and it is unlikely that such measures are possible given the current content of administrative records. For example, measures such as ACOVE or medication reconciliation rely on chart review that is often impractical for most health care systems to produce in a reliable and timely fashion (Wenger and Young, 2003). However, the emergence of performance measurement in this area could potentially serve to foster greater adoption of health information technology, including expansion into postacute and long-term care settings.

Finally practitioners generally lack training on how to execute effective transfers and often do not recognize their role in transition planning. Compounding the problem is the fact that most practitioners have had little exposure to sites of care other than those in which they practice and are therefore unfamiliar with the ability of the receiving institution to manage complex patients. Practitioners require specific training to meet the needs of patients in transition and support systems that facilitate providing treatment, information, durable medical equipment, and other services during a patient's transition. Once again, transitional care performance measurement may represent an effective stimulus for driving greater competency in this area. The SHM example of how professionals can organize to enhance professional competency and performance provided earlier was motivated, in part, to respond to changes in JCAHO accreditation.

RECOMMENDATIONS

This final section attempts to synthesize the earlier sections towards the development of specific performance measurements recommendations for transitional care. Research and quality improvement efforts have predominantly focused on transitions out of institutional settings such as hospitals and skilled nursing facilities and accordingly, the recommendations reflect these advances. In addition, although there has been some investigation to identify those patients at greatest risk for adverse events during care transitions (Coleman et al., 2004a,b), most practice-level initiatives have not preferentially focused on any specific subgroups. As such, these recommendations will not attempt to stratify the measurement population at interest, beyond patients making the transition of interest.

There has been a proliferation of measures in this area. However, this section will only address those measures that are deemed to be ready for "prime time" or in the language of the December 1st 2004 Workshop, "good" or "good enough." As before, the focus remains on the care "hand-offs" that occur at the point of transition across different health care settings. Measures that attempt to capture a patient's care coordination/care integration experience longitudinally are not at a level of sophistication where any recommendations can be made. Further, based on qualitative and quantitative studies on the areas most in need of quality improvement, the measures presented in this section reflect the key domains of patient preparation (both for what to expect and readiness for self-care), information transfer, medication management and/or reconciliation, and follow-up appointments and testing.

Recommendations will be presented using the identical question and answer format requested by the Committee following the December 1st 2004 Workshop.

1. What measures are ready now for immediate implementation or within 1 year?

Criteria for Good/Good Enough:

• Congruent with six aims for quality improvement and rules for redesigning health care articulated in the IOM Chasm report
• Congruent with the key domains identified in qualitative studies as important to patients and family caregivers (i.e., patient/caregiver preparation for self-care and what to expect in next setting, information transfer, medication reconciliation, follow-up appointments and testing)
• Track record for use in "real-world" quality improvement projects
• Formal psychometric testing has been performed
• Items are in the public domain
• Items are actionable at either the clinician level or at the system level
• Items have been tested in more than one "hand-off" or setting
• Items can be incorporated into existing performance measurement activities, where they exist
• Scores have been shown to be associated with other meaningful processes or outcomes
• Scores have been shown to discriminate among different providers

1a. Please suggest a minimum of two that have a sufficient evidence base and have been tested for validity/reliability.

Based on the above criteria and the need for a sufficient evidence base, three measures could potentially be implemented within the upcoming year. All three measures reflect the patient's experiences and rely on self-reported responses to items during either a telephonic or written survey. The exact wording of the items is provided in addition to a description of the measure.

PEP-C-II (see Table I-1) items were developed in partnership with NRC-Picker and were recently used in a survey of 200 hospitals/36,000 patients in California that included public reporting of scores for individual hospitals (California Healthcare Foundation, 2004). These items meet the above-stated criteria with the exception that they are hospital-specific and the NRC-Picker items are proprietary. As this survey focused on the overall hospital care experience, it is not known whether quality improvement projects aimed at transitions out of the hospital have been initiated in Cali-

TABLE I-1   Patients' Evaluation of Performance in California Survey (PEP-C-II)(CHCF)

Did someone on the hospital staff explain the purpose of the medicines you were to take at home in a way you could understand?

Did they tell you what danger signals about your illness or operation to watch for after you went home?

Did they tell you when you could resume your usual activities, such as when to go back to work or drive a car?

fornia. NRC may retain proprietary rights to the items. The items have not been endorsed by NQF.

The development of the CTM (see Table I-2) was explicitly guided by the reported experiences of patients with complex care needs and their family caregivers (Coleman et al., 2004d). Thus the items directly reflect the key patient-centered domains stated earlier. Although the above items include wording for the hospital, CTM items have been used across a variety of care "hand-offs." CTM scores have been shown to predict rates of rehospitalization and return to the emergency department. They have also been shown to discriminate among hospitals known to differ in their commitment to quality improvement in this area. To date, CTM items are being used in at least four quality improvement projects, including one that focuses on pay for performance for transitional care. As noted earlier, the CTM developers have held a series of meetings with JCAHO leaders regarding a possible role for the CTM in assessing the quality of discharge planning as part of the Tracer Methodology initiative. In addition, over 70 requests for the CTM have been received, including 11 different QIOs interested in the CTM for possible implementation in local quality initiatives. A "head-to-head" testing of CTM items and HCAHPS items is under way and results will be available in Spring 2005. In response to comments from NQF, a

TABLE I-2   Care Transitions Measure (CTM)

The hospital staff took my preferences and those of my family or caregiver into account in deciding what my health care needs would be when I left the hospital.

When I left the hospital, I had a good understanding of the things I was responsible for in managing my health.

When I left the hospital, I clearly understood the purpose for taking each of my medications.

next round of testing will soon be under way to test the CTM in more diverse patient populations. To date, 74 requests from this measure have been received from health care delivery systems, QIOs, quality improvement entities and academic researchers from the United States and abroad. The CTM meets the criterion stated above and is being submitted as part of the NQF call for measures under the National Voluntary Consensus Standards for Hospital Performance initiative.

The HCAHPS initiative has great potential for uniform data collection for hospitals nationwide (AHRQ, 2003). The two discharge planning items (see Table I-3) have remained despite tremendous pressure from industry to reduce the number of items. Understandably, HCAHPS are hospital specific. HCAHPS two items were the lowest performers of all of the HCAHPS items in an external validation testing phase (CAHPS II Investigators and AHRQ, 2003). To date, A-CAHPS does not have items specific to care hand-offs. HCAHPS items have been used in public reporting as part of the CHCF initiative described above, but again, it is not clear if any transitional care specific quality improvement initiatives have been implemented as a result. It is also not known whether these items are associated with or predict rehospitalization. Item 1 does not appear to be clearly actionable (i.e., it asks whether a hospital staff member talked to the patient but does not convey whether the staff member acted on this discussion). The items will be submitted for consideration through NQF call for measures to be considered through the Consensus Development Process.

1b. How would you implement them in a way that is feasible?

Currently, nearly every hospital in the country conducts a patient-reported survey of the hospital experience. To date, the area of transitional care has been underrepresented. These items could be incorporated into/supplement these efforts.

2. What measures in your specific area are "nearly there" requiring only modest tweaking?

TABLE I-3   HCAHPS® (AHRQ)

During your hospital stay, did hospital staff talk with you about whether you would have the help you needed when you left the hospital?

During your hospital stay, did you get information in writing about what symptoms or health problems to look out for after you left the hospital?

TABLE I-4   The Assessing Care of Vulnerable Elders Measure (ACOVE)

If a vulnerable elder is discharged from a hospital to home and he or she received a new prescription medication or a change in medication before discharge, then the outpatient medical record should acknowledge the change within 6 weeks of discharge.

If a vulnerable elder is discharged from hospital to home and survives at least 4 weeks after discharge, then he or she should have a follow-up visit or documented telephone contact within 6 weeks of discharge and the physician's medical record documentation should acknowledge the recent hospitalization.

If a vulnerable elder is discharged from hospital to home or to a nursing home, then there should be a discharge summary in the outpatient physician or nursing home record within 6 weeks.

If a vulnerable elder is discharged from hospital to home or to a nursing home, and the transfer form or discharge summary indicates that a test result is pending, then the outpatient or nursing home record should include the test result within 6 weeks of hospital discharge.

If a vulnerable elder is under the outpatient care of >2 or more physicians, and 1 physician prescribed a new prescription medicine or change in medications, then subsequent medical record entries by the nonprescribing physician should acknowledge the medication change.

The measures proposed in the prior section are based on patient report. Transitional care performance measurement would be complemented by the inclusion of process of care measures that examine care processes believed to be associated with high-quality care. ACOVE measures (see Table I-4) were developed for this purpose (Wenger and Young, 2003). Formal psychometric testing is limited and further testing may help "tweak" these items to be almost ready. Further testing might also explore whether these items can discriminate among providers and whether they are associated with outcomes such as recidivism. The primary limitation of these items is that they require chart review.

LOOKING AHEAD: ADDRESSING CURRENT GAPS

Advancing the current "state of the science" with respect to transitional care will require that a number of the current gaps be addressed. The first involves refinement for how an episode of care is defined as it relates to transitional care. Patients with complex care needs frequently make multiple transitions and there is a need to better isolate the episode of care in order to assess performance, particularly as it relates to accountability and potentially financial reward. Similarly, a broader number of care transitions will need to be included, beyond hospital to skilled nursing facilities or hospital to home. Protocols are needed that account for the growing prevalence of cognitive impairment among the population of patients at risk for poor-quality care transitions. Testing in more diverse populations is needed, including for those residing in rural settings where the risks of poor "hand-offs" may be even greater due to geographic distances. With the rapid proliferation of electronic health information systems, new strategies will be needed for how requisite information can be abstracted for the purpose of performance measurement. This will require exploring how to foster greater interoperability to those settings that traditionally have not had electronic health information systems such as nursing homes and home health agencies. As mentioned earlier, it will be particularly important to not only capture whether information is made available but whether the information has been incorporated into the care plan where it would have the potential to positively influence health care outcomes. Finally, throughout this report, the interest and activities among the nation's QIOs have been highlighted. The QIOs are uniquely positioned to play a leadership role in the design and execution of performance measurement efforts that extend beyond a single care setting. The timing appears ideal for CMS to play a leadership role in galvanizing this momentum from a series of individual projects into a nationwide quality improvement effort aimed at expanding the role of performance measurement in improving the quality of transitional care.

REFERENCES

ARHQ (Agency for Healthcare Research and Quality). 1999. *Outcomes by Patient and Hospital Characteristics for All Discharges.* [Online]. Available: *http://www.ahrq.gov/HCUPnet.asp* [accessed June 29, 2004].

AHRQ. 2003. *Update on hospital CAHPS (HCAHPS).* [Online]. Available: *http://www.ahrq.gov/qual/cahps/hcahpsupdate.htm.* [accessed June 29, 2004].

American Academy of Pediatrics. 2003. *What Is a Medical Home? The National Center of Medical Home Initiatives for Children with Special Needs.* [Online]. Available: *http://www.medicalhomeinfo.org/* [accessed January 3, 2005].

Anderson MA, Helms LB. 1995. Communication between continuing care organizations. *Research in Nursing and Health* 18:49–57.

ASTM (American Society for Testing and Materials International), Massachusetts Medical Society, Health Information Management and Systems Society, and American Academy of Family Physicians. 2003. *Continuity of Care Record (CCR) The Concept Paper of the CCR.* [Online]. Available: *http://www.bhtinfo.com/CCR.Concept%20Paper.1.5.doc Version 1.5.* [accessed January 12, 2005].

Bazzoli G, Brewster L, Liu G, Kuo S. 2003. Does U.S. hospital capacity need to be expanded? *Health Affairs* 22:40–54.

Beers M, Sliwkowski J, Brooks J. 1992. Compliance with medication orders among the elderly after hospital discharge. *Hospital Formulary* 27:720–724.

Boockvar K, Fishman E, Kyriacou CK, Monias A, Gavi S, Cortes T. 2004. Adverse events due to discontinuations in drug use and dose changes in patients transferred between acute and long-term care facilities. *Archives of Internal Medicine* 164:545–550.

Brewster LR, Rudell LS, Lesser CS 2001. *Emergency Room Diversions: A Symptom of Hospitals Under Stress.* Issue Brief. Washington, DC: Center for Studying Health System Change.

CAHPS. 2004. *Child Health Plan Survey: Composites for Children with Chronic Conditions.* [Online]. Available: *http://www.cahps-sun.org/Products/Healthplan/HP-CCC-Composite.asp#coc* [accessed January 3, 2005].

CAHPS II Investigators and Agency for Healthcare Research and Quality (AHRQ). 2003. *HCAHPS Three-state Pilot Study Analysis Results.* [Online]. Available: *http:// www.cms.hhs.gov/quality/hospital/3State_Pilot_Analysis_Final.pdf* [accessed January 3, 2005].

California Health Care Foundation. 2004. *California Hospital Experience Survey Executive Summary.* [Online]. Available: *http://www.chcf.org/documents/hospitals/ CAHospitalExpSurvey04ExecSum.pdf* [accessed January 3, 2005].

CMS (Centers for Medicare and Medicaid Services). 2004. Proposed *Summary of Draft 8th Statement of Work for Quality Improvement Group.* [Online]. Available: *http:// www.cms.hhs.gov/qio/2s.pdf* [accessed January 3, 2005].

CMS. 2002. *7th Statement of Work: Joint Commission on Accreditation of Healthcare Organizations. Heart failure: Percent of patients discharged home with written discharge instructions or educational material.* [Online]. Available: *http://www.qualitymeasures.ahrq.gov/ summary/summary.aspx?doc_id=436&string=heart+AND+failure+AND+patients+AND+ discharged+AND+home* [accessed January 3, 2005].

Coleman EA. 2003. Falling through the cracks: challenges and opportunities for improving transitional care for persons with continuous complex care needs. *Journal of the American Geriatric Society* 51:549–555.

Coleman EA, Berenson RA. 2004. Lost in transition: Challenges and opportunities for improving the quality of transitional care. *Annals of Internal Medicine* 141:533–536.

Coleman EA, Boult C. 2003. Improving the quality of transitional care for persons with complex care needs. *Journal of the American Geriatrics Society* 51:556–557.

Coleman EA, Fox PD. 2004. *One Patient, Many Places: Managing Patient Transitions of Care.* [Online]. Available: *http://www.aahp.org/Content/NavigationMenu/Inside_AAHP/ Care_Management1/Care_Management.htm* [accessed October 24, 2004].

Coleman EA, Holthaus D, Johnson MF, Eilertsen TB, Kramer AM. 1999 Development of a quality measurement instrument for post-acute care. 1–17. Office of the Assistant Secretary for Planning and Evaluation, U.S. Department of Health and Human Services.

Coleman EA, Eilertsen TB, Smith JD, Frank J, Thiare JN, Ward A, Kramer AM. 2002. Development and testing of a measure designed to assess the quality of care transitions. *International Journal of Integrated Care Vol. 2.* [Online] Available: *http:// www.ijic.org* [accessed October 15, 2004]

Coleman EA, Foley C, Phillips C. 2003. Falling through the cracks: Practical strategies for reducing adverse events among older patients transferring between sites of care. *Annals of Long Term Care* 11:33–36.

Coleman EA, Min S, Chomiak A, Kramer AM. 2004a. Post-hospital care transitions: patterns, complications, and risk identification. *Health Services Research* 39:1449–1465.

Coleman EA, Smith JD, Raha D, Min S. 2004b. Post-hospital medication discrepancies: Prevalence, types, and contributing system-level and patient-level factors. *Gerontologist* 44[Spec. Issue 1], Abstract #1406.

Coleman EA, Smith JD, Frank JC, Min S, Parry C, Kramer AM. 2004c. Preparing patients and caregivers to participate in care delivered across settings: The Care Transitions Intervention. *Journal of the American Geriatric Society* 52:1817–1825.

Coleman EA, Mahoney E, Parry C. 2004d. Assessing the quality of preparation for post-hospital care from the patient's perspective: The care transitions measure (CTM). *Medical Care* 43(3) 246–255.

Dudas V, Bookwalter T, Kerr KM, Pantilat SZ. 2001. The impact of follow-up telephone calls to patients after hospitalization. *American Journal of Medicine* 111:26S–30S.

Forster A, Murff H, Peterson J, Gandhi T, Bates D. 2003. The incidence and severity of adverse events affecting patients after discharge from the hospital. *Annals of Internal Medicine* 138:161–167.

Gazmararian JA, Baker DW, Williams MV, Parker RM, Scott TL, Green DC, Fehrenbach SN, Ren J, Koplan JP. 1999. Health literacy among Medicare enrollees in a managed care organization. *Journal of the American Medical Association* 281:545–551.

Grimmer K, Moss J. 2001. The development, validity and application of a new instrument to assess the quality of discharge planning activities from the community perspective. *International Journal of Quality in Health Care* 13:109–116.

Grimmer KA, Moss JR, Gill TK. 2000. Discharge planning quality from the care perspective. *Quality of Life Research* 9:1005–1013.

Harrison A, Verhoef M. 2002. Understanding coordination of care from the consumer's perspective in a regional health system. *Health Services Research* 37:1031–1054.

Hendriks A, Vrielink M, Smets E, van Es S, De Haes J. 2001. Improving the assessment of (In)patients' satisfaction with hospital care. *Medical Care* 39:270–283.

Hibbard JH, Stockard J, Mahoney ER,Tusler M. 2004. Development of the patient activation measure (PAM): Conceptualizing and measuring activation in patients and consumers. *Health Services Research* 39:1005–1026.

Institute for Healthcare Improvement. 2004. *Medication Reconciliation Flowsheet.* [Online]. Available: *http://www.ihi.org/IHI/Topics/PatientSafety/MedicationSystems/Tools/Medication+Reconciliation+Review.htm* [accessed January 3, 2005].

IOM (Institute of Medicine). 2000. *To Err Is Human: Building A Safer Health System.* Washington, DC: National Academy Press.

IOM. 2001. *Crossing the Quality Chasm: A New Health System for the 21st Century.* Washington, DC: National Academy Press.

IOM. 2003. *Key Capabilities of an Electronic Health Record System.* Washington, DC: The National Academies Press.

IOM. 2004. *The 1st Annual Crossing the Quality Chasm Summit.* Adams, K, Greiner, AC, Corrigan, JM, eds. Washington, DC: The National Academies Press.

JCAHO (Joint Commission on Accreditation of Healthcare Organizations). 2001. *Standards and Intent Statements-Section 1: Patient-Focused Functions.* Hospital Accreditation Standards. Joint Commission on Accreditation of Healthcare Organizations. Pp. 69–156.

JCAHO. 2004a. *2005 Hospitals' National Patient Safety Goals.* [Online]. Available: http://www.jcaho.org/accredited+organizations/patient+safety/05+npsg/05_npsg_hap.htm [accessed January 1, 2005].

JCAHO. 2004b. *Shared Visions - New Pathways Q&A. New pathway: Tracer methodology.* [Online]. Available: *http://www.jcaho.org/accredited+organizations/svnp/svnp+qa_tracer+methodology.htm* [accessed January 1, 2005].

Katz T, Walke L, Jacobs L. 2000. A geriatric hospitalist program for nursing home residents. *Annals of Long Term Care* 8:51–56.

Kiely DK, Bergmann MA, Murphy KM, Jones RN, Orav EJ, Marcantonio ER. 2003. Delirium among newly admitted postacute facility patients: prevalence, symptoms, and severity. *Journal of Gerontology Series A-Biological Sciences and Medical Sciences* 58:M441–M445.

Kramer A, Eilertsen T, Lin M, Hutt E. 2000. Effects of nurse staffing on hospital transfer quality measures for new admissions. Pp. 9.1–9.22. In *Appropriateness of Minimum Nurse Staffing Ratios for Nursing Homes*. Health Care Financing Administration.

Kramer AM, Bennett R, Fish R, Lin CT, Floersch N, Conway K, Coleman EA. 2004. *Case Studies of Electronic Health Records in Post-Acute and Long-Term Care - Final Report. Office of Disability, Aging, and Long-Term Care Policy*. U.S. Department of Health and Human Services [Contract Number:233-02-0070], 1–141.

Levine C. 1998. *Rough Crossings: Family Caregivers Odysseys Through the Health Care System*. New York: United Hospital Fund of New York.

Moore C, Wisnevesky J, Williams S, McGinn T. 2003. Medical errors related to discontinuity of care from an inpatient to an outpatient setting. *Journal of General Internal Medicine* 18:646–651.

Mor V, Murphy J, Masterson-Allen S, Willey C, Razmpour A, Jackson M, Greer D, Katz S. 1989. Risk of functional decline among well elders. *Journal of Clinical Epidemiology* 42:895–904.

Naylor M, Brooten D, Campbell R, Jacobsen B, Mezey M, Pauly M, Schwartz J. 1999. Comprehensive discharge planning and home follow-up of hospitalized elders: A randomized clinical trial. *Journal of the American Medical Association* 281:613–620.

NCQA (National Committee for Quality Assurance). *Follow-up after Hospitalization for Mental Illness: 7 Days and 30 Days. The State of Health Care Quality: 2004*. [Online]. Available: *http://www.ncqa.org/communications/SOMC/SOHC2004.pdf* [accessed January 3, 2005].

Oregon Health and Science University Center for Ethics and Health Care. 1996. *The Physician Orders for Life-Sustaining Treatment Program (POLST)*. [Online]. Available: *http://www.ohsu.edu/ethics/polst/* [accessed January3, 2005].

Partnership for Solutions. 2002. *Chronic Conditions: Making the Case for Ongoing Care*. Baltimore MD: The Johns Hopkins University.

Reiss J, Gibson R. 2002. Health care transition: Destinations unknown. *Pediatrics*. 110:1307–1314.

Rich MW, Beckham V, Wittenberg C, Leven CL, Freedland KE, Carney RM. 1995. A multidisciplinary intervention to prevent the readmission of elderly patients with congestive heart failure. *New England Journal of Medicine* 333:1190–1195.

Stewart S, Pearson S, Horowitz J. 2000. Effects of a home-based intervention among patients with congestive heart failure discharged from acute hospital care. *Archives of Internal Medicine* 158:1067–1072.

U.S. DHHS (United States Department of Health and Human Services). 2000. *Analysis of Readmissions Under the Medicare Prospective Payment System for Calendar Years 1996 and 1997*. Office of Inspector General, DHHS. [Online]. Available: *http://www.oig.hhs.gov/reports.html* [accessed October 24, 2004].

van Walraven C, Seth R, Austin PC, Laupacis A. 2002a. Effect of discharge summary availability during post-discharge visits on hospital readmission. *Journal of General Internal Medicine* 17:186–192.

van Walraven C, Seth R, Laupacis A. 2002b. Dissemination of discharge summaries. Not reaching follow-up physicians. *Canadian Family Physician* 48:737–742.

vom Eigen K, Walker J, Edgman-Levitan S, Cleary P, Delbanco T. 1999. Carepartner experiences with hospital care. *Medical Care* 37:33–38.

Wachter R, Goldman L. 2002. The hospitalist movement 5 years later. *Journal of the American Medical Association* 287:487–494.

Weaver FM, Perloff L, Waters T. 1998. Patients' and caregivers' transition from hospital to home: Needs and recommendations. *Home Health Care Services Quarterly* 17:27–48.

Wenger NS, Young R. 2003. *Quality Indicators for Continuity and Coordination of Care in Vulnerable Elders.* [Online]. Available: *http://www. acponline. org/sci-policy/acove/* [accessed January 3, 2005].

Wolff JL, Starfield B, Anderson G. 2002. Prevalence, expenditures, and complications of multiple chronic conditions in the elderly. *Archives of Internal Medicine* 162:2269–2276.

TABLE I-5 Potential Measures of Care Transitions

Name of Measure	No. of Items	Data Source	Perspective	Measure Population	Measure Sampling
PEP-C II/ Picker	3	Patient	Patient	Hospitalized patients	All discharges
Care Transitions Measure (CTM)	3	Patient	Patient	Patients in transition *(see section on settings)*	All transfers
HCAHPS	2	Patient	Patient	Hospitalized patients	All discharges
ACOVE	3	Chart	System	Older adults	All discharges
Assessing (In)Patients Satisfaction	4	Patient	Patient	Hospitalized patients	All discharges
PREPARED	NA	Patient	Patient	Hospitalized patients	NA
Referral Data Inventory (RDI)	40	Chart	System	Home care referrals	All referrals
Press Ganey	9	Patient	Patient	Patients in multiple settings *(see section on settings)*	All discharges
NCQA Follow-Up After Hospitalization for Mental Illness	1	Admin or Chart	System	Hospitalized for mental illness	Patients with depression, schizophrenia, attention deficit disorder, personality disorders

Psychometric Testing?	Proprietary or Public Domain?	Prior Use in Quality Improvement?	In What Settings Used?	Are Items Actionable by Clinicians?
Yes (unconfirmed)	Proprietary	Yes	Hospital	Yes
Yes	Public	Yes	Hospital SNF[a] Home Clinic	Yes
Yes	Public	?	Hospital	Yes/No[b]
Yes (unconfirmed)	Public	Yes	Hospital Clinic	Yes
Yes	Public	?	Hospital	Yes/No[b]
Yes	Public	NA	Hospital	?
Yes	Public	?	Home care	Yes
Yes	Proprietary	Yes *unconfirmed*	Hospital Rehab SNF[b] Home care	Yes/No[c]
Yes	Proprietary	Yes	Hospital	Yes

(continued on next page)

TABLE I-5 continued

Name of Measure	No. of Items	Data Source	Perspective	Measure Population	Measure Sampling
CAHPS Patients' Experiences w/Coordination of Their Child's Care	2	Patient	Patient	Children with special care needs	?
JCAHO Accreditation and Patient Safety Items	7	Site visit	System Patient[d]	Hospitalized adults	Patients with predefined diagnoses are selected at random from certain wards
CMS/JCAHO Heart Failure: % of Patients Discharged with Written Discharge Instructions	1 (6 sub-items)	Chart	System	Hospitalized adults with congestive heart failure	All discharges among this patient population

[a]NA = Not available. Details regarding this measure were requested but no response provided.
[b]SNF = skilled nursing facility.
[c]Some items are actionable. The other items are not specific enough to be actionable by clinicians.
[d]JCAHO has recently instiued its "Tracer Methodology" that follows patients through a course of an inpatient illness and includes some patient interviews.

Psychometric Testing?	Proprietary or Public Domain?	Prior Use in Quality Improvement?	In What Settings Used?	Are Items Actionable by Clinicians?
Yes	Public	Yes	Clinic	Yes/No[b]
Unknown	Proprietary	Yes	Hospital	Yes/No[b]
?	Public	Yes	Hospital	Yes

Specific Wording of Items for Measures Included in the Table

Patients' Evaluation of Performance in California Survey (PEP-C-II) (California Health Care Foundation, 2004)

Did someone on the hospital staff explain the purpose of the medicines you were to take at home in a way you could understand?

Did they tell you what danger signals about your illness or operation to watch for after you went home?

Did they tell you when you could resume your usual activities, such as when to go back to work or drive a car?

Care Transitions Measure (Coleman, 2003)

The hospital staff took my preferences and those of my family or caregiver into account in deciding what my health care needs would be when I left the hospital.

When I left the hospital, I had a good understanding of the things I was responsible for in managing my health.

When I left the hospital, I clearly understood the purpose for taking each of my medications.

Hospital CAHPS (AHRQ, 2003)

During your hospital stay, did hospital staff talk with you about whether you would have the help you needed when you left the hospital?

During your hospital stay, did you get information in writing about what symptoms or health problems to look out for after you left the hospital?

The Assessing Care of Vulnerable Elders Measure (ACOVE)(Wenger and Young, 2003)

If a vulnerable elder is discharged from a hospital to home and he or she received a new prescription medication or a change in medication before discharge, then the outpatient medical record should acknowledge the change within 6 weeks of discharge.

If a vulnerable elder is discharged from hospital to home and survives at least 4 weeks after discharge, then he or she should have a follow-up visit or documented telephone contact within 6 weeks of discharge and the physician's medical record documentation should acknowledge the recent hospitalization.

If a vulnerable elder is discharged from hospital to home or to a nursing home, then there should be a discharge summary in the outpatient physician or nursing home record within 6 weeks.

If a vulnerable elder is discharged from hospital to home or to a nursing home, and the transfer form or discharge summary indicates that a test result is pending, then the outpatient or nursing home record should include the test result within 6 weeks of hospital discharge.

If a vulnerable elder is under the outpatient care of >2 or more physicians, and 1 physician prescribed a new prescription medicine or change in medications, then subsequent medical record entries by the nonprescribing physician should acknowledge the medication change.

Assessing (In)Patients' Satisfaction (Hendriks et al., 2001)

How satisfied are you about your exit interview upon discharge?

How satisfied are you about the timing of your discharge from hospital?

How satisfied are you about the information provided regarding further treatment (e.g., diet, working and resting hours, medication)?

How satisfied are you about the way information was passed on to your general practitioner, community care center, etc?

PREPARED (Grimmer and Moss, 2001)

Details about the measures were requested but no response was received

Referral Data Inventory (RDI) (Anderson and Helms, 1995)

40 items divided into the following categories: background data (11 items); psychosocial data (9 items); medical data (10 items); nursing care data (10 items)

Press Ganey (unpublished)

Extent to which you felt ready to be discharged (hospital)

Speed of discharge process after you were told you could go home (hospital)

Instructions given about how to care for yourself at home (hospital)

Help with arranging home care services (if needed) (hospital)

How well the doctor discussed your discharge plans and postdischarge care (inpatient rehabilitation)

How well the nurses instructed you about caring for yourself at home (including medication) (inpatient rehabilitation)

Helpfulness of the social worker in assisting with your discharge plans and posthospital arrangements (inpatient rehabilitation)

Training given to you and your family about your care at home (inpatient rehabilitation)

Degree to which you were included in the planning of your discharge (nursing home)

NCQA Follow-Up After Hospitalization for Mental Illness (National Committee for Quality Assurance, 2004)

Estimates the percentage of health plan members who had a follow-up visit after being discharged from an inpatient mental health stay. The measure includes hospitalizations for depression, schizophrenia, attention deficit disorder, and personality disorders.

CAHPS Patients' Experiences with Coordination of Their Child's Care (CAHPS, 2004)

In the last 12 months, did you get the help you needed from your child's doctors or other health care providers in contacting your child's school or daycare?

In the last 12 months, did anyone from your child's health plan, doctor's office or clinic help coordinate your child's care among these different providers or services?

JCAHO Accreditation and Patient Safety Items (JCAHO) (Joint Commission on Accreditation of Healthcare Organizations, 2001, 2004a)

PF.3.9 Discharge instructions are given to the patient and those responsible for providing continuing care.

CC.3.1 The hospital provides for coordination of care and services among health professionals and settings.

CC.4 Referral, transfer, discontinuation of services, or discharge of a patient to other levels of care, health professionals, or settings is based on the patient's assessed needs and each hospital's capability to provide needed care and services.

CC.4.1 The follow-up process provides for continuing care to meet the patient's needs.

CC.4.1.1 The patient is informed in a timely manner of the need for planning for discharge or transfer to another organization or level of care.

CC.5 Appropriate information related to the care and services provided is exchanged when a patient is accepted, referred, transferred, discontinued service, or discharged to receive further care or services.

CC.3 The hospital provides for continuity over time among the care and services provided to a patient.

(Patient Safety Goal) Develop a process for obtaining and documenting a complete list of the patient's current medications upon the patient's admission to the organization and with the involvement of the patient. This process includes a comparison of the medications the organization provides to those on the list.

(Patient Safety Goal) A complete list of the patient's medications is communicated to the next provider of service when a patient is referred or transferred to another setting, service, practitioner, or level of care within or outside the organization.

CMS 7th SOW and JCAHO—Heart Failure: Percent of Patients Discharged Home with Written Discharge Instructions or Educational Material (Centers for Medicare and Medicaid Services, 2002)

Heart failure patients with documentation that they or their caregivers were given written discharge instructions or other educational materials addressing all of the following: activity level, diet, discharge medications, follow-up appointment, weight monitoring, and what to do if symptoms worsen.

Appendix J

Commissioned Paper

Palliative Care/End-of-Life Measures

Sydney Dy and Joanne Lynn

INTRODUCTION

Recent advances in medical care and expansion of services offer tremendous potential for reducing suffering and improving quality of life for persons with life-threatening illnesses. However, study after study has demonstrated that these advances have not been translated well into clinical practice and that serious quality deficiencies persist for the care of this population (Teno, 2001). Few palliative care performance measures are included in population-based assessments of quality such as the National Healthcare Quality Report, or even in quality reports focused upon settings with high proportions of palliative care patients, such as nursing homes. Measuring quality for palliative care entails many challenges, including defining the denominator, adjusting for risk, accounting for patient preferences, assessing surrogate respondents, adjusting for differences in length of life arising from treatment choices, and evaluating patient-centered outcomes (Rosenfeld and Wenger, 2000). While measurable processes of care should be tightly linked to desirable outcomes, high-quality evidence of that linkage is quite uncommon in end-of-life care, and elements that reflect patient-centered care can be very difficult to measure.

On the other hand, assessing quality in care for the last years of life also has many opportunities for growth, including recent systematic reviews (Higginson et al., 2003; Lorenz et al., 2004), a national consensus project on clinical guidelines (National Consensus Project, 2004), and a large body of literature addressing the important domains and the development of measurement instruments. Palliative and end-of-life care measures must be prominent in any national set of quality measures, since such a high proportion of care occurs in patients with life-threatening illness and since deficiencies in quality may cause particular harm in patients with little time or reserve remaining to recover from adverse effects. A national measurement set must consider the unique priorities and challenges of palliative care patients, as many measures associated with improved outcomes in a healthy population may be inappropriate or even harmful in patients with serious illness and limited prognoses.

For the purposes of this paper, we will use the World Health Organization definition of palliative care as "an approach that improves the quality of life of patients and their families facing the problems associated with life-threatening illness, through the prevention and relief of suffering by means of early identification and impeccable assessment and treatment of pain and other problems, physical, psychosocial and spiritual" (World Health Organization, 2002).

For our conceptual model, we will use the domains of the framework of the Toolkit of Instruments to Measure End of Life Care (Teno, 2000):

- Pain and other symptoms
- Emotional and cognitive symptoms
- Functional status
- Survival time and aggressiveness of care
- Advance care planning
- Continuity of care
- Spirituality
- Grief and bereavement
- Patient-centered reports and rankings (aka satisfaction) with the quality of care
  - Caregiver well-being
  - Quality of life

For each domain, where appropriate, we have also organized measures into those applicable to assessment, management, and outcome. We have listed topics in this order in the text and Table J-1, and compared the results of our searches to these categories to determine where there are particular gaps in performance measurement for palliative care.

METHODS AND SOURCES

We limited our review to measurement sets particularly relevant to palliative care, as more general sets are under review in other parts of this project. We considered information from recent systematic reviews and consensus statements in palliative care, as well as previous reviews of quality indicators for palliative care, relevant reports from the Institute of Medicine (Lunney et al., 2003; Teno et al., 2001), and other pertinent books and reports. We also reviewed articles and Web sites from recent RAND initiatives to define performance indicators. We performed Medline searches using the terms "quality indicator" and "performance measure" with the terms "palliative" and "end of life." Finally, we reviewed Web sites for palliative care standards or indicator initiatives in other countries, including Canada, Australia, and the United Kingdom.

MEASURE SETS

Palliative Care

Leading measurement sets in palliative care are described below, and pertinent measures are included in Table J-1.

Dartmouth Atlas

Wennberg and colleagues (1999, 2004) have used Medicare administrative data to evaluate a number of potential performance measures and to compare them across geographic regions defined by political division or hospital referral region. For the end-of-life measures, they have tabulated the services that Medicare recipients used in the last 6 months of life, showing wide variation by region and provider. Their measures include the number of days spent in the hospital; number of days spent in the intensive care unit; percentage of patients seeing 10 or more physicians; percentage ever enrolled in hospice; percentage of deaths occurring in the hospital; and percentage of deaths occurring in association with an intensive care unit. We describe several of these measures in more detail in Table J-1. Although the variation in these measures is striking, it is unclear whether those variations correlate with the quality of the end-of-life experience. Fisher et al. (2003a,b) did find that higher levels of resource utilization in the last 6 months of life were not associated with improved mortality or satisfaction for Medicare patients with serious illnesses, measuring regional satisfaction with the Medicare Current Beneficiary Survey. Drawbacks of retrospective analyses of patients who have died are discussed in the section below on challenges of measurement in end-of-life care.

Brown Atlas of Dying

The Brown Atlas (Teno, 2004) has extended the work of the Dartmouth group by using several additional data sources to examine regional variation in end-of-life care. The Atlas includes site of death information for

TABLE J-1   Selected Potential Performance Measures for Palliative/
End-of-Life Care

Domain Category Name of Measure	Description	Numerator Denominator
Pain		
Assessment		
Pain measurement UHC	Chart review	Numerator: Patients who had any pain measurement within 48 hours of admission Denominator: Palliative care population hospital admissions
Use of numeric pain scale **UHC, Brown-QIO, VHA-QIO**	Chart review	Numerator: Patients who had a numeric pain scale used Denominator: Palliative care or other population admissions with a pain score within 48 hours
Pain as 5th vital sign **VHA-QIO**	Across all settings Chart review	Numerator: Patients who had pain assessed when other vital signs taken Denominator: All patients (unless lesser frequency indicated and documented in chart)
Appropriate pain assessment **Brown-QIO**	Assessment of pain intensity, 4 other elements	Numerator: Patients with appropriate pain assessment Denominator: All NH residents with pain
Treatment		
Pain medication prescribed **Brown-QIO**	Any pain medication	Numerator: Any pain medication prescribed Denominator: All NH residents with pain
Nonpharmacological treatment **Brown-QIO**	Any nonpharmacological treatment in plan of care	Numerator: Nonpharmacological treatment Denominator: All NH residents with pain
Change in pain medication **Brown-QIO**	Change in pain medication for uncontrolled pain	Numerator: Change in pain medication Denominator: NH residents with daily pain and documented moderate-severe pain

Psychometric Testing (Validity/ Reliability)	Prior Use	References
N	Benchmarking Multiple settings	
N	Benchmarking	Baier et al., 2004; Cleeland et al., 2003
N	Improvement	Cleeland et al., 2003
Y—e.g., Brief Pain Inventory	Improvement	Baier et al., 2004; Lorenz et al., 2004
N	Improvement	Baier et al., 2004
N	Improvement	Baier et al., 2004
N	Improvement	Baier et al., 2004

(continued on next page)

TABLE J-1 continued

Domain *Category* **Name of Measure**	Description	Numerator Denominator
Adherence to guidelines **Du Pen**	Adherence to "best practice" pain guidelines, defined as score of 2.5 on score of 0–3	Numerator: Adherence Denominator: Community oncology patients with pain of 3 or greater on 10-point scale
Outcome Rate of pain **VHA-IHI**	% of patients with moderate-severe pain; various settings Patient perspective	Numerator: % of patients with moderate or severe pain Denominator: All patients in setting
Rate of pain in nursing homes **Brown Atlas**	% of patients with moderate-severe pain; Collected from Minimum Data Set (MDS)	Numerator: % of patients with moderate or severe pain over 7-day lookback period Denominator: All nursing home patients
Persistent pain in nursing homes **Brown Atlas**	% of nursing home patients with persistent pain	Numerator: patients who still have moderate or excruciating pain on 2nd assessment 60–180 days after admission Denominator: Nursing home patients with pain on 1st assessment. Subgroups: persons with documented terminal illness; persons cognitively intact and able to report on their pain; patients with cancer
Comfortable dying **NDS**	% of patients whose pain was brought to a comfortable level within 48 hours of admission to hospice	Numerator: patients answering that pain was brought to a comfortable level within 48 hours Denominator: patients uncomfortable due to pain on admission, able to self-report, and ≥18 years of age
Pain relieved/reduced **UHC**	Hospital Chart review	Numerator: Pain relieved/ reduced to <3/10 within 48 hours of admission Denominator: Palliative care population reporting pain on hospital admission
Satisfaction **Du Pen**	Satisfaction with current pain treatment; patients who would choose to have similar treatment again	Numerator: Patients satisfied with current pain treatment Denominator: Patients treated for pain

Psychometric Testing (Validity/ Reliability)	Prior Use	References
N	Improvement. Adherence was greater in intervention group and associated with reduced pain scores	Du Pen et al., 1999
N	Improvement	Cleeland et al., 2003
MDS pain reporting has substantial validity issues. Currently undergoing further development as a CMS demonstration project	Reporting, Improvement	Teno et al., 2004; Baier et al., 2004
N	Benchmarking	Teno et al., 2002; Teno, 2004
N	Benchmarking	Connor et al., 2004
N		
Y	Improvement. Rates higher in intervention group	Du Pen et al., 1999

(continued on next page)

TABLE J-1   continued

Domain Category Name of Measure	Description	Numerator Denominator
Dyspnea **Assessment** Dyspnea assessment **UHC**	Dyspnea assessment within 24 hours of admission Hospital Chart review	Numerator: Patients assessed for dyspnea within 24 hours of admission Denominator: Palliative care population admissions
Outcome Dyspnea relieved/ reduced **UHC**	Dyspnea relieved/ reduced within 48 hours of admission Hospital Chart review	Numerator: Patients with dyspnea reduced/ relieved to ≤3 within 48 hours of admission Denominator: Patients with documented dyspnea
Constipation **Treatment** Bowel regimen **UHC**	Bowel regimen within 24 hours of opioid administration Hospital Chart review	Numerator: Patients with bowel regimen ordered within 24 hours or bowel regimen contraindicated Denominator: Palliative care population admissions started on opioids
Emotional and cognitive symptoms **Assessment** Depression and comorbid disease **ACOVE Depression**	Screening for depression with new onset of serious comorbid conditions Community	Numerator: Patient asked about or treated for depression or referred to mental health professional within 2 months of diagnosis of condition Denominator: Vulnerable elders who present with new onset of serious comorbid conditions, including malignancy
Treatment Recognizing depression **ACOVE Depression**	Evaluation/treat- ment for depression if presents with depressive symptoms Community	Numerator: Patient asked about or treated for depression or referred to mental health pro- fessional within 2 weeks of presentation Denominator: Vulnerable elders who present with new onset of symptoms of potential depression

Psychometric Testing (Validity/ Reliability)	Prior Use	References
N		
N		
N		
Tested in managed care organizations as part of ACOVE measurement set	Benchmarking	Nakajima and Wenger, 2003
		Nakajima and Wenger, 2003

(continued on next page)

TABLE J-1 continued

Domain Category Name of Measure	Description	Numerator Denominator
Care planning **Process** Documentation of patient status **UHC**	Documentation of all 4 aspects of patient status within 48 hours of admission: prognosis, functional status, psychosocial symptoms, symptom distress	Numerator: Patients with all 4 aspects documented within 48 hours Denominator: Palliative care admissions
Patient/family meeting **UHC**	Patient/family meeting within 1 week of admission. Defined as documented discussion of patient preferences/plans for discharge disposition Hospital Chart review	Numerator: Patients with patient/family meeting documented within 1 week of admission Denominator: Palliative care admissions
Discharge planning **UHC**	Plan for discharge disposition documented within 4 days of admission Hospital Chart review	Numerator: Patients with discharge disposition documented within 4 days of admission Denominator: Palliative care population admissions
Use of discharge planner **UHC**	Discharge planner/ social services arranged services required for discharge Hospital Chart review	Numerator: Patients where discharge planner/ social services arranged services required for discharge Denominator: Palliative care population admissions
Advance directives and surrogates— outpatient **ACOVE EOL**	Surrogate decision-maker should be documented in outpatient charts Chart review Community	Numerator: Outpatient chart includes: (1) Advance directive indicating surrogate decision maker, (2) documentation of discussion of who would be surrogate or search for surrogate, or (3) indication that there is no identified surrogate Denominator: Vulnerable elders

Psychometric Testing (Validity/ Reliability)	Prior Use	References
	Prognosis was least frequently documented, followed by functional status and psychosocial symptoms	
N	Benchmarking	
N	Benchmarking	
	Benchmarking	
The ACOVE indicators have been tested in managed care settings; further research is addressing quality improvement	Research	Wenger et al., 2003

(continued on next page)

TABLE J-1 continued

Domain Category Name of Measure	Description	Numerator Denominator
Advance directives and surrogates – hospital **ACOVE EOL**	Advance directives in hospital chart for patients admitted with dementia, coma, or altered mental status Chart review Hospital	Numerator: Same as above, except documentation in hospital medical record within 48 hours of admission Denominator: Vulnerable elders admitted to hospital with dementia, coma, or altered mental status, who survive 48 hours
Documentation of care preferences— dementia **ACOVE EOL**	Documentation of preferences for patients hospitalized with severe dementia Chart review Hospital	Numerator: Within 48 hours of admission, medical record documents that patient's prior preferences for care either have been considered or could not be elicited or are unknown Denominator: Vulnerable elders with severe dementia admitted to the hospital and surviving 48 hours
Site of death	% of patients who died where death occurred in (1) home; (2) hospital; or (3) nursing home. Adjusted for age and gender. Subgroups include patients with cancer and the elderly (Dartmouth Atlas)	Numerator/Denominator: All persons 15 years of age or older who died of any non-traumatic or external cause in a state.[a] Patients listed as "other" are included in denominator (this would include inpatient hospice)
Outcome Self-determined life closure **NDS**	Rate of unwanted hospitalizations and resuscitations (NHPCO) Hospice	Numerator: Patients not hospitalized or not discharged concurrent with a hospital admission Denominator: Discharged patients whose most recently recorded preference was to avoid hospitalization (may be via legal representative/advance directive). Excludes patients without recorded preference. CPR measure is equivalent

Psychometric Testing (Validity/ Reliability)	Prior Use	References
	Research	Wenger et al., 2003
	Research	Wenger et al., 2003
Y	Benchmarking Improvement	Teno 2004
N	Benchmarking	Connor et al., 2003

(continued on next page)

TABLE J-1 continued

Domain Category Name of Measure	Description	Numerator Denominator
Satisfaction After-death bereaved family interview	3 versions: hospice, hospital, and nursing home. Up to 8 domains and 133 items. Telephone survey with family member 3–6 months after death Family perspective	Numerators: Family members who reported that: (1) overall assessment of quality was excellent; (2) sufficient desired physical comfort and emotional support provided to patient; (3) shared decision making supported; (4) patient treated with respect; (5) needs of family attended to; (6) care coordinated. Denominator: Deaths
NHPCO FEHC NDS	Family Evaluation of Hospice Care: Core survey, 43 items; 17 optional items. Sent 2 months after death. Bereavement satisfaction survey sent 13 months after death Family perspective	3 numerators: Family members who reported—(1) Safe dying (caregiver confidence in providing safe care) (2) Effective grieving (emotional support to loved ones before and after death) (3) Family evaluation of hospice care (willingness to recommend hospice care) Denominator: Hospice deaths
Continuity Identify source of care ACOVE Continuity	All vulnerable elders should be able to identify a provider or clinic that they would call in need of medical care	Numerator: Patient who can identify provider/clinic to call if needs health care Denominator: Vulnerable elders

aDeath certificates that listed death as a result of any of the following were excluded: pregnancy and childbirth-related causes, motor vehicle accidents, all other accidents, suicide, assault homicide, and all other external causes. Foreign residents and those with an unknown site of death were also excluded. Death certificates that listed a site of death as other than a nursing home, hospital, or home were included in the denominator for all calculations.

For UHC data, palliative care population admissions were defined as: Adult patients with 2 previous admissions (any DRG) within 12 months of the target admission; and target admission with >4 days length of stay for DRGS for heart failure (127), cancer DRG pool (82, 203, 172, 274, 346, 10), HIV (489), or respiratory DRG pool (483, 475).

Psychometric Testing (Validity/ Reliability)	Prior Use	References
Y (Teno et al., 2001)	Home care/hospice, hospital, nursing home; National norms are available for comparisons in all 3 settings (Teno et al., 2004)	Teno et al., 2004
N Ceiling effects	Benchmarking, although no evidence of substantial variation among hospices or across time	Connor et al., 2004
ACOVE testing in managed care plans	Benchmarking Improvement	Wenger and Young, 2003

For ACOVE, "vulnerable elders" are defined as persons 65 years of age and older who are at increased risk for death or functional decline. A scoring tool, the Vulnerable Elders Survey (VES-13), is available to identify vulnerable elders in the community.

All measures are from the patient perspective and in the public domain unless otherwise noted.

decedents older than 15 years of age, as well as data on a number of measures in nursing homes, including 12 measures for pain, advance directive use, do not resuscitate orders, and feeding tubes. Several of these are summarized in Table J-1.

After-Death Bereaved Family Interview

This is a set of measures developed for an interview with a family member after a patient's death (Teno et al., 2001; Teno, 2004). The measures arose from a review of professional guidelines and a series of focus groups of bereaved family members. Versions are available for different settings of care, and a national study has demonstrated feasibility and differences by the type of care provided. Growing evidence also provides a baseline for benchmarking. Unlike most other satisfaction measures, ceiling effects do not limit its utility. The instrument measures quality across various domains, reflecting the priorities of the patients' family members. The response rate was acceptable (58 percent), the instruments are in the public domain, and various researchers are using them in a variety of settings. The developers require users to contribute to a database intended to aid organizations in benchmarking their data. Measures are summarized in Table J-1 under "satisfaction" and include: physical comfort and emotional support; shared decision-making; treating dying person with respect; attending to the emotional needs of the family; and coordinating care.

National Hospice and Palliative Care Organization National Hospice Data Set (NDS)

This industry wide, voluntary data collection includes five outcome categories: comfortable dying (comfort 48 hours after admission); self-determined life closure (unwanted hospitalizations and resuscitations); safe dying (caregiver confidence in providing safe care); effective grieving (emotional support); and family evaluation of hospice care (willingness to recommend hospice care). The last three categories are obtained from the NHPCO Family Satisfaction Survey (Connor et al., 2004). The NHPCO Web site includes a comprehensive summary of the numerators, denominators, and measures that were considered and pilot-tested in the development of these measures, as well as the protocols for the current measures (Ryndes et al., 2000). The final measures are in Table J-1.

Assessing Care of Vulnerable Elders (ACOVE) Quality of Care Assessment System

The ACOVE project developed quality indicators relevant to the comprehensive care of vulnerable elders, including outpatient, hospital, and nursing home care. They also developed measurement tools to document performance on each of the indicators. Wenger et al. reported applying the indicators to measure quality in two managed care organizations, and ongoing research involves testing interventions to determine whether they improve performance. One of the domains in ACOVE is End-of-Life Care, which includes 14 quality indicators. The indicators overall have excellent reliability from repeated chart abstraction (97 percent agreement) (Wenger et al., 2003). Nine of the end-of-life indicators relate to advance care planning; the other four are management of ventilator withdrawal, treatment of pain, treatment of dyspnea, and attention to spiritual issues. These indicators are included in Table J-1.

Solomon et al. (2003) reported on an evaluation of all 203 ACOVE quality indicators by a committee of geriatric experts for appropriateness for use in patients with advanced dementia or poor prognosis. They concluded that 120 of the indicators were appropriate for use in patients with advanced dementia, and 130 were appropriate for patients with a prognosis of 6 months or less. We have included several of the ACOVE indicators that apply to the elderly generally in Table J-1 under "depression" and "continuity." Minor but important modification of many of the ACOVE measures would improve their appropriateness for the population nearing death. For example, the indicator for continuity states that patients should know whom to call if they have a health care need. Due to the high needs and acuity in palliative care, a higher standard may be needed, such as 24-hour availability of a provider who can coordinate their care and respond to urgent situations without relying only upon emergency hospitalization. A recent review of the ACOVE indicators also found that experts in Britain approved 86 percent for use there (Steel et al., 2004).

University Health System Consortium—Palliative Care Benchmarking 2004

The purpose of this project was to identify institutions with better performance in order to provide benchmarks. This project involved 35 university hospitals and reviewed 1,597 charts. The palliative care performance measures, bundled together, were associated with reduced length of stay. The performance measures identified five better performing sites. The benchmarks are undergoing revisions; current versions are listed in Table J-1.

RAND Quality Assessment Tools: Quality of Care for Oncologic Conditions and HIV

Two chapters have indicators particularly relevant to the end of life: Chapter 7, Lung Cancer, and Chapter 11, Cancer Pain and Palliation. The lung cancer chapter includes indicators for the palliative treatment of brain metastases in both small-cell and non-small-cell lung cancer, and for treatment of bone pain in small-cell lung cancer. For pain management, three indicators are included: (1) patients with metastatic cancer to bone should have the presence or absence of pain noted at least every 6 months; (2) cancer patients whose pain is uncontrolled should be offered a change in pain management within 24 hours of the pain complaint; and (3) patients with painful bony metastases, who are noted to be unresponsive to or intolerant of narcotic analgesia, should be offered one of the following within one week of the notation of pain: radiation therapy to the sites of pain, or radioactive strontium therapy (Asch et al., 2000). These measures have been used as part of the QA tools to evaluate quality in nationwide studies and in the Veterans Health Administration health system (Asch et al., 2004). As these measures are specific to particular issues in cancer, they have not been included in Table J-1.

QUALITY IMPROVEMENT

A number of palliative care measures have also been used in large quality improvement projects. The Veterans Health Administration—Institute for Healthcare Improvement (VHA-IHI) initiative used the IHI rapid change "Breakthrough Series Model" (Cleeland et al., 2003). Over 9 months, 73 teams improved pain management in several settings, including ambulatory care, inpatient rehabilitation, oncology, and long-term care. The assessment measure was screening documentation (use as the fifth vital sign), the treatment measures included documented care plans for patients with pain scores >3 and distribution of pain educational materials, and the outcome measure was a reduction in the percentage of patients with moderate-severe pain.

In Rhode Island, a collaborative between the state Quality Improvement Organization and Brown University was able to achieve improvements in a number of process and outcome measures in pain management in 21 nursing homes (Baier et al., 2004), although the project was limited by many structural factors, such as nursing turnover. The IHI and the RAND/Washington Home for Palliative Care Studies have also conducted end-of-life collaboratives with promising results (Lynn et al., 2000). Two collaboratives that are ongoing are the National Medicaring Quality Improvement Collaborative (www.medicaring.org) and the United Hospital Fund's Palliative Care Quality Improvement Initative. The measures developed in quality improvement work generally have face validity and the test of usefulness inherent in that work, but they have not often had formal testing of reliability and validity.

We also describe measures in Table J-1 used in a randomized, clinical trial of implementing pain guidelines (Du Pen et al., 1999) in cancer patients in clinical oncology practices that resulted in a statistically significant reduction in usual pain intensity, as well as improved satisfaction with pain.

Special Populations

Several ongoing projects are addressing the development of measures for pediatrics, intensive care, and cancer.

Pediatrics

A recent review of quality measures for children for the Institute of Medicine (Beal et al., 2004) found that 19 health care quality measure sets with 396 quality measures for children did not include any measures particularly relevant for the end of life. The Initiative for Pediatric Palliative Care (Dokken et al., 2001) has developed a set of quality domains, goals, and indicators for children living with life-threatening conditions, as well as an institutional assessment tool that is being field-tested, but measures are not yet ready for use as quality indicators.

Intensive Care

The Robert Wood Johnson Foundation Critical Care End-of-Life Peer Workgroup (Clarke et al., 2003) has developed a set of 7 proposed end-of-life quality domains and 53 quality indicators, as well as a set of clinician and organizational interventions and behaviors that might address these indicators in the intensive care unit. Performance measures that may be relevant for validation and adoption by organizations are under development.

Cancer

In addition to the QA tools, Earle et al. (2003) conducted a recent project to explore potential end-of-life cancer quality indicators that could be monitored using administrative data. They used a literature review to identify indicators that would be feasible with current Medicare data and then identified those that would be acceptable, using focus groups of patients and family members and an expert panel. The final list included 7 indicators, several of which are also part of the Dartmouth Atlas. Others include a short interval between last chemotherapy dose and death; frequent emergency room visits; and a short interval between starting a new chemotherapy regimen and death. Additional indicators that some care provider organizations may monitor include clinical trial participation, use of multidisciplinary care, and physician continuity. Indicators not currently amenable to administrative data included communication, shared decision-making, advance directives, and pain and symptom management.

The National Quality Forum (NQF) also has started a cancer initiative relative to palliative care, described below under "ongoing initiatives."

International Efforts

Many other countries are working on developing and implementing standards, indicators, and/or performance measures concerning palliative care, including Canada, Australia, and the United Kingdom, where palliative care is a regular part of care and evaluation.

Gold Standards Framework—United Kingdom

More than 1000 (Murray, 2004) primary care practices in the United Kingdom have adopted the Gold Standards Framework, a quality monitoring and improvement process that addresses care system performance in supporting people with serious and eventually fatal conditions. Current performance measures in the palliative care population include assessment of pain; assessment of the preferred place of death and congruence between the actual and preferred place of death; and number of crises or hospitalizations. Evaluation of validity, reliability, and effectiveness of these measures is ongoing. Time series data from the practices show responsiveness of these measures to improved care processes.

Ongoing Initiatives

Several current initiatives will provide further insight into measures that may be applicable to the end of life. The NQF, in partnership with other organizations, has launched several relevant initiatives on measuring quality of care for cancer: Symptom Management/End-of-Life, funded by CDC, National Care Institute (NCI), Agency for Healthcare Research and Quality (AHRQ), and CMS; Palliative Care, funded by the Robert Wood Johnson Foundation; and Long-Term Care. As part of the Symptom Management/End-of-Life Project, the Southern California Evidence-Based Practice Center will perform a systematic review of the literature on evidence for measures for depression, pain, dyspnea, and advance care planning. The NQF will also issue a broad appeal for measures of symptom management/end-of-life care. NQF will be weighing many of the measures identified in these ways for potential endorsement.

Other Measurement Sets

Many other measurement sets, including Nursing Home Compare (Centers for Medicare and Medicaid Services, 2004), Home Health Compare, and measures for specific conditions, such as depression, contain measures that are relevant to palliative care and the end of life.

MEASUREMENT RECOMMENDATIONS

Areas with Measures That Are Ready for Implementation

Our criteria for choosing measures included evidence for reliability, validity, association with outcomes, ability to be improved in research studies or quality improvement, feasibility, and applicability across health care settings and across possible definitions of palliative care. We propose measures in the two domains that others have also often proposed as being nearly ready for implementation: care planning and pain management. While most indicators of quality have started with assessment of the patient's situation, actual improvement requires assessment, appropriate initial response, and reassessment and repeated response as needed.

High-quality care planning involves many elements, including ensuring that patients have an accurate understanding of the meaning of their illness and of potential interventions; ensuring that care plans are consistently applied through transitions between providers and settings; and communicating about potential changes in care plans with changes in patients' clinical situations. Depending on the situation, care planning may involve addressing various issues, including designation of a surrogate and future care preferences and addressing preferences for resuscitation and other aggressive treatments. As recent systematic reviews (Lorenz et al., 2004; Wenger and Rosenfeld, 2001) have described in detail, little high-quality evidence links higher rates of care planning to improved outcomes. Observational and prospective time-series studies provide some evidence of the linkage, qualitative studies support the claim that care planning is important to patients and families, and studies have shown that interventions can increase the rate of care planning. In many situations, care plans may need to be more detailed in order to be effective in shaping care, as in addressing whether a terminally ill nursing home patient should be hospitalized. Care plans often need to address particularly important and complicated situations, such as withdrawal of mechanical ventilation, rather than just stating broad approaches. Finally, care planning should not just address what should be avoided, but positive elements as well, such as designating and planning for the preferred place of death.

The measurement of care planning has mostly relied upon simple rates: completed plans, divided by eligible patients. Few studies have attempted to measure the appropriateness, completeness, utility, or actual use of the care plans, and those few have also relied upon straightforward, unadjusted rates. Controlled trials of interventions to improve care planning have sometimes shown small increases in the rates of advance directives, but the gains have been small and have not generally included testing of the effectiveness of the care plan in shaping the care. Some evidence indicates that care planning makes the task of the family surrogate somewhat easier. Observational reports from quality improvement projects demonstrate remarkable improvements in the rate of documented care planning and show care delivery being in accord with the plan (Hammes and Rooney, 1998; Lynn et al., 2000).

Measuring care planning requires specifying the content and process required to count as an advance care plan and specifying the denominator population carefully. The stability of the denominator population is especially problematic if it relates to a particular setting of care and part of the care planning creates biases in the future composition of the population of patients who use that setting. For example, if care planning in the hospital results in much lower use of the hospital among nursing home patients nearing death, the rate of care planning might stay stable among those continuing to use the hospital although the intervention was actually quite successful in removing patients from that environment.

The advance care planning indicators of quality would seem to be that patients facing serious complications and death have had the opportunity to plan in advance of emergency or incompetence for the likely scenarios, including designating a surrogate decision maker, forgoing undesired interventions, ensuring desired interventions (including setting of care), and having these plans reliably available and implemented in various settings and circumstances. Measurement of these aspects of care can be rolled up into a composite measure that sums over a number of steps, as the Gold Standards Framework in Britain does with its "dying in the preferred place of choice" measure. Most often, measurement of advance care planning simply reflects adding up advance directive documents and dividing by the number of eligible persons in a particular setting. The Veterans Administration initiative to increase advance care planning also specified that advance care plans had to include designation of a surrogate decision maker, a decision about resuscitation, and a decision about aggressive symptom management, in order to count as a completed advance care plan. The report from La Crosse, Wisconsin tallied regional experience with aggressive education and encouragement and not only tallied completed documents but also whether they were available at the time of death and whether they were followed (Hammes and Rooney, 1998). The options for measures thus include:

1. Rate of documented plans of care, perhaps requiring designation of a surrogate, decisions about resuscitation, and whatever specific issues are salient in the population (resuscitation in hospitalized persons, tube feeding in dementia, etc.);
2. Rate at which documented plans of care are available when needed;
3. Rate at which available plans of care are implemented;
4. Rate of a composite measure of patients getting what they have designated as preferred, such as the preferred place of death.

Improving pain management also requires numerous steps. Again, a recent systematic review found little high-quality evidence that pain can be improved on a population level, although quality improvement collaboratives (Baier et al., 2004; Cleeland et al., 2003; Lynn et al., 2000) have shown promising results. As in advance care planning, qualitative studies have demonstrated that recognition and treatment of pain are important priorities for patients receiving palliative care. High-quality pain assessment needs to include a number of elements: providers need to be knowledgeable about and comfortable with the treatment of pain; systems of care must support quality pain management; and reassessment and adjustment of medications are often necessary to maintain pain control. Pain is a multifactorial experience, and assessment usually has to specify whether to address such differing concepts as worst pain, average pain, pain before or after treatment, meaning of pain in terms of activity or emotional impact, and character of the pain. Detailed pain improvement projects have measured a number of other process elements, including the use of opioids (correct dosing, rotation, conversion, escalation). Some measures have addressed outcomes, such as the NHPCO measure of "comfortable dying"; however, this measure is best adapted for internal quality improvement, due to validity issues related to risk adjustment and patient preference. The pain measures most nearly ready for implementation, with evidence of reliability and validity, are:

1. Assessment.
   Numerator: Patients with a high-quality pain assessment with a validated instrument, including intensity, location, what makes it better, what makes it worse, and effects of medications.

   Denominator: A defined population at risk, stable over the period of inquiry.

   Settings: Admission to a nursing home, hospital, home care organization, hospice, or new outpatient provider. Every shift in a hospital, every day in hospice, every week in home care.

Further development should include evaluating which elements of assessment are most associated with outcomes; consensus on defining the denominator; and evaluating evidence of applicability across settings. In addition, since few information systems can currently provide this data, the number of medical records to be reviewed will need to be defined.

    2. Response.

    Numerator: Patients who have a change in their pain management program, or the number with a change that is within defined quality parameters.

    Denominator: Palliative care patients, as described above under assessment, or patients with certain diagnoses or severity of illness associated with particular diagnoses, with uncontrolled pain (e.g., patients with pain score of 5 or greater on a 10-point scale).

    Settings: as above.

Further development, in addition to those mentioned for assessment, should include refining the definition of uncontrolled pain and the definition of a change in pain management. Ideally, future research and development of data assessment tools and systems would allow longitudinal measurement of patients' experience, especially with new pain syndromes or worsening of chronic pain. Leaders in palliative care claim that rates of moderate and severe physical pain should diminish to a very small fraction of at-risk patients in systems offering good care; however, demonstrations of that claim in any sizable populations are remarkably rare or absent.

Areas with Measures That Show Promise, but Require Further Development

    A number of measures deserve mention for potential inclusion in the future, including the After-Death Bereaved Family Interview and many other elements of pain management and care planning, including the preferred place of death. The After-Death Interview has been carefully developed and rigorously tested in a national population, shows differences by the type of care provided, is not limited by ceiling effects, and includes measures in a number of different domains. Although the Interview addresses surrogates' perceptions of care, which may have variable correlation with patients' perceptions, surrogates' perspectives are valued independently in palliative care and their experience may affect the future bereavement and health. The Interview would require further development for use as a measure, including adaptation to a paper survey, shortening, summarizing into a small number of key dimensions, demonstration of broad applicability (region, type of illness, approach to care services, ethnic background), and demonstration that scores improve when processes of care improve (Teno et al., 2001; Teno, 2004).

Many other potential measures of pain management and care planning are listed in Table J-1 and have some evidence to support their use.

Areas with Measures That Need to Be Developed

Many domains relevant to palliative care lack measures with sufficient supporting evidence for confidence even about whether further development of current approaches would yield useful measures. These include the treatment and prevention of most symptoms other than pain in patients who are very sick and nearing death. Measurement tools are available to address other physical and emotional symptoms, but insufficient work has yet been done to translate these into performance measures for this population. Measures for some symptoms have been developed for other populations, such as nausea in cancer treatment or depression in the elderly, but these do not have sufficient supporting evidence and have not been evaluated in the palliative care population. Many other areas, such as spirituality, life closure, and caregiver burden and bereavement, have measurement tools available, but generally research has not tested whether these vary with better care, whether they have ceiling effects, whether routine measurement is feasible, or most of the other attributes of useful measures of care system quality.

Caregiving and caregiver concerns are areas with particular needs for further development. Caregivers are vital to many elements of the end-of-life experience, including psychosocial distress, life closure, and site of death. The quality and quantity of caregiving can affect many other measurement domains, including symptom management and advance care planning. In addition, the impact of caregiving on the caregivers can have consequences for their physical and emotional health. We identified no performance measures specific to caregiving. Although the After-Death Bereaved Family Interview is an interview of caregivers, it is oriented towards the caregiver's perception of the patient's experience rather than towards caregiver issues. In our systematic review of the end-of-life literature (Lorenz et al., 2004), we found that, although many measurement instruments have been developed to examine caregivers' experiences, interventions for caregivers have had little consistent effect on these outcomes. Outcome measures also differed widely across studies; although caregiver burden was frequently studied, other outcomes included stress, depression, anxiety, satisfaction, caregiver morbidity and mortality, unmet needs, and institutionalization.

The domain of grief and bereavement also has many available measurement instruments (Lorenz et al., 2004), but little is available to guide performance measurement. Bereavement may have significant impact on significant others' health, including depression and suicidality, particularly for parents of children and widowed elders. However, recent systematic reviews have found that, despite a large number of interventions in the literature, there is no clear evidence that interventions are effective in improving the experience of a sizable population, except for the pharmacological treatment of depression (Forte et al., 2004). Much of the reason for the lack of demonstrated efficacy is the low quality and variability in measurement and interventions in the literature (Forte et al., 2004).

As documented in our recent evidence report (Lorenz et al., 2004), many domains do not even have well-developed measurement tools for use in palliative care; in particular, continuity of care, dignity, and autonomy require further work on every stage—concepts, factors influencing the domain, reliability and validity, generalizability, and evidence that care system improvement affects the measures. Finally, few measurement tools have records of use across diverse populations, including pediatrics, and further research in performance measures will need to address differences among fatal diagnoses, ethnic groups, and age groups.

Key Gaps in the Evidence Base

Our recent systematic review of the end-of-life literature (Lorenz et al., 2004) summarized the major gaps in the palliative care evidence base, and many of these deficiencies affect the development of measures. The lack of research on the implications of alternative definitions of the end-of-life population hinders convergence on a routine denominator in palliative care research or improvement activities. The lack of palliative care measures (such as symptom levels) in most research on specific diseases also limits our ability to define populations with unmet palliative care needs. Although research has developed many measurement tools for different domains in palliative care, these measures have rarely been tested in different settings or populations, which limits their applicability for use in performance measurement. Performance measures in symptom management await studies on symptom prevalence in noncancer populations; on associations between processes and outcomes; and on how interventions can improve symptoms across populations. Some sustained research has developed better pain management, but research for other symptoms is mostly nonexistent. In advance care planning, the key issue is to understand how various interventions actually have impacts on achieving patients' goals, an outcome that has mostly evaded assessment. Finally, little research is available to inform performance measures in continuity, spirituality, or caregiver issues.

Gaps in Understanding How Population Measures Need to Be Altered for the Palliative Care/End-of-Life Population

Existing measures may apply to an elderly population or one defined by a particular diagnosis, but these need testing and adaptation to be sure that they will apply well to the palliative care population. For example, in ACOVE, a panel of geriatric experts found that only 130/203 of the indicators intended for vulnerable elders were still appropriate for patients with a prognosis of 6 months of less, and many of the general measures could be more useful if specifically adapted to the palliative care population (Solomon et al., 2003). Walter et al. (2004) found that not accounting for the seriousness of underlying illness, patient preferences, or clinician judgment can seriously compromise the performance of a quality measure. In populations with high proportions of patients who are ill or do not want aggressive care, high rates of screening may reflect badgering and imprudent decisions rather than quality, and low rates may be perfectly appropriate.

Measure sets addressing populations with high proportions of palliative care patients need to include measures relevant to palliative care issues. For example, Mitchell et al. (2004) found that the 6-month mortality among newly admitted nursing home residents with advanced dementia was over 30 percent. However, measure sets in these settings often do not include appropriate elements of palliative care. For example, elements such as documentation of proxy decision makers, decisions to forgo resuscitation or hospitalization, or prognosis and symptoms might greatly improve the appropriateness of MDS for the high proportion of nursing home patients who need palliative care (American Academy of Hospice and Palliative Medicine, 2004).

CHALLENGES TO APPLYING THESE MEASURES FOR THE PURPOSES OF QUALITY IMPROVEMENT, PAY FOR PERFORMANCE, AND PUBLIC REPORTING

Challenges of Outcomes in Palliative Care

Two major challenges to using outcome measures in palliative and end-of-life care are validity and adjustment for patient characteristics and preferences. Although many potential measures are objective (such as site of death) or have undergone careful development and extensive psychometric testing (such as the After-Death Bereaved Family Interview), the validity of these measures as indicators of the overall quality of palliative care has not been well established.

Site of death is a good example of concerns about validity. Increasing the numbers of patients who die at home appears, at first glance, to be a laudable objective. Site-of-death information can generally be reliably obtained from death certificate or Medicare data. However, measuring whether dying at home is an important outcome may depend on how the question is asked. One national survey found that more than 60 percent of the elderly and more than 80 percent of seriously ill patients would prefer to die at home. However, in another national survey of seriously ill patients, in a list of nine attributes of what was important at the end of life, dying at home was ranked last (Steinhauser et al., 2000). Only 35 percent of patients and 30 percent of bereaved family members agreed that dying at home was important (Steinhauser et al., 2000). Whether a patient dies at home may depend on patient and caregiver preferences, and the patient's perceptions of caregiver burden. For example, Fried et al. (1999) found that the primary concern of patients who preferred to be at home was the desire to be with their family members, while those who chose other settings were more concerned about their families' ability to care for them and burden on their families. One would expect that the element that would be more important than the location at the time of death would be the patient's preference as to where to live when near to death, but that question has not yet been asked in a research context.

Dying at home may also be strongly dependent on whether supportive resources are available in that locality. Pritchard et al. (1998) found that in-hospital death increased with greater hospital bed availability and use and decreased with greater nursing home and hospice availability and use. Hospital bed availability was the most powerful predictor, far outstripping patient preference. However, Pritchard et al. also pointed out that the arrangements for care in a locality enmeshed a broad array of social patterns and expectations, including the behavior of the police and the neighbors, making it difficult to handle any one patient's situation in a novel or customized way. Temkin-Greener and Mukamel (2002) found that the percentage of deaths that occurred at home among patients enrolled in the program of all-inclusive care for the elderly (PACE) varied from 25 to 76 percent, depending on the PACE site where patients received care. In a study in 8 counties, Tang and McCorkle (2003) found that patients who died in the county with the most resources available were most likely to die in their preferred location. Tang (2003) also found that many of these same factors, including family caregivers' ability to provide care at home, might also predict the use of hospice care. These complex issues defy straightforward adjustment, since we have no tools that account for the effects of such factors as the availability of family caregivers or community resources.

Broad use of a measure such as site of death, hospital length of stay, hospice referral, or length of hospice use could have adverse consequences. Working to decrease the number of persons who die within a hospital setting without increasing resource availability at home or in the nursing home may lead to discharges with uncontrolled symptoms, untrained and over-burdened caregivers, and increased readmissions, or misuse of hospice. In addition, neither palliative care interventions nor those specifically targeted towards improving the rate of home death have shown significant impact on increasing the rate of home death (Higginson et al., 2003). In one trial of hospital at home for the terminally ill, an intent-to-treat analysis showed no effects; but those who actually received the intervention had much higher rates of home death. Hospice in the United States also delivers very high rates of dying at home (50 percent at a private home), compared to the national rate of only 23 percent, but estimating the effect of selection bias would be difficult and has not been done.

Denominator Issues/Population Definition

A recent systematic review of the end-of-life literature (Lorenz et al., 2004) details the numerous challenges in defining the palliative care population. Most of the practical definition of "end of life" in the United States has relied upon the concept underlying the Medicare hospice benefit, which requires that eligible people would have a discernible phase of dying that reliably lasted less than 6 months. However, other concepts did arise in the literature review: e.g., "readiness" for death, "active dying," and serious and eventually fatal illness. While many articles address the plausibility of prognosticating the timing of death, the summation of them is that no approach reliably distinguishes those who will die soon from those who will manage to survive for much longer. Most prognoses are ambiguous at a time that turns out to be within a week or two of dying. The inability to create categories by prognostic models affects all of the major causes of death except perhaps the most relentless of cancers. Yet, the other strategies for labeling a group as being at "the end of life" have almost no research base. Quality improvement work has tended to use either an arbitrary category that combines service utilization with diagnosis (e.g., all cancer patients seen in our clinic, or all heart failure patients admitted to the hospital) or the "surprise question," which requires asking a clinician who knows the patient whether the patient is sick enough that it would be no surprise for the patient to die within 6 months or a year. The "surprise question" captures a much larger population that those thought appropriate for hospice referral, since it focuses upon a high risk of dying, rather than near certainty, and since it does not require also attending to the question of whether the patient will still be under life-prolonging treatment.

The measures selected in Table J-1 use a number of different denominator definitions, all of which suffer from lack of validity testing. These include "vulnerable elderly," or those at high risk of death or reduced functional status; "poor prognosis," or prognosis of 6 months or less; patients considered to be "terminally ill" (MDS); patients currently receiving hospice care; and patients where a provider states that they would not be surprised if the patient died within the next year. Some measures also use denominators identifying all nontraumatic deaths retrospectively. This denominator is particularly problematic for use in performance measures, as many of these patients might not have been identified prospectively as being part of a palliative care population (Bach et al., 2004).

Settings

We identified two major issues related to the use of measures in different settings. First, due to the fractured nature of our health care system, measures have often been developed specifically for certain settings, often for nonpalliative care measure sets, and therefore cannot be compared across settings. For example, OASIS (home care), MDS (nursing homes), and NDS (hospice) all have very different pain performance measure methodology. Since important portions of palliative care occur in hospitals, providers' offices, nursing homes, home care, and hospice, and patients will often make multiple transitions among settings, standardization of key measures would be critical to assessing performance and improving care across the continuum. If the hospital or its professionals are not performing well on the treatment of pain, for example, patients admitted to hospice will have a higher frequency and severity of pain on admission, which might affect the hospice's performance measures adversely. Improving the overall care of these patients would require improvements by nonhospice providers. In working with a population that routinely changes settings often, and for whom improvements might well change the way that different settings are used, measures that are tied to particular settings are likely to be misleading.

Use of Surrogates/Missing Data

Issues related to the collection of data in palliative care have also been summarized in the recent systematic review (Lorenz et al., 2004) and need further research. Patients who are seriously ill or near the end of life are often unable to report on symptoms or other patient-centered elements of care. Measurement either resorts to proxy measures (such as after-death surveys of families), which often have only moderate congruence with patient reports, or carry high proportions of missing data and are therefore subject to bias. Further research will have to determine how and when to combine patient and proxy reporting and how to account for missing data through methods such as adjustment or repeat assessments.

The Effect of Altering Survival Time

Survival time has a troublesome interaction with most of the other elements that one might measure to estimate quality of care. With many outcome indicators of quality care, the patient is more at risk of adverse experience with longer survival, both from longer exposure and from more fragile health. Thus, for example, a care pattern that secured two months longer survival with emphysema would seem to have higher rates of dyspnea, more caregiver burnout, higher costs, and generally more adverse indicators. Since policymakers and researchers do not pay attention to this possibility and do not have metrics that would allow adjustment, this acts as an unmeasured confounder. This potential effect is one that is particularly difficult to discuss, since putting it into words risks allegations of having interest in foreshortening life (or, for that matter, of prolonging dying and inflicting suffering while increasing the bills).

CONCLUSION

While the costs of care at the end of life probably use about one-third of Americans' lifetime health care, and while disapproval of the quality and reliability of that care is widespread, the indicators of quality, the measures to estimate quality, and the benchmarks and practical approaches to ensuring quality show longstanding inattention. Within a year, the NQF could probably field measures of physical pain and advance care planning that would be good enough for comparing health care delivery systems as to the quality of care. With more deliberate development over just a few years, life closure, caregiver experience, and some other symptoms (depression, dyspnea, chemotherapy-associated nausea and vomiting, for example) could be in the field. Some composite measures like knowing and delivering on the preferred place of death show promise precisely because high rates require a number of generally beneficial steps to have been taken. Having practical approaches to identifying the "end of life" population more usefully will require focused attention; finding clinical and administrative triggers that can concurrently identify the patients who face serious illness through to death is a task that will be essential for improvement activities. A recent State of the Science conference documented research priorities for end of life care (http://consensus.nih.gov/ta/024/EndofLifeStatementDRAFThtml.htm).

REFERENCES

American Academy of Hospice and Palliative Medicine and Americans for Better Care of the Dying. 2004. *Testimony Concerning MDS 3.0*. [Online]. Available: *http://www3.cms.hhs.gov/quality/mds30/* [accessed January 4, 2005].

Asch SM, Kerr EA, Hamilton EG, Reifel JL, McGlynn EA, eds. 2000. *Quality Of Care for Oncologic Conditions and HIV: A Review of the Literature and Quality Indicators.* MR-1281-AHRQ, 2000. [Online]. Available: *http://www.rand.org/publications/MR/MR1281/* [accessed January 3, 2005].

Asch SM, McGlynn EA, Hogan MM, et al. 2004. Comparison of quality of care for patients in the Veterans Health Administration and patients in a national sample. *Annals of Internal Medicine* 14(12):938–945.

Bach PB, Schrag D, Begg CB. 2004. Resurrecting treatment histories of dead patients: A study design that should be laid to rest. *Journal of the American Medical Associaton* 292(22): 2765–2770.

Baier RR, Gifford DR, Patry G, Banks SM, Rochon T, DeSilva D, Teno JM. 2004. Ameliorating pain in nursing homes: A collaborative quality-improvement project. *Journal of the American Geriatrics Society* 42:1988–1995.

Beal AC, Co JPT, Dougherty D, Jorsling T, Kam J, Perrin J, Palmer RH. 2004. Quality measures for children's health care. *Pediatrics* 133:199–209.

Centers for Medicare and Medicaid Services' National Nursing Home Quality Initiative (NHQI). 2004. *Nursing Home Compare.* [Online]. Available: *http://www.medicare.gov/nhcompare/home.asp* [accessed January 3, 2005].

Clarke EB, Curtis JR, Luce JM, Levy M, Danis M, Nelson J, Solomon MZ. 2003. Robert Wood Johnson Foundation Critical Care End-of-Life Peer Workgroup Members. Quality indicators for end-of-life care in the intensive care unit. *Critical Care Medicine* 31(9): 2255–2262.

Cleeland CS, Reyes-Gibby CC, Schall M, Nolan K, Paice J, Rosenberg JM, Tollett JH, Kerns RD. 2003. Rapid improvement in pain management: The Veterans Health Administration and the Institute for Healthcare Improvement Collaborative. *Clinical Journal of Pain* 19(5):298–305.

Connor SR, Tecca M, LundPerson J, Teno J. 2004. Measuring hospice care: The National Hospice and Palliative Care Organization National Hospice Data Set. *Journal of Pain and Symptom Management* 28(4):316–328.

Dokken DL, Heller KS, Levetown, M, et al. for The Initiative for Pediatric Palliative Care (IPPC). 2001. *Quality Domains, Goals, and Indicators of Family-Centered Care of Children Living with Life-Threatening Conditions.* Newton, MA: Education Development Center, Inc., 2001. [Online]. Available: *http://www.ippcweb.org* [accessed December 27, 2004].

Du Pen SL, Du Pen AR, Polissar N, Hansberry J, Kraybill BM, Stillman M, Panke J, Everly R, Syrjala K. 1999. Implementing guidelines for cancer pain management: Results of a randomized controlled clinical trial. *Journal of Clinical Oncology* 17:361–370.

Earle CC, Park ER, Lai B, Weeks JC, Ayanian JZ, Block S. 2003. Identifying potential indicators of the quality of end-of-life cancer care from administrative data. *Journal of Clinical Oncology* 21(6):1133–1138.

Fisher ES, Wennberg DE, Stukel TA, Gottlieb DJ, Lucas FL, Pinder EL. 2003a. The implications of regional variations in Medicare spending. Part 1: The content, quality, and accessibility of care. *Annals of Internal Medicine* 138(4):273–287.

Fisher ES, Wennberg DE, Stukel TA, Gottlieb DJ, Lucas FL, Pinder EL. 2003b. The implications of regional variations in Medicare spending. Part 2: Health outcomes and satisfaction with care. *Annals of Internal Medicine* 138(4):288–298.

Forte AL, Hill M, Pazder R, Feudtner C. 2004. Bereavement care interventions: A systematic review. *BioMed Central Palliative Care* 3(1):3.

Fried TRE, O'Leary JH, Drickamer MA. 1999. Older persons' preferences for site of terminal care. *Annals of Internal Medicine* 131:109–112.

Hammes BJ, Rooney BL. 1998. Death and end-of-life planning in one Midwestern community. *Archives of Internal Medicine* 158(4):383–390.

Higginson IJ, Finlay IG, Goodwin DM, Hood K, Edwards AG, Cook A, Douglas HR, Normand CE. 2003. Is there evidence that palliative care teams alter end-of-life experiences of patients and their caregivers? *Journal of Pain and Symptom Management* 25(2): 150–168.

Lorenz K, Lynn J, Morton SC, Dy S, Mularski R, Shugarman L, Sun V, Wilkinson A, Maglione M, Shekelle PG. 2004. *End-of-Life Care and Outcomes*. Evidence Report/Technology Assessment No. 110. (Prepared by the Southern California Evidence-based Practice Center, under Contract No. 290-02-0003). AHRQ Publication No. 05-E004-2. Rockville, MD: Agency for Healthcare Research and Quality, 2004.

Lunney JR, Foley KM, Smith TJ, Gelband H, eds. 2003. *Describing Death in America: What We Need to Know*. Washington, DC: The National Academies Press.

Lynn J, Schuster JL, Kabcenell A. 2000. *Improving Care for the End of Life: A Sourcebook for Heatlh Care Managers and Clinicians*. New York: Oxford University Press.

Mitchell SL, Kiely DK, Hamel MB, Park PS, Morris JN, Fries BE. 2004. Estimating prognosis for nursing home residents with advanced dementia. *Journal of the American Medical Association* 291(22):2734–2740.

Murray SA, Boyd K, Sheikh A, Thomas K, Higginson IJ. 2004. Developing primary palliative care. *British Medical Journal* 329(7474):1056–1057. [Online]. Available: *http://www.macmillan.org.uk/healthprofessionals/disppage.asp?id=6875* [accessed January 8, 2005].

Nakajima GA, Wenger NS. 2003. *Quality Indicators for the Care of Depression in Vulnerable Elders*. [Online]. *Available: http://www.rand.org/health/tools/vulnerable.elderly.html* [accessed January 7, 2005].

National Consensus Project for Quality Palliative Care. 2004. *Clinical Practice Guidelines for Quality Palliative Care*. [Online]. Available: *http://www.nationalconsensusproject.org* [accessed December 15, 2004].

Pritchard RS, Fisher ES, Teno JM et al. 1998. Influence of patient preferences and local health system characteristics on the place of death. *Journal of the American Geriatric Society* 46:1242–1250.

Rosenfeld K, Wenger NS. 2000. Measuring quality in end-of-life care. *Clinical Geriatric Medicine*; 16(2):387–400.

Ryndes T, Connor S, Cody C, Merriman M, Bruno S, Fine P, Dennis J. 2000. *Report on the Alpha and Beta Pilots of End Result Outcome Measures Constructed by the Outcomes Forum*. A joint effort of the National Hospice and Palliative Care Organization and the National Hospice Work Group. [Online]. Available: *http://www.nhpco.org* [accessed January 3, 2005].

Solomon DH, Wenger NS, Saliba D, et al. 2003. Appropriateness of quality indicators for older patients with advanced dementia and poor prognosis. *Journal of the American Geriatric Society* 51:902–907.

Steel N, Melzer D, Shekelle PG, Wenger NS, Forsyth D, McWilliams BC. 2004. *Quality and Safety of Health Care* 13(4):260–264.

Steinhauser KE, Christakis NA, Clipp EC, McNeilly M, McIntyre L, Tulsky JA. 2000. Factors considered important at the end of life by patients, family, physicians, and other providers. *Journal of the American Medical Association* 284:2476–2482.

Tang ST. 2003. Determinants of hospice home care use among terminally ill cancer patients. *Nursing Research* 52:217–225.

Tang ST, McCorkle R. 2003. Determinants of congruence between the preferred and actual place of death for terminally ill cancer patients. *Journal of Palliative Care* 19:230–237.

Temkin-Greener H, Mukamel DB. 2002. Predicting place of death in the program of all-inclusive care for the elderly (PACE): Participant versus program characteristics. *Journal of the American Geriatric Society* 50:125–135.

Teno JM. 2000. *TIME: Toolkit of Instruments to Measure End-of-Life Care.* [Online]. Available: *http://www.chcr.brown.edu/pcoc/toolkit.htm* [accessed January 7, 2005].

Teno JM. 2001. Quality of care and quality indicators for end-of-life cancer care: Hope for the best, yet prepare for the worst. In: Foley KM, Gelband H, eds. *Improving Palliative Care for Cancer.* Washington, DC: National Academy Press. Pp. 96–131.

Teno, JM. 2004. *The Brown Atlas of Dying.* Brown University Center for Gerontology and Health Care Research. [Online]. Available: *http://www.chcr.brown.edu/dying* [accessed December 27, 2004].

Teno JM, Clarridge B, Casey V, Edgman-Levitan S, Fowler J. 2001. Validation of toolkit after-death bereaved family member interview. *Journal of Pain and Symptom Management* 22(3):752–758.

Teno JM, Weitzen S, Wetle T, Mor V. 2002. Persistent pain in nursing home residents. *Journal of the American Medical Association* 285(16):2081.

Teno JM, Clarridge BR, Casey V, Welch LC, Wetle T, Shield R, Mor V. 2004. Family perspectives on end-of-life care at the last place of care. *Journal of the American Medical Association* 291(1):88–93.

Walter LC, Davidowitz NP, Heineken PA, Covinsky KE. 2004. Pitfalls of converting practice guidelines into quality measures: Lessons learned from a VA performance measure. *Journal of the American Medical Association* 291(20):2466–2470.

Wenger NS, Rosenfeld K. 2001. Quality indicators for end-of-life care in vulnerable elders. *Annals of Internal Medicine* 135(8 Pt. 2):677–685.

Wenger NS, Young RT. 2003. *Quality Indicators of Continuity and Coordination of Care for Vulnerable Elder Persons.* [Online]. Available: http://www.rand.org/health/tools/vulnerable.elderly.html [accessed January 7, 2005].

Wenger NS, Solomon DH, Roth CP, et al. 2003. The quality of medical care provided to vulnerable community-dwelling older patients. *Annals of Internal Medicine* 139(9): 740–747.

Wennberg JE, Cooper MM, eds. 1999. *The Quality of Medical Care in the United States: A Report on the Medicare Program. The Dartmouth Atlas of Health Care 1999.* Chicago, IL: American Hospital Association Press.

Wennberg JE, Fisher ES, Stukel TA, Skinner JS, Sharp SM, Bronner KK. 2004. Use of hospitals, physician visits, and hospice care during last six months of life among cohorts loyal to highly respected hospitals in the United States. *British Medical Journal* 328:607.

World Health Organization (WHO). 2002. *Summary Measures of Population Health: Concepts, Ethics, Measurement and Application.* Geneva, Switzerland: World Health Organization.

LIST OF ABBREVIATIONS

ACOVE   Assessing Care of Vulnerable Elders
CMS   Center for Medicare and Medicaid Services
EOL   end of life
ICU   intensive care unit
IHI   Institute for Healthcare Improvement
LOS   length of stay
MDS   Minimum Data Set (CMS)
NDS   National Discharge Sample (NHPCO)
NHPCO   National Hospital and Palliative Care Organization
UHC   University Health Consortium
VHA   Veterans Health Administration

Appendix K

Biographical Sketches

Main Committee on Redesigning Health Insurance, Performance Measures, Payment and Performance Improvements Programs* and the Performance Measures Subcommittee†

Steven A. Schroeder, M.D., *Chair—Main Committee*,* is distinguished professor of health and health care, Division of General Internal Medicine, Department of Medicine, University of California, San Francisco (UCSF), where he also heads the Smoking Cessation Leadership Center. The Center, funded by the Robert Wood Johnson Foundation, works with leaders of American health professional organizations and health care institutions to increase the rate at which patients who smoke are offered help to quit. Between 1990 and 2002 he was president and Chief Executive Officer of the Robert Wood Johnson Foundation. During his term of office the Foundation made grant expenditures of almost $4 billion in pursuit of its mission of improving the health and health care of the American people. During those $12\frac{1}{2}$ years the foundation developed new programs in substance abuse prevention and treatment, care at the end of life, and health insurance expansion for children, among others. In 1999, it reorganized into health and health care groups, reflecting the twin components of its mission. Dr. Schroeder graduated from Stanford University and Harvard Medical School, and trained in internal medicine at the Harvard Medical Service of Boston City Hospital and in epidemiology as an EIS Office of the Centers for Disease Control and Prevention (CDC). He held faculty appointments at Harvard, George Washington, and UCSF. At both George Washington and UCSF he was founding medical director of a university-

---

*Member of the Main Committee on Redesigning Health Insurance Performance Measures, Payment and Performance Improvement Programs.

sponsored HMO, and at UCSF he founded its division of general internal medicine. He has published extensively in the fields of clinical medicine, health care financing and organization, prevention, public health, and the work force, with over 260 publications.

He currently serves as chairman of the American Legacy Foundation and of the International Review Committee of the Ben Gurion School of Medicine, is a member of the editorial board of the *New England Journal of Medicine*, the Harvard Overseers, and a director of the James Irvine Foundation, the Save Ellis Island Foundation, and the Charles R. Drew University of Medicine and Science. Dr. Schroeder is a member of the Institute of Medicine (IOM). He has six honorary doctoral degrees and numerous awards.

Bobbie Berkowitz, Ph.D., R.N., F.A.A.N.,* is the alumni endowed professor of nursing at the University of Washington (UW) School of Nursing and adjunct professor in the School of Public Health and Community Medicine. She directs the "Turning Point" initiative funded by the Robert Wood Johnson Foundation and the Center for the Advancement of Health Disparities Research funded by the National Institute of Nursing Research. She is a member of the board of trustees for Group Health Cooperative, a fellow in the American Academy of Nursing and a member of the Institute of Medicine (IOM). She served as co-chair of the IOM Committee Using Performance Monitoring to Improve Community Health and as vice-chair of the IOM/Transportation Research Board Committee on Physical Activity, Health, Transportation, and Land Use. She holds a Ph.D. in Nursing Science from Case Western Reserve University.

Donald M. Berwick, M.D., M.P.P., *Co-chair PM Subcommittee,** † is president and CEO of the Institute for Healthcare Improvement (IHI), a not-for-profit organization helping to accelerate the improvement of health care throughout the world. He is clinical professor of pediatrics and health care policy at the Harvard Medical School and professor of health policy and management at the Harvard School of Public Health. He is also a pediatrician, an associate in pediatrics at Boston's Children's Hospital, and a consultant in pediatrics at Massachusetts General Hospital. Dr. Berwick has published over 110 scientific articles in numerous professional journals on subjects relating to health care policy, decision analysis, technology assessment, and health care quality management. Dr. Berwick serves on the National Advisory Council of the Agency for Healthcare Research and

---

*Member of the Main Committee on Redesigning Health Insurance Performance Measures, Payment and Performance Improvement Programs.

†Member of the Performance Measures Subcommittee.

Quality (AHRQ), the IOM's Governing Council and the IOM's Board on Global Health. He is also a member of several editorial boards, including that of the *Journal of the American Medical Association*. A summa cum laude graduate of Harvard College, Dr. Berwick holds a master of public policy degree from the John F. Kennedy School of Government and an M.D. cum laude from the Harvard Medical School.

Bruce E. Bradley, M.B.A.,* is director of Health Plan Strategy and Public Policy, Health Care Initiatives, for General Motors Corporation in Pontiac, Michigan. He is responsible for health care-related strategy and public policy with a focus on quality measurement and improvement, consumer engagement and cost effectiveness. General Motors provides health care coverage for over 1.1 million employees, retirees and their dependents with an annual expense of $5.2 billion. Mr. Bradley joined General Motors in June 1996 after five years as corporate manager of Managed Care for GTE Corporation. In addition to his health care management experience at GTE, he spent nearly 20 years in health plan and health maintenance organization's (HMO) management. From 1972 to 1980 he was executive director of the Matthew Thornton Health Plan, Nashua, New Hampshire. From 1980 to 1990 he was president and CEO of the Rhode Island Group Health Association in Providence, Rhode Island, a staff model HMO. He was co-founder of the HMO Group (now the Alliance of Community Health Plans), a national corporation of 15 non-profit, independent group practice HMOs, and the HMO Group Insurance Co., Ltd. Mr. Bradley has gained recognition for his work in achieving health plan quality improvement and for his efforts in developing the Health Employer Data and Information Set (HEDIS) measurements and processes. He is a board member of the National Quality Forum, past member of the board of the Foundation for Accountability, board member of the American Board of Internal Medicine Foundation, a past board member of the Academy for Health Services Research and Policy, and a founding member and past chair of the Leapfrog Group board. A native of Pelham, New York, Mr. Bradley holds a bachelor's degree in psychology from Yale University (1967) and master's degree in business and health care administration from the Wharton School at the University of Pennsylvania (1972).

Janet M. Corrigan, Ph.D.,* is president and CEO of the National Committee for Quality Health Care (NCQHC), a nonprofit, nonpartisan education and research institute. Prior to joining NCQHC in June 2005, she was senior board director at the IOM, where she was responsible for the Board on

---

*Member of the Main Committee on Redesigning Health Insurance Performance Measures, Payment and Performance Improvement Programs.

Health Care Services portfolio of initiatives on quality and safety, health services organization and financing, and health insurance issues. She provided leadership for IOM's Quality Chasm Series which produced ten reports during her tenure including: *To Err Is Human: Building a Safer Health System* and *Crossing the Quality Chasm: A New Health System for the 21st Century.*

Prior to joining IOM in 1998, Dr. Corrigan was the executive director of the President's Advisory Commission on Consumer Protection and Quality in the Health Care Industry. Dr. Corrigan serves on the boards of the Baldrige Board of Overseers and the National Center for Healthcare Leadership. She received both her doctorate in health services research and master of industrial engineering degrees from the University of Michigan, and master's degrees in business administration and community health from the University of Rochester.

Karen Davis, Ph.D.,* is president of the Commonwealth Fund, a national philanthropy engaged in independent research on health and social issues. A nationally recognized economist, has had a distinguished career in public policy and research. She served as deputy assistant secretary for health policy in the U.S. Department of Health and Human Services from 1977-1980, and holds the distinction of being the first woman to head a U.S. Public Health Service agency. Prior to her government career, Dr. Davis was a senior fellow at the Brookings Institution in Washington, D.C., a visiting scholar at Harvard University, and an assistant professor of economics at Rice University. She was chair of health policy and management at the Johns Hopkins Bloomberg School of Public Health from 1981-1992. She also serves on the board of Geisinger Health System. She is the recipient of the 2000 Baxter-Allegiance Foundation Prize for Health Services Research and the 2006 Academy Health Distinguished Investigator Award. She is a former president of Academy Health. Dr. Davis received her doctorate in economics from Rice University, and was awarded an honorary doctorate in humane letters from Johns Hopkins University in 2001.

Nancy-Ann Min DeParle, J.D.,* is a senior advisor to JPMorgan Partners, LLC, and adjunct professor of health care systems at the Wharton School of the University of Pennsylvania. From 1997 to 2000, she served as administrator of the Health Care Financing Administration (HCFA), which is now the Centers for Medicare and Medicaid Services (CMS). Before joining HCFA, Ms. DeParle was associate director for health and personnel at the White House Office of Management and Budget. From 1987 to 1989 she

---

*Member of the Main Committee on Redesigning Health Insurance Performance Measures, Payment and Performance Improvement Programs.

served as the Tennessee Commissioner of Human Services. She has also worked as a lawyer in private practice in Nashville, Tennessee, and Washington, DC. She is a member of the Medicare Payment Advisory Committee, a trustee of the Robert Wood Johnson Foundation, and a board member of Cerner Corporation, DaVita Guidant Corporation, Triad Hospitals, and the National Quality Forum. Ms. DeParle received a B.A. degree from the University of Tennessee; B.A. and M.A. degrees from Oxford University, where she was a Rhodes Scholar; and a J.D. degree from Harvard Law School.

Elliott S. Fisher, M.D., M.P.H., *Co-chair PM Subcommittee,** † is professor of medicine and community and family medicine, where he is the director of the Institute for the Evaluation of Medical Practice at the Center for the Evaluative Clinical Sciences, Hanover, NH, and senior associate of the VA Outcomes Group, Veterans Administration Medical Center, White River Junction, VT Center for the Evaluative Clinical Sciences. He is a general internist and former Robert Wood Johnson clinical scholar who has broad expertise in the use of administrative databases and survey research methods in health systems evaluation. His research has focused on exploring the causes and consequences of variations in clinical practice and health care spending across U.S. regions and among health care providers.

Richard G. Frank, Ph.D., * is the Margaret T. Morris Professor of Health Economics in the Department of Health Care Policy at Harvard Medical School. He is also a research associate with the National Bureau of Economic Research. Dr. Frank is a member of the IOM. He advises several state mental health and substance abuse agencies on issues related to managed care and financing of care. He also serves as co-editor for the *Journal of Health Economics*. Dr. Frank was awarded the Georgescu-Roegen prize from the Southern Economic Association for his collaborative work on drug pricing, the Carl A. Taube Award from the American Public Health Association for outstanding contributions to mental health services and economics research, and the Emily Mumford Medal from Columbia University's Department of Psychiatry. In 2002 Dr. Frank received the John Eisenberg Mentorship Award from National Research Service Awards.

Patricia A. Gabow, M.D., † is the CEO and medical director of Denver Health and Hospital Authority, one of the nation's most efficient, highly regarded, extensive and integrated health care systems that includes the Denver Health Medical Center, a regional Level I trauma center, the 911

---

*Member of the Main Committee on Redesigning Health Insurance Performance Measures, Payment and Performance Improvement Programs.
†Member of the Performance Measures Subcommittee.

system, a system of family health centers, school-based clinics, Denver Public Health, the Rocky Mountain Poison and Drug Center, a correctional health care program, the Rocky Mountain Center for Medical Response to Terrorism, and more. She has been nationally recognized for her work to increase access to basic health care for all Coloradoans, especially the underserved, most of whom are women and children. In seeking to improve sustainability of the mission, Dr. Gabow led the effort to convert the hospital from part of the city to an independent governmental authority. She joined the staff in 1973 as chief of the Renal Division. During her tenure in that role and as director of medical services, she became internationally known for her scientific work in polycystic kidney disease. Her current research relates to health services for the underserved. Author of over 150 articles and book chapters, Dr. Gabow is also professor of medicine in the Division of Renal Disease at the University of Colorado School of Medicine. She received her medical degree from the University of Pennsylvania School of Medicine, trained in internal medicine at the Hospital of the University of Pennsylvania and Harbor General Hospital in Torrance, California and received further training in nephrology at San Francisco General Hospital and the Hospital of the University of Pennsylvania. She has been awarded the Florence Rena Sabin Award for medical education and public health advocacy and elected to the Colorado Women's Hall of Fame for her commitment to Colorado's health care safety net. She was named one of the top 25 Women in Health Care by *Modern Health Care Magazine* in 2005.

Robert S. Galvin, M.D.,* is the director of Global Health Care for General Electric (GE). He is in charge of the design and performance of GE's health programs, totaling over $3 billion annually, and oversees the 1 million patient encounters that take place in GE's 220 medical clinics in over 20 countries. Drawing on his clinical expertise and training in Six Sigma, Dr. Galvin has been an advocate and leader in extending the benefits of this methodology to health care. He has focused on issues of market-based health policy and financing, with a special interest in promoting transparency and reforming the payment system. He is a past member of the Strategic Framework Board of the National Quality Forum and is currently on the board of the National Committee for Quality Assurance. He is a co-founder of the Leapfrog Group, founder of Bridges to Excellence, and member of the Advisory Group of the Council on Health Care Economics and Policy. Dr. Galvin is widely published on issues affecting the purchaser side of health care. He is professor adjunct of medicine at Yale, where he directs the seminar series

---

*Member of the Main Committee on Redesigning Health Insurance Performance Measures, Payment and Performance Improvement Programs.

on the private sector for the Robert Wood Johnson Clinical Scholars fellowship. He is a fellow of the American College of Physicians.

Lillee Smith Gelinas, R.N., M.S.N.,[†] is a member of Veterans Health Administration's (VHA's) clinical performance leadership team, where she supports VHA's efforts to help members improve their clinical and economic performance. She works extensively with VHA's 2,400 member health care organizations and 18 local offices to help hospitals measure and improve clinical quality. Ms. Gelinas is a national champion for VHA's well-recognized efforts to help members achieve clinical excellence. In addition, she supports programs, products, and services which impact VHA's nurses and nursing leaders through clinical improvement, education, networking and research activities—key responsibilities since 1986. She has published findings for VHA Inc. on the changing role of nursing leaders since 1993 and is a nationally recognized speaker on clinical, health care management and nursing issues.

Ms. Gelinas attended Louisiana State University, earned her bachelor's degree in nursing from the University of Louisiana at Lafayette and a master's degree in nursing, with honors, from the University of Pennsylvania where she also studied at the Wharton School of Business.

For the Joint Commission on Accreditation of Healthcare Organizations, she serves as a member of the National Nursing Council as well as the Hospital Standards Advisory Group and has been a John M. Eisenberg Patient Safety and Quality Award judge for two years. She co-chaired the 2003 National Quality Forum project to establish national voluntary consensus measures for nursing sensitive care. For the IOM, she served on the Crossing the Quality Chasm 2004 Summit committee and chaired the agenda subgroup. She was inducted as a fellow in the American Academy of Nursing in November 2005. In addition, she is a member of the Board of Directors for Exempla Healthcare, Denver, Colorado.

David H. Gustafson, Ph.D.,[*] is a research professor at the University of Wisconsin, Madison, where he directs the Center of Excellence in Cancer Communications (designated by the National Cancer Institute) and the Network for the Improvement of Addiction Treatment (supported by the Robert Wood Johnson Foundation and the federal government's Center for Substance Abuse Treatment). His research focuses on the use of systems engineering methods and models in individual and organizational change. Much of his research centers on the development and evaluation of health

---

*Member of the Main Committee on Redesigning Health Insurance Performance Measures, Payment and Performance Improvement Programs.

†Member of the Performance Measures Subcommittee.

systems to support people facing serious health problems such as cancer. His randomized controlled trials and field tests help understand acceptance, use and impact of eHealth on quality of life, behavior change and health services utilization. His research also contributes to organizational improvement with a particular attention to models that predict and explain organizational change. Dr. Gustafson is a fellow of the Association for Health Services Research and of the American Medical Informatics Association, a fellow and past vice-chair of the board of the Institute for Healthcare Improvement. He also chaired the recently completed Federal Science Panel on Interactive Communications in Health and is chair of the eHealth Institute. He is a member of the University of Wisconsin Athletic Board.

Margarita P. Hurtado, Ph.D., M.H.S., M.A.,[†] is principal research scientist at the American Institutes for Research (AIR) and a health services researcher with expertise in quality of care measurement and primary care. On CAHPS II, funded by AHRQ and CMS, she is task leader for quality improvement (QI), task leader for cultural comparability, and a member of the instrumentation and core teams for the development of the Ambulatory CAHPS survey. Her CAHPS II work focuses on consumer survey development, survey translation and cultural adaptation, QI based on patient reports of care, and cross-cultural issues related to measurement and reporting. She is also task leader on a project to develop a tool kit of classroom- and clinic-based interventions to promote child health through health centers located in elementary schools. Previously, she was PI on a project with Center for Naval Analysis (CNA) to support the CMS Doctor's Office Quality project by developing composite measures of quality of chronic disease care taking into account clinical aspects and patient reports of care. She was also project director for the evaluation of National Heart, Lung, and Blood Institute's "Your Heart, Your Health Program" that examined the effectiveness of lay health educators in promoting behavior change among Latinos. She was senior advisor on an Office of Minority Health project to promote patient-centered care through the development of Cultural Competency Curriculum Modules for Family Physicians. Before joining AIR, Dr. Hurtado was with the IOM where she was study director for AHRQ's National Healthcare Quality Report. Previous to that, she worked as a consultant for the Pan American Health Organization on primary care and health system reform and with the Ministry of Health in Colombia. She was the recipient of a National Research Service Award from National Institutes of Health, a primary care fellow at the Johns Hopkins School of Public Health, and a recipient of the Marilyn Bergner Award for Health Services Research and

---

[†]Member of the Performance Measures Subcommittee.

the John Hume Award for her dissertation research. She is an associate at the Johns Hopkins University School of Public Health and a member of the editorial board of the *International Journal for Quality in Health Care*. She served on the AHRQ Special Emphasis Panel on Practice-Based Research Networks and the Translation of Research into Practice in July 2004. Dr. Hurtado holds a Ph.D. in Health Services Research, a Master in Health Sciences, and a Master of Arts in International Relations, all from the Johns Hopkins University.

George J. Isham, M.D.,[†] is medical director and chief health officer for HealthPartners, a large health plan in Minnesota, representing nearly 630,000 members. He is responsible for quality improvement and utilization management, health professional education, and research. Before his current position, Dr. Isham was medical director of MedCenters Health Plan in Minneapolis. In the late 1980s, he was executive director of University Health Care, an organization affiliated with the University of Wisconsin, Madison. His practice experience as a primary care physician included eight years at the Freeport Clinic in Freeport, Illinois, and three and half years as clinical assistant professor in medicine at the University of Wisconsin. Dr. Isham was chair of the IOM committee that produced the report, *Priority Areas for National Action: Transforming Health Care Quality*. Dr. Isham received his medical degree from the University of Illinois and served his internship and residency in Internal Medicine at the University of Wisconsin Hospital and Clinics in Madison. He also has a Master of Science in Preventive Medicine/Administrative Medicine from the University of Wisconsin, Madison.

Brent C. James, M.D., M. Stat,[†] is vice president for medical research and executive director of Intermountain Health Care's (IHC) Institute for Health Care Delivery Research. IHC is an integrated system of 21 hospitals, more than 80 clinics, a 400+ member physician group, and an HMO/PPO insurance plan jointly responsible for more than 1,000,000 covered lives. IHC is widely recognized for its work in clinical quality improvement and electronic clinical decision support systems. Dr. James also leads IHC's clinical improvement efforts.

Dr. James received an undergraduate degree in computer science, a Master of Statistics degree, and an M.D. degree from the University of Utah, with subsequent training in general surgery from that institution. An interest in cancer led him to spend several years with the American College of Surgeons, where he helped support the Commission on Cancer and de-

---

[†]Member of the Performance Measures Subcommittee.

signed and staffed the College's first in-house main frame computer system. He later served as a biostatistician in the Eastern Cooperative Oncology Group, while an assistant professor in the Department of Biostatistics at the Harvard School of Public Health.

Dr. James presently holds joint adjunct professorships in the University of Utah School of Medicine's Department of Family and Preventive Medicine and the Department of Medical Informatics. He is a visiting lecturer in the Department of Health Policy and Management at the Harvard School of Public Health, and an adjunct professor at Tulane University. He served on the IOM's National Roundtable on Healthcare Quality and its committee on Quality of Healthcare in America. He is a past member of the National Quality Forum's Strategic Framework Board, and sits on the board of trustees of the National Patient Safety Foundation. He serves on a number of other boards for not-for-profit health care institutions with missions directed at measuring and improving the quality and availability of health care services.

Mary Anne Koda-Kimble, Pharm.D.,* is dean of the School of Pharmacy at the UCSF, where she teaches and has cared for patients at the UCSF Diabetes Center. She holds the Thomas J. Long Endowed Professorship in Chain Pharmacy Practice and has previously served as chairwoman of the Department of Clinical Pharmacy. Dr. Koda-Kimble received her Pharm.D. from UCSF and joined its faculty in 1970, where she was involved in developing an innovative clinical pharmacy curriculum. Dr. Koda-Kimble is a member of the United States Pharmacopoeia board of trustees and is vice chair of the Accreditation Council of Pharmaceutical Education Board of Directors. She was a past president of the American Association of Colleges of Pharmacy and has served on the California State Board of Pharmacy, the Food and Drug Administration's (FDA) Nonprescription Drugs Advisory Committee, and many other boards and task forces of national professional associations. Dr. Koda-Kimble is frequently invited to address national and international groups and has many publications, the best known of which is Applied Therapeutics, a text widely used by health professional students and practitioners throughout the world.

Arthur A. Levin, M.P.H.,† is director of the Center for Medical Consumers, a New York City–based nonprofit organization committed to informed consumer and patient health care decision-making, patient safety, evidence-based, high-quality medicine and health care system transparency. The

---

*Member of the Main Committee on Redesigning Health Insurance Performance Measures, Payment and Performance Improvement Programs.
†Member of the Performance Measures Subcommittee.

Center publishes a monthly newsletter HealthFacts, which offers a critique of medical and health practices based on the available scientific evidence and expert opinion.

Mr. Levin was a member of the IOM's Committee on the Quality of Health Care that published the *To Err Is Human* and *Crossing the Quality Chasm* reports. He also served as a member of the IOM committee that evaluated the federal quality effort and made recommendations to Congress in its report *Leadership by Example*.

Mr. Levin spent more than 10 years as a public member of an Institution Review Board at a New York State hospital and research center aligned with a large academic medical center. He also was a member of a Department of Health task force that reviewed special concerns about research and healthy normal volunteers.

He is currently a member of the FDA Consumer Nominating Workgroup that recommends consumer representatives for FDA Advisory Committees and of the New York State Department of Health statewide workgroup that has redesigned the state's hospital incident reporting and adverse event tracking system known as NYPORTS. Mr. Levin has also served as a guest expert on risk management at several FDA Drug Advisory Committee meetings and currently serves as the consumer member on the FDA's Drug Safety and Risk Management Advisory Committee (DSaRM). Mr. Levin is a member of the Committee on Performance Measures of the National Committee for Quality Assurance and of the National Quality Forum's Standardizing Cardiac Surgery Measures Steering Committee. He earned his Master of Public Health degree from Columbia University School of Public Health and his Bachelor of Arts degree in philosophy from Reed College.

Glen P. Mays, Ph.D., M.P.H.,[†] recently joined the faculty of the University of Arkansas for Medical Sciences (UAMS) College of Public Health after four years at Mathematica Policy Research as a senior health researcher. He currently serves as an associate professor of health policy and director of research for the college's department of health policy and management. Dr. Mays' research focuses on strategies for organizing and financing public health services, health insurance, and medical care services for underserved populations. Much of his work has explored the institutional and economic forces that shape public health and medical care systems and their interface. He led a series of CDC-supported studies examining how public health services are organized, financed, and delivered across local communities, and what factors influence the performance of essential public health services. This work has included the development of instruments and analytic techniques used to measure public health system performance in improving

[†]Member of the Performance Measures Subcommittee.

population health. Dr. Mays' work in health insurance has included economic evaluations of state strategies to expand health insurance coverage, and studies of health promotion and disease prevention activities pursued by private health insurers and employers. As part of this work, he serves as a senior researcher on the Center for Studying Health System Change's *Community Tracking Study*, where he analyzes the decisions of insurers and employers regarding health benefits.

Dr. Mays also studies systems of health care for the uninsured and other vulnerable populations. He led a national study for AHRQ evaluating the effects of managed care contracting arrangements on community health center performance in delivering care for the uninsured, and currently directs a HRSA-sponsored evaluation of a pharmacy-based disease management demonstration program targeted to low-income patients with chronic diseases. With colleagues at Mathematica Policy Research, Dr. Mays is conducting a study to identify best practices in delivering cardiovascular screening and health promotion services to uninsured women served through CDC's WISEWOMAN demonstration program. Dr. Mays has published more than 40 journal articles, books, and chapters on issues involving public health systems, health insurance, and safety-net health care programs for the uninsured. He received Ph.D. and M.P.H. degrees in health policy and administration from the University of North Carolina at Chapel Hill, and completed a postdoctoral fellowship in health economics at Harvard Medical School.

Elizabeth A. McGlynn, Ph.D.,[†] is an associate director for RAND Health and director of the Center for Research on Quality in Health Care. She holds the RAND Corporate Chair in Health Care Quality. Dr. McGlynn is an internationally known expert on methods for assessing and reporting on quality of health care delivery at different levels within the health care system. She has led the development of QA Tools, a comprehensive system for assessing the effectiveness of care for children and adults. The system has been used to evaluate the quality of care delivered by individual physicians, in medical groups, managed care plans, and at the community and national levels. She is currently leading a project to evaluate the methodological and policy implications of measuring effectiveness and efficiency at the individual physician level. She is also directing a project to evaluate a variety of health reform options. Dr. McGlynn is currently a member of the National Committee for Quality Assurance's Committee on Performance Measurement and she chairs the technical Advisory Group to this committee. She is a member of the advisory committee for the National Board of Medical Examiners' Center for Innovation. She is a member of an advisory commit-

---

[†]Member of the Performance Measures Subcommittee.

tee on quality for the American Board of Internal Medicine Foundation. Dr. McGlynn serves on the editorial boards for *Health Services Research* and the *Milbank Quarterly* and is a reviewer for many leading journals. Dr. McGlynn received her Ph.D. in public policy analysis in 1988 from the RAND Graduate School.

Arnold Milstein, M.D.,[†] is the medical director of the Pacific Business Group on Health (PBGH) and the chief physician at Mercer Human Resource Consulting. PBGH is the largest health care purchasers coalition in the United States.

Dr. Milstein's work and publications focus on health care purchasing strategy, clinical performance measurement, and the psychology of clinical performance improvement. He co-founded both the Leapfrog Group and the Consumer-Purchaser Disclosure Project and heads performance measurement activities for both initiatives. He also serves as the private sector representative on the Medicare Payment Advisory Commission.

Educated at Harvard (B.A. Economics), Tufts (Medical Degree), and University of California, Berkeley (M.P.H. Health Services Evaluation and Planning), he is an associate clinical professor at University of California, San Francisco.

Alan R. Nelson, M.D.,[*] is an internist-endocrinologist who was in private practice in Salt Lake City, Utah, until becoming chief executive officer of the American Society of Internal Medicine (ASIM) in 1992. Following the merger of ASIM with the American College of Physicians (ACP) in 1998, Dr. Nelson headed the Washington Office of ACP-ASIM until his semi-retirement in January 2000, and currently serves as special advisor to the executive vice-presicent/CEO of the College. He was president of the American Medical Association and currently serves as a member of the Medicare Payment Advisory Commission, which advises congress on Medicare issues. A member of the IOM, he was chair of the IOM Committee on Ethnic and Racial Disparities in Health Care and is a co-editor of the study report, *Unequal Treatment: Confronting Racial and Ethnic Disparities in Health Care.* Dr. Nelson attended Utah State University, and received his M.D. degree from Northwestern University in 1958.

Sharon-Lise Normand, Ph.D.,[†] is professor of health care policy (biostatistics) in the Department of Health Care Policy at Harvard Medical School and professor in the Department of Biostatistics at the Harvard School of

---

*Member of the Main Committee on Redesigning Health Insurance Performance Measures, Payment and Performance Improvement Programs.
†Member of Performance Measures Subcommittee.

Public Health. Her research focuses on the development of statistical methods for health services and outcomes research, primarily using Bayesian approaches to problem solving, including methods for causal inference, provider profiling, item response theory analyses, meta-analyses, and evaluation of medical devices in randomized and nonrandomized settings. She serves on several task forces for the American Heart Association and the American College of Cardiology, is a member of the FDA Circulatory System Devices Advisory Panel, the Massachusetts Cardiac Care Quality Advisory Commission, and is Director of Mass-DAC, a data coordinating center that monitors the quality of cardiac surgeries and coronary interventions in Massachusetts' acute care hospitals. Dr. Normand earned her Ph.D. in biostatistics from the University of Toronto, and holds M.S. and B.S. degrees in statistics. She is a fellow of the American Statistical Association as well as a fellow of the American College of Cardiology.

Barbara R. Paul, M.D.,[†] is senior vice president and chief medical officer of Beverly Enterprises, a leading provider of elder care headquartered in Fort Smith, Arkansas. She was previously director of the Quality Measurement and Health Assessment Group for CMS in Baltimore, Maryland. While at CMS, she led the launch of Health and Human Services Secretary Tommy G. Thompson's Nursing Home Quality Initiative and Home Health Quality Initiative, and played a key role in the agency's overall quality measurement and public reporting work. She represented the agency on the boards of the National Quality Forum and the Leapfrog Group.

Dr. Paul is an internist who was in full-time practice in Napa, California, from 1987 to 1999, in a small group practice affiliated with Queen of the Valley Hospital, and with Kaiser Permanente. She served as director of women's health services and chairperson of the Department of Medicine at Queen of the Valley Hospital, and was active with the California Medical Association where she chaired their Council on Ethical Affairs and served on their board of trustees.

Dr. Paul earned a B.S. degree in biochemistry from the University of Wisconsin, Madison, and her M.D. from Stanford University School of Medicine.

Norman C. Payson, M.D.,[*] retired as chairman and CEO of Oxford Health Plans, Inc., in November of 2002. Oxford Health Plans is a prominent greater New York health plan with 1.5 million members. Dr. Payson was recruited to the CEO position in 1998 after Oxford experienced severe

---

[*]Member of the Main Committee on Redesigning Health Insurance Performance Measures, Payment and Performance Improvement Programs.
[†]Member of Performance Measures Subcommittee.

operational and financial challenges and then led its successful turnaround. Prior to joining Oxford, Dr. Payson was co-founder and CEO of Healthsource, Inc., from its inception in 1985 until its sale to CIGNA Corporation in 1997. During his tenure, Healthsource grew to 3 million members in 15 states.

Dr. Payson is a graduate of the Massachusetts Institute of Technology and received his M.D. at Dartmouth Medical School.

William A. Peck, M.D.,* became the Alan A. and Edith L. Wolf Distinguished Professor of Medicine and director of the Washington University Center for Health Policy in 2003. From 1989 to 2003 he served as dean of Washington University School of Medicine and vice chancellor for medical affairs (executive vice chancellor from 1993-2003), and president of the Washington University Medical Center. Dr. Peck was awareded an honorary Doctor of Science from the University of Rochester in 2000. His academic activities include original investigations in bone and mineral metabolism, extensive clinical teaching and patient care experience. Major scientific contributions include the first method for studying directly the structure, function and growth of bone cells, demonstration of mechanisms whereby hormones regulate bone cell function, and examination of causes of osteoporosis. Dr. Peck served as founding president of the National Osteoporosis Foundation. He serves on the boards of Allied Health Care Products, Angelica Corporation, TIAA-CREF Trust Company, Research!America (vice chair) and a trustee of the University of Rochester. Dr. Peck is past chairman of the American Association of Medical Colleges. Dr. Peck has served on the editorial boards of major pharmaceutical companies.

Neil R. Powe, M.D., M.P.H., M.B.A.,* is professor of medicine, professor of health policy and management and professor of epidemiology at the Johns Hopkins University School of Medicine and the Johns Hopkins Bloomberg School of Public Health. He also is director of the Welch Center for Prevention, Epidemiology and Clinical Research, an interdisciplinary research and training center at the Johns Hopkins Medical Institutions focused on population-based and health services research. Dr. Powe's research has involved clinical epidemiology, technology assessment, patient outcomes research and health services research in many areas of medicine. He has also studied physician decision making and other determinants of use of medical practices including payers' decisions about insurance coverage for new medical technologies, the effect of financial incentives on the use of technology, efficiency and outcomes in for-profit versus non-profit health

---

*Member of the Main Committee on Redesigning Health Insurance Performance Measures, Payment and Performance Improvement Programs.

care institutions, and the relation between hospital volume, technology and outcomes. He has extensive experience in developing and measuring outcomes and quality in chronic kidney disease and is author of more than 230 articles. Dr. Powe received his M.D. degree from Harvard Medical School, M.P.H. degree from Harvard School of Public Health, and M.B.A. from the University of Pennsylvania. He completed his residency at the Hospital of the University of Pennsylvania where he was also a Robert Wood Johnson Clinical Scholar and fellow in the Division of General Internal Medicine. Dr. Powe is a member of the American Society of Clinical Investigation, the Association of American Physicians, and American Society of Epidemiology.

Christopher Queram, M.A.,* has been CEO of the Employer Health Care Alliance Cooperative (The Alliance) of Madison, WI, since 1993. The Alliance is a health care purchasing cooperative owned by more than 160 member companies that contracts with providers, collects and reports cost and utilization data, conducts consumer education and advocacy initiatives, and designs employer quality initiatives and reports. In addition to his responsibilities at The Alliance, Mr. Queram is a member of the board of the Leapfrog Group and currently serves as treasurer. He is a member and vice chair of the Wisconsin Board on Health Information. In addition, he is a member of the "Principals" for the American Hospital Association/CMS National Voluntary Hospital Reporting Initiative, a board member of the Wisconsin Collaborative for Healthcare Quality, and a member of the steering committee for the Wisconsin Hospital Association's CheckPoint quality reporting initiative. He served as a member of the Planning Committee for the National Quality Forum and continues as chair of the Purchaser Council and board member of the Forum. He also served as a member of the IOM's Committee on the Consequences of Uninsurance and President Clinton's Advisory Commission on Consumer Protection and Quality in the Health Care Industry. Prior to his current position, Mr. Queram was a hospital executive in Madison and Milwaukee, WI. Mr. Queram holds a Master of Arts degree in health services administration from the University of Wisconsin, Madison and is a fellow in the American College of Healthcare Executives.

Robert D. Reischauer, Ph.D.,* is the president of the Urban Institute, a nonprofit, nonpartisan policy research and education organization that examines the social, economic, and governance problems facing the nation. He served as the director of the Congressional Budget Office (CBO) between 1989 and 1995 and was CBO's assistant director for human resources and deputy

---

*Member of the Main Committee on Redesigning Health Insurance Performance Measures, Payment and Performance Improvement Programs.

director of CBO during the 1977 to 1981 period. Dr. Reischauer has been a senior fellow in the Economic Studies Program of the Brookings Institution (1986 to 1989 and 1995 to 2000) and the senior vice president of the Urban Institute (1981 to 1986). He is an economist with an undergraduate degree from Harvard and a Ph.D. in economics and Masters in International Affairs from Columbia University. Dr. Reischauer is a member of the Harvard Corporation and serves on the boards of several educational and nonprofit organizations. He is vice-chair of the Medicare Payment Advisory Commission and served as chair of the National Academy of Social Insurance's project "Restructuring Medicare for the Long Term" from 1995 through 2004.

William C. Richardson, Ph.D.,* is president and CEO of the W.K. Kellogg Foundation of Battle Creek, Michigan. Before joining the foundation in August 1995, Dr. Richardson was president of the Johns Hopkins University, a position he had held since 1990. In addition, Dr. Richardson was professor of health policy and management at the university. He has been appointed professor and president emeritus. Dr. Richardson is a member of the IOM of the National Academies and is a fellow of the American Academy of Arts and Sciences and a member of the American Public Health Association. Dr. Richardson has served on the boards of the Council of Michigan Foundations and the Council on Foundations (trustee and chairman). He also serves on the board of directors of the Kellogg Company, CSX Corporation, and the Bank of New York. Dr. Richardson is a graduate of Trinity College and the University of Chicago.

Cheryl M. Scott, M.H.A.,* is currently the president emerita for Group Health Cooperative (GHC). From 1997-2004, she was its president and CEO. GHC is one of the the nation's largest consumer-governed, nonprofit health care systems. Prior to assuming her position in 1997, Scott served as GHC's executive vice president/chief operating officer. Ms. Scott is a clinical professor in the Department of Health Services at the University of Washington. At the national level, Ms. Scott served on the board of the Alliance of Community Plans (trustee and chair) and the board of America's Health Insurance Plans. She currently serves as the board chair for the Health Technology Center and is a trustee for the Washington State Life Sciences Discovery Fund. Ms. Scott received a bachelor's degree in communications and a master's degree in health administration from the University of Washington.

---

*Member of the Main Committee on Redesigning Health Insurance Performance Measures, Payment and Performance Improvement Programs.

Stephen M. Shortell, Ph.D., M.P.H.,* is a prominent researcher in health policy and organization behavior at the University of California, Berkeley and is dean of the School of Public Health. Dr. Shortell is known as a leading academic voice advocating reform of the nation's health system. His research has helped establish determinants of health outcomes and quality of care for health care organizations. As the Blue Cross of California Distinguished Professor of Health Policy and Management, Shortell holds a joint appointment at UC Berkeley's School of Public Health and the Haas School of Business. He also is affiliated with UC Berkeley's Department of Sociology and UC San Francisco's Institute for Health Policy Studies. Dr. Shortell is an elected member of the IOM of the National Academies. Dr. Shortell has received the Baxter-Allegiance Prize, considered the highest honor worldwide in the field of health services research. He also has received the Distinguished Investigator Award from the Association for Health Services Research and the Gold Medal award from the American College of Healthcare Executives for his contributions to the field. He serves on the boards of the Health Research and Educational Trust (HRET) and the National Center for Healthcare Leadership (NCHL). Dr. Shortell received his bachelor's degree from the University of Notre Dame, his master's degree in public health from UCLA and his Ph.D. in behavioral science from the University of Chicago. Before coming to UC Berkeley in 1998, Shortell held teaching and research positions at Northwestern University, the University of Washington, and the University of Chicago.

Samuel O. Thier, M.D.,* † is professor of medicine and professor of health care policy at Harvard Medical School. He was president and CEO of Partners HealthCare System from 1996-2002. From 1994-1997 he was president of the Massachusetts General Hospital, and was Brandeis University's president during the previous three years. He served six years as president of the IOM, the National Academies and eleven years as chairman of the Department of Internal Medicine at Yale University School of Medicine, where he was sterling professor. Dr. Thier is an authority on internal medicine and kidney disease and is also known for his expertise in national health policy, medical education and biomedical research. Born in New York, he attended Cornell University and received his medical degree from the State University of New York at Syracuse in 1960. He served on the medical staff of Massachusetts General Hospital, as an intern, resident, chief resident in medicine and chief of the renal unit, and held a faculty appointment at Harvard. Prior to joining the faculty of Yale in 1975, he was professor and

---

*Member of the Main Committee on Redesigning Health Insurance Performance Measures, Payment and Performance Improvement Programs.
†Member of Performance Measures Subcommittee.

vice chairman of the Department of Medicine at the University of Pennsylvania. He has received several honorary degrees and the UC Medal of the University of California, San Francisco. He has served as president of the American Federation of Clinical Research and chairman of the American Board of Internal Medicine and is a master of the American College of Physicians, a fellow of the American Academy of Arts and Sciences, and a member of the American Philosophical Society. Dr. Thier is a director of Charles River Laboratories, Inc., the Commonwealth Fund (Chairman), Federal Reserve Bank of Boston, and Merck & Co., Inc., and a member of the Board of Overseers of TIAA-CREF and the Board of Overseers of Cornell University Medical College.

Paul J. Wallace, M.D.,[†] is executive director of Kaiser Permanente Care Management Institute (CMI), Oakland, California, and serves on Kaiser Permanente's Interregional New Technologies, Guidelines, Research and Diversity committees. Dr. Wallace is a member of the National Advisory Council for AHRQ, a member of the Committee on Performance Measurement for the National Committee for Quality Assurance, and a board member for the Disease Management Association of America. Previously, he was the director for the Clinical Practice Guidelines Program at the Northwest Region Permanente Medical Group, Portland, Oregon, and clinical oncology studies investigator at the Center for Health Research, Kaiser Permanente Northwest Region.

Dr. Wallace is board certified in internal medicine and hematology, and practiced for several years within the Northwest Permanente Medical Group. He combines past experiences in academic medicine and clinical medical oncology and hematology practice with work in quality improvement, especially in the areas of guideline development and evaluation of emerging medical technologies. He has conducted extensive research in these areas and published several articles. He participates in both national and community professional associations. A graduate of Drake University, Dr. Wallace holds an M.D. from the College of Medicine, University of Iowa.

Gail R. Wilensky, Ph.D.,[*] is a senior fellow at Project HOPE, an international health education foundation, where she analyzes and develops policies relating to health reform and to ongoing changes in the medical marketplace. Dr. Wilensky testifies frequently before Congressional committees, acts as an advisor to members of Congress and other elected officials, and speaks nationally and internationally before professional, business and con-

---

*Member of the Main Committee on Redesigning Health Insurance Performance Measures, Payment and Performance Improvement Programs.
†Member of Performance Measures Subcommittee.

sumer groups. From 2001 to 2003, she co-chaired the President's Task Force to Improve Health Care Delivery for Our Nation's Veterans, which covered health care for both veterans and military retirees. From 1997 to 2001, she chaired the Medicare Payment Advisory Commission, which advises Congress on payment and other issues relating to Medicare, and from 1995 to 1997, she chaired the Physician Payment Review Commission. Previously, she served as deputy assistant to President (GHW) Bush for policy development, advising him on health and welfare issues. Prior to that, she was administrator of the HCFA, overseeing the Medicare and Medicaid programs. Dr. Wilensky is an elected member of the IOM and its Governing Council, and serves as a trustee of the Combined Benefits Fund of the United Mineworkers of America, the American Heart Association, and is on the Advisory Board of the National Institute of Health Care Management. She is an advisor to the Robert Wood Johnson Foundation and The Commonwealth Fund, immediate past chair of the Board of Directors of Academy Health, and is a director on several corporate boards. Dr. Wilensky received a bachelor's degree in psychology and a Ph.D. in economics at the University of Michigan.

Institute of Medicine Staff Biographies

Rosemary A. Chalk, is the director of Board on Children, Youth and Families (BCYF) and also serves as the director of the Committee on Redesigning Health Insurance Performance Measures, Payment, and Performance Improvement Programs at the IOM. She has been a senior staff member of the IOM and the Division of Behavioral and Social Sciences and Education at the National Academies for almost 19 years, directing studies on vaccines and immunization finance, educational finance, family violence, child abuse and neglect, and research ethics. She took on the role of BCYF director in September 2003 and began directing the Redesigning Health Insurance project in April 2005.

For three years (2000 to 2003), Ms. Chalk was a half-time study director at the IOM and also directed the child abuse/family violence research area at Child Trends, a nonprofit research center in Washington, D.C., where she conducted studies on the development of child well-being indicators for the child welfare system. Over the past decade, Ms. Chalk has directed a range of projects sponsored by the William T. Grant Foundation, the Doris Duke Charitable Foundation, the Carnegie Corporation of New York, the David and Lucile Packard Foundation, and various agencies within the U.S. Department of Health and Human Services.

Earlier in her career, Ms. Chalk was a consultant and writer for a broad array of science and society research projects. She has authored publications on issues related to child and family policy, science and social responsibility, research ethics, and child abuse and neglect. She was the first program head of the Committee on Scientific Freedom and Responsibility of the American Association for the Advancement of Science from 1976 to 1986 and is a former section officer for the same organization. She served as a science policy analyst for the Congressional Research Service at the Library of Congress from 1972 to 1975. She has a B.A. in foreign affairs from the University of Cincinnati.

Karen Adams, Ph.D., M.T. (A.S.C.P.), was a senior program officer at the IOM in Washington, D.C. until February 2006. She was lead staff on the Performance Measures Subcommittee and the Pay for Performance Subcommittee of the IOM congressionally mandated study Redesigning Health Insurance Performance Measures, Payment, and Performance Improvement Programs. Her prior work at the IOM includes serving as study director of the IOM report *Priority Areas for National Action: Transforming Health Care Quality* and co-study director of the report *The 1st Annual Crossing the Quality Chasm Summit: A Focus on Communities.* Before coming to the IOM, she held the rank of assistant professor in the Department of Medical and Research Technology, University of Maryland School of Medicine and also was the academic coordinator of the undergraduate medical technology program. She received her undergraduate degree in medical technology from Loyola College, a master's degree in management from the College of Notre Dame, and a doctorate degree in health policy from the University of Maryland. During her doctoral studies she was awarded an internship at AHRQ where she researched over 30 years of innovations in medical informatics. She is also certified as a medical technologist by the American Society of Clinical Pathologists.

Samantha M. Chao, M.P.H., is a senior health policy associate for the Board on Health Care Services of the IOM. She recently completed her master's degree in health policy at the University of Michigan School of Public Health. In completing her studies, she interned with both the Michigan Department of Community Health and the American Heart Association to promote the study of chronic disease and disease prevention.

Contessa Fincher, Ph.D., M.P.H., was a program officer with the Board on Health Care Services of the IOM from 2004 until July 2005. She is a recent graduate from the University of Alabama at Birmingham in administration-health services with a focus in outcomes research. She has a Master of Public Health from the University of Texas School of Public Health at Houston with a concentration in health services research. Her postdoctoral work was completed at Wyeth Research, in the department of Global Health Outcomes and Pharmacoeconmic Assessment. She designed cost-effectiveness models at Wyeth as a part of her postdoctoral work in the area of cardio-vascular disease. Before joining IOM, she briefly worked as a pharmaco-economist at the FDA and Abt Associates, a government and pharmaceutical consulting company. She has published articles in journals such as *New England Journal of Medicine*, *American Journal of Cardiology*, and *Ethnicity & Disease*.

Tracy A. Harris, D.P.M., M.P.H., joined the Board on Health Care Services of the IOM in 2004 as a program officer. Her work background includes clinical experience and health policy work. Previously, she was trained in podiatric medicine and surgery and spent several years in private practice. In 1999, Dr. Harris was awarded a congressional fellowship with the American Association for the Advancement of Science. She spent one year working in the U.S. Senate on many issues including elder fraud, telemedicine, national practitioners data bank, health professional shortage areas, stem cell research, and malpractice caps. While earning her master's degree, she worked on various projects including Medicaid disease management and the uninsured. She has a Doctor of Podiatric Medicine degree from the Temple University School of Podiatric Medicine and a Master of Public Health degree with a concentration in health policy from the George Washington University.

Dianne Miller Wolman is lead staff on a Congressionally mandated evaluation of the Quality Improvement Organization Program of Medicare, part of the IOM's Redesigning Health Insurance Project. Prior to this she co-directed a 3-year study of the Consequences of Uninsurance, which produced a series of six reports: *Insuring Health*. She also directed the study that resulted in the IOM report, *Medicare Laboratory Payment Policy: Now and in the Future*, released in 2000. She joined the IOM Health Care Services Division in 1999 as a senior program officer. Her previous work experience in the health field has been varied and focused on finance and payment in insurance programs. She came from the General Accounting Office, where she was a senior evaluator on studies of the HCFA and its management capacity. Previously, she was a policy specialist at a national association representing nonprofit providers of long-term care services. Her earlier positions included policy analysis and management with the office of the secretary, DHHS; a peer-review organization; a governor's task force on access to health care; and a third-party administrator for very large health plans. In addition, she was policy director for a state Medicaid rate setting commission. She has a master's degree in government administration from Wharton Graduate School, University of Pennsylvania.

Index

A